I0110217

Everyone Else is Lying to You

How our medical establishment weaponized doubt to spread COVID, normalize quackery, and undermine public health

Jonathan Howard, M.D.

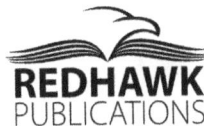

REDHAWK
PUBLICATIONS

Everyone Else is Lying to You

Copyright © 2025 Jonathan Howard, M.D.

All rights reserved. No part of this publication may be reproduced, distributed, or transmitted in any form or by any means, including photocopying, recording, or other electronic or mechanical methods, without the prior written permission of the publisher, except in the case of brief quotations embodied in critical reviews and certain other noncommercial uses permitted by copyright law. For permission requests, write to the publisher, addressed "Attention: Permissions Coordinator," at the address below.

See page 8 for indemnity legal disclaimers.

ISBN: 978-1-959346-99-9 (Paperback)

Library of Congress Control Number: 2025941256

Cover Design (Art):Erin Mann
Book Design:Robert T Canipe

Printed in the United States of America.

First printing 2025.

Redhawk Publications
The Catawba Valley Community College Press
2550 Hwy 70 SE
Hickory NC 28602
https://redhawkpublications.com

We are at a critical point in the history of public health. Anti-science, anti-vaccine activists are poised to take over the institutions responsible for ensuring the safety of the American people. Dr. Jonathan Howard shows us how we ended up in this situation, unpacks the reckless plans to undermine trust in public health and science in the United States, and explains just how much is at stake. This is a crucial book to help navigate a dangerous time.

—Adam Ratner, MD, MPH New York University Langone School of Medicine

As health disinformation accelerated across America during our time of Covid, NYU-Langone psychiatrist, Jonathan Howard MD, emerged as one of our pandemic heroes. Dr. Howard has chronicled the depravity of the pandemic disinformation machine like few others, paying special attention to the self-appointed health experts and contrarians who promoted an alternate universe - one that downplayed the seriousness of COVID-19, pushed discredited accounts of herd immunity, convinced Americans to shun vaccines, and even blame the scientists for creating or leaking the Covid virus. His latest book provides us with an important historical record, which will be examined by science historians for years to come.

—Dr. Peter Hotez, Dean for the National School of Tropical Medicine Baylor College of Medicine

While I was reading Jonathan Howard's latest book, a few phrases and cliches came to mind: "Idiot savants;" "a little knowledge is a dangerous thing;" "hoisted on one's own petard." I say this because the book focuses on a small but vociferous group of academics who were mostly on the fringes of their fields before the Covid-19 pandemic. The social and traditional media interest in what was happening gave these individuals bully pulpits to spread misinformation and, frankly, garbage. Howard calls them out by the highly effective tactic of using their own words against them, showing how their utterances were inconsistent over time - many social media posts aged particularly poorly. While the scientists and physicians acting in this way were not necessarily unintelligent, they displayed appalling judgment, and in doing so they betrayed the trust the public should have in those who have faculty appointments at leading universities.

—Dr. John Moore, Professor of Microbiology and Immunology, Cornell University

We live in a time where *Everyone Else is Lying to You* is more needed than ever to help us understand how the anti-vaccine movement has infiltrated and undermined public health. Dr. Jonathan Howard lived and breathed the ravages of the Covid-19 pandemic on the frontlines along with countless health professionals who had their efforts thwarted by pseudoscientific ideas promoted in the wellness industry and perhaps more perniciously by fringe scholars existing within our academic and health institutions. Drawing on his wealth of clinical and scientific expertise as a neurologist, psychiatrist, and science communicator, Howard incisively and meticulously details the precise way in which anti-vaccine misinformation insidiously has become politicized and popularized to gravely threaten our health and the health of those we love. This book documents and exposes the naked truth about how contrarian ideology and the egoistic interests of some physicians came to trump scientific consensus and a duty to save lives

—Jonathan N. Stea, Ph.D., R. Psych. Clinical Psychologist, University of Calgary

In this important book, Dr. Jonathan Howard continues the work he did in his book *We Want Them Infected*, documenting the work of respected, well-credentialed doctors to undermine public health efforts and misinform people about vaccines. Besides providing additional information, this book shows how the tactics of misinforming doctors were similar to other misinformers, in other contexts. The book is incisive, well-researched, and paints a frightening picture of doctors that should have known and done better, but did not. Any public health and public health law scholar, as well as citizens, would do well to read this book and arm themselves against future misinformation efforts.

—Dorit Reiss, Professor of Law University Of San Francisco

A comprehensive and sober fact-checking of a disturbing phenomenon: the rise of the COVID contrarian doctor. *We Want Them Infected* deconstructs the revisionist history and failed predictions of the physicians repeatedly caught prioritizing wishful thinking over data. Dr. Howard has kept the receipts that show these contrarian doctors' crystal balls are badly broken.

—Jonathan Jarry, MSc Science Communicator for McGill University's Office for Science and Society

Jonathan Howard is an invaluable help in making sense of what has gone so deeply wrong since COVID. He brings meticulous receipts on the fringe doctors who opportunistically exploited the pandemic crisis to boost their personal profiles, while deranging medical science discourse. For some, this has now led to powerful positions at the very top of hugely consequential medical science agencies. Howard's voice is an antidote to the now normalized, and institutionalized, toxic pseudoscience misinformation of MAHA. Essential reading.

—Julian Walker, Co-author of *Conspirituality: How New Age Conspiracy Theories Became a Health Threat.*

People are going to be hurt, and they are going to die. Liberalism tried to avert this situation but thanks to docility by the Democratic Party, dishonesty by the mainstream media, and thuggery from the right, we are here anyway. Our role? To tell everyone involved, including the public who went along with it, that we told you so.

—Oliver Willis,
November 24, 2024

Author's Disclaimer

The views, thoughts, and opinions expressed in this book belong solely to the author and do not necessarily reflect those of the author's employer, affiliated institutions, or any other organization the author is or has been associated with. The information provided is for general informational purposes only and is not intended as professional or institutional advice.

Publisher Disclaimer

The Author agrees to indemnify, defend, and hold harmless the Publisher—including its officers, employees, affiliates, agents, and representatives—from any claims, liabilities, losses, costs, or damages arising out of the content of this work. This includes, but is not limited to, claims of defamation, copyright infringement, invasion of privacy, or any other legal issues that may arise from the Author's words or ideas.

If any such claim is made against the Publisher, the Publisher reserves the right to choose legal counsel and to manage the defense. The Author agrees to cooperate in this process entirely. After consulting with the Author, the Publisher may settle any claim on terms it deems appropriate. The Author will be responsible for any costs, settlements, or damages resulting from such claims.

FOREWORD

Have you noticed that almost nobody talks about COVID anymore? At least not in the mainstream press, and certainly not as an ongoing problem. That ended sometime after the deadly omicron wave killed roughly 210,000 Americans. It's strange really, this post-pandemic reality.

The worst public health crisis in a century sweeps the nation leaving more than one million dead and millions more suffering lingering health issues. The virus itself continues to circulate, mutate, kill, and disable as it goes, and we simply ignore it.

Stranger is the fact that functionally, we changed very little as a society in the wake of the virus and all the destruction it has wrought. There are no new workplace safety requirements to protect workers and customers; no new laws on the books to hold disinformation-spreading doctors accountable for causing harm. It's just back to normal with more than a sprinkling of denial. In fact, public health authorities say that in terms of pandemic preparedness, we are worse off today than we were prior to COVID.

But it didn't start that way. In fact, the pandemic initially looked like a historic moment of change, which promised to catapult us into the 21st century—a great leap forward into a more humane future for the nation and the world.

The challenges the crisis presented had laid bare the inadequacies of the calcified neoliberal ideology that had dominated the western world for the better part of a century. The capabilities of the free markets were so grossly mismatched to the needs of the moment that everyone could see it. We needed government—a New Deal-scale response.

Senate Republicans and the Trump administration, eyeing the critical 2020 census-year election in November, must have realized it too because it was not long before the president was signing historically generous relief bills. There was generous pandemic unemployment relief, a program to expand broadband internet access, an eviction moratorium, a freeze on student loan debt repayment, an expanded child tax credit, and even direct cash payments in the form of stimulus checks.

All told, it was the largest expansion of the American social safety net in a generation, made possible by incredible bipartisanship unseen in years.

Perhaps an unintended consequence of government largess was a shift in the balance of power between labor and employers. With the new threat of the novel airborne SARS-CoV-2 virus dropping bodies by the thousands, low-wage workers at gas stations, supermarkets, fast food restaurants, and other frequented businesses were no longer low achievers who simply needed to boot-straps themselves into a bachelor's degree and more gainful employment. Suddenly, they were "essential workers"— the brave citizens risking their health, and that of their families, to keep American society thrumming. Where would we be without them and why shouldn't they enjoy a greater share of the wealth they create? After all, how hard did corporate executives really work in comparison?

These questions were impossible to ignore and gave workers new leverage in their dealings with their employers. Many began leaving their jobs and others started organizing.

For the major corporate interests and power players behind the modern conservative movement, whose political project over the past 50 years has been shrinking government programs and eroding public goods, the situation was untenable. As long as Americans believed the crisis was real, ongoing, and serious, not only were Republicans imperiled in November, but every victory conservatives had scored since the Reagan Era was potentially at risk as well.

Something had to be done.

It wasn't long before the gears of the right-wing messaging machine

Jonathan Howard   11

began to turn. Its goal was simple: Reopen America as quickly as possible. To that end, right-wingers would run every playbook in their arsenal to politicize the pandemic. Former Tea Party groups began promoting anti-lockdown protests and demonstrations. Conservative think tanks began churning out commentaries questioning how serious the situation really was and urging restraint by public health authorities. Right-wing media personalities warned about societal panic.

The virus wasn't killing *that* many people, claimed the late Rush Limbaugh. The pandemic shouldn't be used to promote progressive policy reforms, cautioned Hoover Institution Senior Fellow Richard Epstein. Government should allow businesses to "continue to adapt and innovate," argued Emily Seidel, CEO of billionaire Charles Koch's flagship political group, Americans for Prosperity. Pandemic relief programs were impeding back-to-work efforts, and the answer was weakening unions and worker protections, proposed a Heritage Foundation report.

Novel as the crisis was the underlying right-wing strategy for dealing with it was decades old—borrowed straight from the fossil fuel and tobacco industries: Sow doubt in science to undermine government.

Aiding in the sabotage of the COVID response was a cadre of fringe medical doctors and scientists willing to leverage their voices, credentials, and often prestigious university affiliations to add a veneer of legitimacy to what was ultimately an unscientific economic position supported by some of the wealthiest individuals and most powerful corporate interests in the country.

These voices were rewarded with attention, honoraria, and ultimately influence, amplified by a sprawling network of business-aligned, right-wing media outfits and dark money groups from the Heritage Foundation and Hoover Institution to newer outfits like the so-called Brownstone Institute. Several were tapped for high-level public health positions in the new Trump administration.

In his seminal work, "How the failed quest for herd immunity led doctors to embrace the anti-vaccine movement and blinded Americans to the threat of COVID," Dr. Howard, who served on the front line of the COVID pandemic, treating patients, meticulously chronicled the various contradictory, false, and misleading statements and rosy predictions of many of these modern-day merchants of doubt. The book, which presented their remarks with minimal commentary, was an essential reference guide for those of us who look back for posterity—and to seek accountability, if not now, then hopefully in the future.

This new project expands on the previous one, exploring the success of the campaign to undermine public health—a campaign that I have spent years covering in my capacity as a journalist. *Everyone Else Is Lying to You* is critical reading for anyone wishing to understand how it is that Donald Trump, a man who presided over 400,000 American COVID deaths during his first term, could ultimately return to power with the popular vote behind him—and why he brought anti-vax and herd immunity-promoting cranks with him. It explores the tactics and victories of one of the most pernicious, damaging movements in the history of public health.

In this fraught environment, rife with distrust and disinformation, we have to fight for every ounce of truth. We cannot allow a single lie to be absorbed into the bloodstream of the national discourse. That is why Dr. Howard's book is so important: It fights back. Its accurate retelling of the last few critical years is itself an act of defiance against a hungry maw that threatens to engulf not just American democracy, but democracy across the globe.

—Walker Bragman

Table of Contents

Introduction

It's been a tough period, absolutely, and especially … for me.
— Dr. Jay Bhattacharya

In December 2022, Dr. Jay Bhattacharya, then a health economist at Stanford University, tweeted that he "would have" done many impressive things regarding COVID if only social media companies and the National Institutes of Health (NIH) were not in his way. He posted:

> *Imagine there hadn't been an @NIH-led "devastating takedown" of the @gbdeclaration in Oct 2020. Imagine no media/social media suppression. We would have won the policy argument. Schools would have opened. We would have prioritized protection of the vulnerable. Instead, lockdowns.*[1]

Dr. Bhattacharya became a widely admired celebrity based on these entirely hypothetical accomplishments, and he used them to catapult himself to head the NIH. However, actually doing things is more challenging than boasting about what he "would have" done in a fantasy world.

On May 5th, 2025, just one month into his tenure as NIH director, Dr. Bhattacharya gave a revealing interview to *Science* with Jocelyn Kaiser, who said, "The encounter was brief, sometimes confrontational, and even personal."[2] Even at this early point, things were not going well at the NIH. Over 1,000 NIH workers were fired on April 1, 2025—his first day in office. The headline in *Nature* read "'One of the Darkest Days': NIH Purges Agency Leadership Amid Mass Lay-offs," which also stated:

> *In shock move, four institute directors at the US biomedical agency are removed from their posts.*[3]

Appropriately, Dr. Bhattacharya's picture appeared immediately below these words.

In addition to saying what he "would have" done, Dr. Bhattacharya achieved fame by portraying himself as a free speech warrior and censored scientific dissident. Though this supposed "censorship" was entirely about a small amount of social media content, Dr. Bhattacharya did not mince words about his perceived victimhood. For example, in 2023 he tweeted to epidemiologist Dr. Marc Lipsitch:

> *You work for an administration that runs a vast censorship regime to suppress scientific discussion. Most authoritarian policy I've seen from an American government. You wash your hands of the CDC's failures, though you were in a high position. You should be ashamed of yourself. I call it like I see it.*[4]

Yet, under his leadership, articles have appeared with titles like "Leading Nutrition Scientist Departs N.I.H., Citing Censorship," which said:

> *For the past two decades, Kevin Hall, a nutrition and metabolism scientist at the National Institutes of Health, has devoted his career to studying how people's diets affect their health. He has led some of the world's most important research on ultraprocessed foods, including one study that demonstrated, for the first time, that they caused people to overeat. This linked ultraprocessed foods to chronic conditions like Type 2 diabetes and obesity.*
> *Dr. Hall had planned to keep doing this work for many years — and hoped it might accelerate under the health secretary, Robert F. Kennedy Jr., who has said that fixing the nation's food supply is a priority. But now, at 54, he is retiring early.*
> *In an interview with* The New York Times, *Dr. Hall said his decision was driven in part by several instances in which federal officials censored his work. In one, he said he was barred from*

speaking freely with reporters about a study that might have been
seen as contradicting Mr. Kennedy's stance on the addictive na-
ture of ultraprocessed foods, which include products like chicken
nuggets, hot dogs, packaged cookies and chips. [...]

To have federal officials interfere with how the study was por-
trayed to a news outlet was "galling" and "a huge red flag," Dr.
Hall said.

At the end of March, Dr. Hall emailed Mr. Kennedy and Dr. Jay
Bhattacharya, the director of the N.I.H., expressing his concerns
about the censorship and informing them that he was considering
leaving his post. He also described how his research had been
"hobbled" in recent months because of spending and hiring
freezes that made it difficult to bring on research assistants and
to buy food and other supplies for his clinical trials.

"The future of our studies seems bleak," he wrote in the email.

Mr. Kennedy and Dr. Bhattacharya have not responded.[5]

People remaining at the NIH spoke about chaos and poor morale, and
every news report on the topic contained quotes from scientists who "requested anonymity out of fear of professional retribution from the federal
government"[6] and "asked not to be identified because they still depend on
the institution for funding."[7]

NIH employees refused to clap when Dr. Bhattacharya was introduced at his first town hall, and dozens walked out in protest after he
blamed them for starting the pandemic. According to an article by Walker
Bragman titled "'Out of His Depth,' 'Sold His Soul,' 'Clueless': NIH
Staffers Speak Out About Director Bhattacharya":

"It's a total shit show," one agency staffer told Important Context, *explaining that Bhattacharya seemed unaware of how NIH*

*operated when he arrived. They said he had been promising
reforms that were already part of the agency's work.*

*"His attitude coming in has just been so condescending, and so
like, 'Oh, we're going to make NIH great'... and 'we're going to
make... science transparent, and we're going to introduce all of
these programs' that, mind you, already exist," the staffer said.*

*"Like, these are things we actively do... You fired people that do
those things that you say you want to do." [...]*

*Insiders described Bhattacharya as "arrogant," "in over his
head," "out of his league," "out of his depth," "clueless,"
"weak," and "full of shit." The NIH director did not respond to
our requests for comment.*

*"In some ways, I do feel vaguely sorry for him, because he is
clueless, and he clearly does not know what he's doing," one
staffer said. "But he's also arrogant, and he thinks that he can
just come in and tell us how to do our jobs, when he has no idea
how science actually works." [...]*

*The program officer speculated that Bhattacharya might be rely-
ing on "a lot of mental gymnastics to contort himself into believing he's doing the right/best thing," but said it ultimately did not
matter because "either way, he is at fault."*

*"No matter what he tells himself to sleep at night, people will
suffer and potentially die because of the policies he's allowing at
NIH under his leadership," they said. [...]*

*Another said that while Bhattacharya had once been "respect-
ed," "now he sounds like a joke, an ignorant political hack,
every time he speaks... he comes across as someone who has sold
his soul."[8]*

Despite the purges, censorship, and dysfunction at the NIH, Dr. Bhattacharya centered himself in his *Science* interview. "It's been a tough period, absolutely, and especially … for me," he said.[2] He complained that Dr. Harold Varmus, a Nobel Prize winner and previous NIH director, had "attacked me pretty viciously."

He seemed to have little idea what was happening at the agency he was leading. He scolded Ms. Kaiser for "spreading rumors" and "panic" that the NIH planned to suspend grants for foreign collaborations. However, just hours later, the NIH announced exactly that, calling it a policy change. Whether Dr. Bhattacharya deceived Ms. Kaiser or was in the dark about it himself is unclear.

When he was not denying reality or feeling sorry for himself for having to fire scientists and dedicated federal employees, Dr. Bhattacharya was eager to absolve himself from any problems at the NIH. While he expected credit for imaginary achievements regarding COVID, he refused to accept responsibility for actual calamities at the NIH. "I had nothing to do with it. […] It's not me personally […] Those decisions are not up to me," he said. The *Science* interview reported:

> **On NIH's cancellation of more than 800 grants, many on HIV research:**
> *I don't personally review grant lines and say, "I cancel this grant. Don't cancel that grant." That's not what I do. … There's a process. It's not me personally, but I mean, the best I can tell, most of those were canceled before I even got into office.*
> **On Trump-imposed freezes on NIH grants to Columbia University and other institutions because of alleged antisemitism:**
> *Those decisions are not up to me, but I do notice these institutions ought to obey the civil rights laws, and I think eventually*

they will. ... There's a lot of excellent science that goes on in these places. It's very difficult to do excellent science, though, in a place that doesn't have basic civil rights laws.

On morale on the NIH campus:

It's been a tough period, absolutely, and especially ... for me. I arrived the day that the RIF [reduction in force] happened. ... I had nothing to do with it. But in the month I've been here, I think things have turned around pretty significantly.

All this from a doctor—the *Director* of the NIH no less—who accused *others* of trying to "wash their hands"[4] of problems within the government.

Even if Dr. Bhattacharya was somehow blameless for purges at the start of his tenure, the day after bragging about turning things around "pretty significantly," the headlines read, "National Institutes of Health Lays Off Hundreds More Staff, Including at Cancer Research Institute." The article said:

> *The National Institutes of Health has laid off hundreds more staff, multiple current and laid-off employees of the health agency told CBS News, including at its cancer research institute.*
>
> *Around 200 employees began receiving layoff notices Friday evening, said three people who spoke on the condition of anonymity. The move surprised NIH officials, since the department previously claimed no further cuts were planned at the agency.*
>
> *"We thought the worst was behind us, and we were transitioning into this new phase, and the rug was just pulled out from underneath us," one laid-off employee said.*
>
> *A spokesperson for the NIH did not comment on why NIH Director Dr. Jay Bhattacharya sought the additional layoffs, referring*

an inquiry to the Department of Health and Human Services, which oversees the NIH.[8]

In contrast to Dr. Bhattacharya, these scientists lost much more than a YouTube video and some tweets. In his article "Inside the Bloodbath at the NIH," Dr. Gregg Gonsalves wrote:

> *Yet, over a month into his tenure, Bhattacharya hasn't complained or pushed back against what is happening at the NIH. In fact, he seems happy and at home after the institutes' Red Wedding and its continuing aftermath: hundreds of fired employees; hundreds of grants terminated and hundreds more in limbo falling afoul of a list of trigger words for conservatives; thousands of careers around the US and the world up in smoke; a lost generation of biomedical research in this country; and, most tragically, the cures now delayed or forever deferred.*
>
> *As a former NIH-funded researcher himself, one could have envisioned him as the hero of this tale—fighting back and creating a better NIH for our times. I held out that hope for a week or so myself, thinking he must surely see and know what is going on and would soon call a stop to it. Yet now here he sits among the rubble, surveying his kingdom of dust, and one can't help but think he's gotten what he wanted all along. The rest of us will have to live—and yes, die and suffer—with his legacy and the legacy of these men who would destroy the NIH.*[9]

Dr. Bhattacharya's interview ended early. His kingdom of dust beckoned. Ms. Kaiser wrote:

> *Twenty minutes in, NIH Principal Deputy Director Matthew Memoli, who had served as acting director until Bhattacharya arrived, opened the door to say: "Hey, Jay, I need you right now.*

I got a call from downtown." The interview was over.[2]

This book is about doctors who gained power by posting online about all the amazing, incredible, wonderful things they "would have" done, the harm they actually did, and the harm they are currently doing now that they are the medical establishment.

Jonathan Howard
May 2025

Chapter 1: 'One of the Darkest Days': NIH Purges Agency Leadership Amid Mass Lay-offs

There are adverse events from the vaccine. It does cause deaths every year. It causes all the illnesses that measles itself causes.
— Robert F. Kennedy Jr.

Chronologically, I am going to start at the end. Except for the introduction and this chapter, I wrote most of this book before January 1, 2025. In the book's conclusion, I predicted things were likely to get worse before they got better, and indeed, they have gotten much worse. Anti-vaxxers are winning, and science is under attack as never before. Had the election turned out differently, many people would have dismissed this book as hysterical fear-mongering. Instead, a massive propaganda campaign has succeeded, and we are witnessing the disastrous consequences.

At the time of this writing, headlines read, "Measles Cases Reach 1,046 in US as Infections Confirmed in 30 States."[1] As measles hospitalizes and kills unvaccinated children for the first time since 1991,[2] Robert F. Kennedy Jr.—America's #1 spreader of anti-vaccine disinformation for 20 years and the current Secretary of the U.S. Department of Health and Human Services (HHS)—is going hiking and blaming the outbreak on poor nutrition.[3] He said, "If you're healthy, it's almost impossible to die from an infectious disease in modern times."[4] He is responsible for the headline "Dozens of Free Measles Vaccine Clinics Close in Texas as Federal Funding is Cut"[5] and is trying to contain the outbreak with vitamin A and cod liver oil,[6] saying doctors have obtained "almost miraculous and instantaneous"[7] recoveries with such quackery.

After a second child died in Texas, he attended her funeral, and according to one news report, "Kennedy spent most of his time in Texas celebrating parents who refuse to vaccinate, highlighting how many kids they have who didn't die."[8] He praised anti-vax doctors there, saying they had "treated and healed some 300 measles-stricken Mennonite children using aerosolized budesonide and clarithromycin."[9]

Unfortunately, trusting parents are listening to this nonsense. One article quoted Katherine Wells, the director of public health in Lubbock, who said:

> *I'm worried we have kids and parents that are taking all of these other medications and then delaying care. Some seriously ill children had been given alternative remedies like cod liver oil. If they're so, so sick and have low oxygen levels, they should have been in the hospital a day or two earlier.*[10]

These "treatments" have harmed other children. According to the article "Remedy Supported by Kennedy Leaves Some Measles Patients More Ill":

> *Physicians at Covenant Children's Hospital in Lubbock, Texas, say they've now treated a handful of unvaccinated children who were given so much vitamin A that they had signs of liver damage.*[11]

Kennedy has predictably fearmongered about the measles vaccine. He falsely claimed it contained "aborted fetus debris"[12] and asked that we acknowledge "vaccine-injured kids and look them in the eye."[7] During an interview with Fox News in March 2025, he said, "There are adverse events from the vaccine. It does cause deaths every year. It causes — it causes all the illnesses that measles itself causes, encephalitis and blindness, et cetera."[13] None of this is true.

However, Kennedy has made some tepid statements encouraging

getting the measles vaccine. Predictably, this enraged his supporters, convincing none of them. Kennedy spent 20 years telling them that anyone who makes accurate statements on vaccines is a dishonest pharma shill, and he has now become involuntarily woven into the conspiracy he has worked so hard to create. The article "Health Secretary RFK Jr. Endorses the MMR Vaccine — Stoking Fury Among His Supporters" reported:

> *"I'm sorry, but there is no defense for this poorly worded statement," wrote Dr. Sherri Tenpenny, a prominent anti-vaccine activist who once claimed during a legislative hearing in Ohio that the COVID vaccine could cause patients to become magnetized, allowing them to stick "spoons and forks" all over their bodies. Del Bigtree, a prominent anti-vaccine activist who supported Kennedy's presidential run and recently co-founded a non-profit with him called MAHA Action, also questioned the health secretary's endorsement. Bigtree suggested that Kennedy's post had "got cut off." He then went on to make unproven claims about vaccines and autism, and linked to a documentary he had made on the topic.*
>
> *"We voted for challenging the medical establishment, not parroting it," posted Dr. Mary Talley Bowden, a Texas-based physician who has opposed COVID vaccines and is currently fighting a complaint from Texas's medical board over hospital admitting privileges.*[14]

Meanwhile, many of the techniques doctors used to minimize COVID—which were plagiarized from pre-pandemic anti-vaccine balderdash—are being recycled to minimize measles. The myths that healthy children don't *suffer* from measles; that children suffer *with* measles, not *from* measles; that measles is just a little rash and fever; and that doctors are misdiagnosing measles patients or are responsible for their demise have all returned.

Something else that has returned is pro-virus rhetoric. Kennedy falsely claimed:

> There's a lot of studies out there that show that if you actually do get the wild infection, you're protected later. It boosts your immune system later in life against cancers, atopic diseases, cardiac disease, etc.[15]

An article titled "RFK Jr.: It Would Be Better If 'Everybody Got Measles'" quoted him as saying:

> It used to be that everybody got measles. And the measles gave you lifetime protection against measles infection. The vaccine doesn't do that. The vaccine is effective for some people for life, but for many people it wanes. […] It used to be that very young kids were protected by breast milk. Women who get vaccinated do not provide that level of immunity.[16]

This comment is very similar to what Allison Krug and Dr. Vinay Prasad wrote in their February 2022 article, "Should We Let Children Catch Omicron?" during the pandemic's most severe wave for children. They said:

> When it comes to infectious disease, normality means a world where they are routinely exposed to, and overcome, viral illness. For children, getting sick and recovering is part of a natural and healthy life. Dropping masks, quarantines, distancing, and all other mitigations will allow children to develop the kind of broad immunity gained by living a normal life. Shielding kids from exposure only increases their future risk. […] It's time to allow children to resume normal life, not simply because their

exclusion is unfair or hurts them socially and psychologically, but because it is immunologically in their best interest. Parents must consider that exposures are how we best protect our children against the variants of the future. In fact, it is reckless to let children age into a more serious encounter with a disease best dealt with while younger.[17]

Doctors in this book helped normalize this sort of pro-virus thought.

"HHS Taps Anti-Vaccine Activist to Look at Debunked Links Between Autism and Vaccines, Sources Say"
— NBC News headline

While scientists and doctors are horrified, anti-vaxxers are ecstatic. Anti-vaxxers have long fantasized about punishing the "medical establishment," and this is the moment they've been waiting for. Vaccine rates are slipping,[18] pertussis and measles are spreading,[19] public health is endangered, and prominent scientists need bodyguards,[20] exactly as they intended. Kennedy is making their dreams a reality, and they are eager for more results. In April 2025, Mary Holland, the CEO of Children's Health Defense, Kennedy's anti-vaccine organization, said, "I really feel like we're riding a wave right now. We have Bobby Kennedy as HHS secretary. No one could have predicted that."[21] She continued:

He hasn't backed down on vaccines. For people who are disappointed that he hasn't ended the childhood schedule or that he said, you can take an MMR. He has not backed down. He is saying, we're going to look at this. We're going to look at everything. So he's up against a lot.

I think we're blessed that Bobby's in office, and I think those of us in this movement have every good reason to support what he's doing. If it turns out in one year he's got nothing done, which I can't imagine, well then, OK, then let's get somebody else. But we've got to give this guy a chance.

Indeed, Kennedy's war on vaccines and infectious-disease research and prevention isn't just limited to measles. Our medical establishment unilaterally decided not to authorize new COVID vaccines for millions of Americans unless they show their value in randomized placebo-controlled trials (RCTs), which may take several years to complete and be prohibitively expensive to perform. Other headlines from his first couple of months in office include:

- A Texas Child Who Was Not Vaccinated Has Died of Measles, a First for the US in a Decade[22]
- RFK Jr. Minimizes Measles Outbreak in Texas[23]
- RFK Jr. Says Federal Vaccine Advisers Are Beholden to Industry. The Evidence Does Not Support Him[24]
- Measles is Back — And RFK Jr. Isn't Taking it Seriously[25]
- Texas Children Poisoned After RFK Jr. Touts Vitamin A as Measles Treatment[26]
- Measles Outbreak in Texas Hits 481 Cases, with 59 New Infections Confirmed in Last 3 Days[27]
- Second Unvaccinated Child Dies After Contracting the Measles[28]
- NIH To Terminate or Limit Grants Related to Vaccine Hesitancy and Uptake[29]
- FDA Annual Flu Vaccine Meeting and CDC's 'Wild to Mild' Campaign Canceled[30]
- RFK Jr. Pauses Peninsula Company's Oral Covid Vaccine Clinical Trial[31]

- CDC Will Research Widely Debunked Link Between Vaccines and Autism[32]
- Scientists Say NIH Officials Told Them to Scrub mRNA References on Grants[33]
- Kennedy's Alarming Prescription for Bird Flu on Poultry Farms[34]
- Experts Concerned as NIH Axes Critical Vaccine Study Funds[35]
- NIH to Ax Grants on Vaccine Hesitancy, mRNA Vaccines[36]
- Long Covid Office 'Will Be Closing,' Trump Administration Announces[37]
- Vaccine Skeptic Hired to Head Federal Study of Immunizations and Autism[38]
- Saying 'Pandemic is Over,' NIH Starts Cutting COVID-19 Research[39]
- Vaxart Lays Off 10% of Staff After HHS Unexpectedly Demands Halt to COVID Vaccine Trial[40]
- CDC is Pulling Back $11B in Covid Funding Sent to Health Departments Across the U.S.[41]
- Trump Cuts Damage Global Efforts to Track Diseases, Prevent Outbreaks[42]
- U.S. to End Vaccine Funds for Poor Countries[43]
- CDC Layoffs Strike Deeply at its Ability to Respond to the Current Flu, Norovirus and Measles Outbreaks and Other Public Health Emergencies[44]
- Trump Administration Says It Will Pull Back Billions in COVID Funding from Local Health Departments[45]
- A Federal Lab That Tracked Rising S.T.I.s Has Been Shuttered[46]
- HHS Orders CDC to Halt Some Vaccine Ads, Saying RFK Jr. Wants Message Focused on 'Informed Consent'[47]

- RFK Jr. Lays Off Staffers Who Run FDA's Vaccine Expert Panel[48]
- HHS Taps Anti-Vaccine Activist to Look at Debunked Links Between Autism and Vaccines, Sources Say[49]
- As Measles Continues to Rise, CDC Muffles Vaccine Messaging[50]
- Measles Cases in Texas Rise to 400 as U.S. Total Reaches Nearly 500 Amid Worsening Outbreak, Officials Say[51]
- Robert F Kennedy Jr Claims Anti-Vax Physicians Healed 'Some 300 Measles-Stricken Children'[52]
- Anti-Vaccine Sentiment May Derail Vaccines Already Awaiting FDA Approval, Experts Fear[53]
- What RFK Jr. Told Grieving Texas Families About the Measles Vaccine[54]
- FDA Lays Off Bird Flu Leadership, Among Steep Cuts to Senior Veterinarians[55]
- Gavi, the Vaccine Alliance, Has Its Billion Dollar Grant Cut by Trump Administration[56]
- H.H.S. Scraps Studies of Vaccines and Treatments for Future Pandemics[57]
- Vaccine Critic's Apparent Selection to Head HHS Autism Study Shocks Experts[58]
- Trump Administration at 'War' With mRNA Technology: Scientists Alarmed Vaccine Skeptics Could Kill Research[59]
- Ex-Official Says He Was Forced Out of FDA After Trying to Protect Vaccine Safety Data from RFK Jr.[60]
- Deep Cuts to HIV Research Could Halt Decades of Progress, Scientists Say[61]
- Kennedy Draws from Misinformation Playbook by Touting an Inhaled Steroid to Treat Measles[62]

- RFK Jr. Cuts CDC Labs Investigating Outbreaks of STDs and Hepatitis[63]
- Trump's War Against HIV Research and Care[64]
- Trump Administration Cuts FDA Staff Handling Bird Flu Outbreaks[65]
- Trump Team Guts AIDS-Eradication Programme and Slashes HIV Research Grants[66]
- Washington State Vaccination Clinic Canceled After CDC Funding Cuts[67]
- "The Country is Less Safe": CDC Disease Detective Program Gutted[68]
- The CDC Buried a Measles Forecast That Stressed the Need for Vaccinations[69]
- Doctors Blast RFK Jr After Vaccine Chief Forced Out: 'Gutting of Expertise'[70]
- US FDA Commissioner Makary Was Sworn In, Knew of Plan to Push Out Marks, Sources Say[71]
- Top Trump FDA Official Brenner Hits Pause on Novavax Covid-19 Vaccine Decision[72]
- Fauci Allies, Covid Vaccine Officials Get Ax at NIH[73]
- RFK Jr. Suggests Some Vaccines Are Risky or Ineffective, Downplays Measles Threat[74]
- RFK Jr.'s Purge of FOIA Staff at FDA Spares People Working on Covid Vaccine Lawsuits[75]
- FDA's Top Vaccine Scientist is Out, Citing Kennedy's 'Misinformation and Lies'[76]

That last article, about Dr. Peter Marks, a vaccine expert who was vital to the development of the COVID vaccines, reported:

In a resignation letter to acting FDA Commissioner Sara Brenner, Marks wrote that undermining confidence in vaccines is "irresponsible, detrimental to public health, and a clear danger to our nation's health, safety, and security."

He said he had been willing to work with Kennedy to address any concerns about vaccine safety and transparency.

"However, it has become clear that truth and transparency are not desired by the secretary, but rather he wishes subservient confirmation of his misinformation and lies," Marks wrote.

Another article titled "Ousted Vaccine Chief Says RFK Jr.'s Team Sought Data to Justify Anti-Science Stance" reported:

In early March, Marks said, Kennedy's team requested that Marks turn over data on cases of brain swelling and deaths caused by the measles vaccine—data that Marks said doesn't exist because there have been no such confirmed cases in the U.S.

"I can only come to a single conclusion that there was not an appreciation for having somebody who was rigorously science-driven within the organization," Marks said.[77]

They broke something without real plans to fix it, because the people who were doing the breaking didn't have any idea.

— *Dr. Peter Marks*

That same article also quoted Dr. Marks as saying:

They broke something without real plans to fix it, because the people who were doing the breaking didn't have any idea. They took the place apart without having an instruction manual of how to put it back together.

Indeed, reminiscent of Lysenkoism in the Soviet Union, science itself is under attack. Scientists are being fired, universities and medical journals are being targeted, research is being halted, words are being banned, and thoughts are being policed. Scientists are reasonably wondering if they have a future in the U.S. Today's headlines speak of purges, chaos, wrecking balls, and bloodbaths:

- Staff at CDC and NIH Are Reeling as Trump Administration Cuts Workforce[78]
- RFK Jr. Says He'll Cut 20,000 Positions from Health and Human Services Workforce[79]
- 'Chaos and Confusion' at the Crown Jewel of American Science[80]
- FDA Tobacco Official Is Removed from Post in Latest Blow to Health Agency's Leadership[81]
- Massive Layoffs, Purge of Leadership Underway at U.S. Health Agencies[82]
- RFK Jr. Purges CDC and FDA's Public Records Teams, despite "Transparency" Promises[83]
- 'One of the Darkest Days': NIH Purges Agency Leadership Amid Mass Lay-offs[84]
- Doctor Behind Award-Winning Parkinson's Research Among Scientists Purged From NIH[85]
- NIH Hit with Chaos, Cuts, and Contractor Purge[86]
- We Are Witnessing the Destruction of Science in America[87]
- 'No Guidance and No Leadership': Chaos and Confusion at CDC After Mass Firings[88]
- CDC Cuts Key Smoking Programs Despite Success in Curbing Smoking Rates[89]
- DOGE Moves to Gut CDC Work on Gun Injuries, Sexual Assault, Opioid Overdose Data, and More[90]
- HHS Starts Layoffs of Thousands of Workers Across Its Agencies[91]
- CDC Faces Backlash for Cutting Sickle Cell, Adult Disability Programs[92]
- Trump Cuts Target Next Generation of Scientists and Public Health Leaders[93]

- Trump Officials Will Screen NIH Funding Opportunities[94]
- F.D.A. Layoffs Could Raise Drug Costs and Erode Food Safety[95]
- FDA Planning for Fewer Food and Drug Inspections Due to Layoffs, Officials Say[96]
- Trump Admin Cancels NIH Scientific Integrity Policy[97]
- Decimation of HHS Comms, FOIA Offices Will Leave Americans in the Dark About Urgent Health Matters[98]
- NIH Funding Is Drying Up. Drug Discovery Could Go with It[99]
- New York City's Health Department Just Lost $100 Million In Federal Funds. That Has Consequences[100]
- At CDC, Trump Administration's Job Cuts Wipe Out Wide Array of Specialists[101]
- Gold-Standard Maternal Mortality Database in Limbo as CDC Staff Placed on Leave[102]
- NIH Scientists Have a Cancer Breakthrough. Layoffs Are Delaying It[103]
- How Kennedy Is Already Weakening America's Childhood Vaccine System[104]
- FDA Layoffs Described As "Devastating" As Mass Cuts Ensue Across Government Agencies[105]
- Mass Layoffs Begin at HHS Agencies Responsible for Research, Tracking Disease and Regulating Food[106]
- 'It's A Bloodbath': Massive Wave of Job Cuts Began at US Health Agencies[107]
- RFK Jr. Vowed to Upend American Health Care. It's Happening Faster Than Expected[108]
- FDA Staff Left 'Scrambling' to Complete Product Reviews After DOGE Layoffs[109]
- More NIH Job Cuts Coming? Agency's Scientists Already Reeling After Week of Firings[110]
- 5 High-Level CDC Officials Are Leaving in the Latest Turmoil for the Agency[111]

- Here Are the Words Putting Science in the Crosshairs of Trump's Orders[112]
- The CDC Has Been Gutted[113]
- RFK Jr. Says 20% Of Health Agency Layoffs Could Be Mistakes[114]
- 'Taking Away Years of Experience': NIH Probationary Employees Fired Friday[115]
- 'Bloodbath' at NIH and Elsewhere at HHS Begins[116]
- Global Science Bodies Pivot to Capitalize on US Brain Drain[117]
- Overseas Universities See Opportunity in U.S. 'Brain Drain'[118]
- Trump Administration Eviscerates Maternal and Child Health Programs[119]
- After RFK Jr.'s 'Radical Transparency' Pledge, HHS Shutters Much of Its Communications, FOIA Operations[120]
- After April Fools' Day Purge, U.S. Health Agencies Spiral into Chaos[121]
- Trump Team Removes Senior NIH Chiefs in Shock Move[122]
- Trump Administration Fires Workers at NIH's Alzheimer's Research Center, Including Incoming Director[123]
- CDC's Population Health Office Is Gone[124]
- Attempts to Slash NIH Funding Continue, Threatening the Future of Scientific Research[125]
- Trump White House Directs NIH To Study 'Regret' Following Gender Transition Treatments[126]
- NIH Sued Over 'Ideological Purge' Of DEI, Covid and Vaccine Research[127]
- Inside Yesterday's Anxiety-Inducing, 'Crude and Callous' HHS Cuts[128]
- Robert F Kennedy Jr's Proposal to Remove Public Commentary from US Health Policy Is a Threat to Science and Public Health[129]
- Top Scientists Warn of 'Climate of Fear' Under Trump, Urge the Public to Act[130]

- CDC's Office of Smoking and Health Eliminated[131]
- RFK Jr. Cuts 4,700 FDA and NIH Jobs as HHS Eliminates 'An Entire Alphabet Soup of Departments'[132]
- Staff Working on Childhood Lead Exposure and Cancer Clusters Fired From CDC[133]
- FDA Cuts Threaten Medical Product Review Programs[134]
- Trump Administration Orders NIH To Eliminate $2.6 Billion In Federal Contracts[135]
- The Expert Who Kept Eye Drops from Blinding You Was Fired Yesterday[136]
- 'Wrecking Ball': RFK Jr. Moves to Fire Thousands of Health Agency Employees[137]
- More Than 1000 NIH Employees Terminated in Latest Round of Federal Layoffs[138]
- Widespread Firings Start at Federal Health Agencies Including Many in Leadership[139]
- Trump Administration Has Begun a War on Science, Researchers Say[140]
- 75% of US Scientists Who Answered *Nature* Poll Consider Leaving[141]
- FDA Is 'Finished' Amid HHS Firings. Drug Stocks Are Falling[142]
- Young Scientists See Career Pathways Vanish as Schools Adapt to Federal Funding Cuts[143]
- NIH Cuts Will Devastate Disease Research, Say Senators and Scientists[144]
- NIH Removing Outside Scientific Advisers Who Evaluate Research[145]
- CDC Division Responsible for Asthma Control and Lead Poisoning Prevention Effectively Eliminated[146]
- At NIH, 'Everyone Is on Edge' as They Brace for Deep Cuts and More Centralized Control[147]
- 'All This Is in Crisis': US Universities Curtail Staff, Spending as Trump Cuts Take Hold[148]

- RFK Jr.'s HHS Just Dismantled a Center Focused on Efficiency[149]
- Inside the "Vital" Office for Reproductive Health Gutted by Mass HHS Firings[150]

The decimation of research funds threatens several universities that turned a blind eye to or even promoted disinformation spread by faculty members. Recent headlines read: "Johns Hopkins University to Slash 2,000 Jobs After $800M In Federal Cuts,"[151] "Stanford to Lose $160 Million In NIH Funding Change,"[152] and "UCSF 'Borders on Panic' Facing Potential Trump Funding Slash."[153] That's a steep price to pay for "institutional neutrality."

Dr. Gregg Gonsalves summed up the destruction in his article "Trump and RFK Jr. are Destroying a Generation of Knowledge":

What we are seeing is a purge—of the administrative state, of the universities, of expertise—that is consistent with events like the Cultural Revolution in China in the 1960s and '70s, or the dismantling of the tsarist civil service after the Bolshevik Revolution in 1917. Just because this moment isn't associated with the intense political bloodshed of those eras doesn't make the comparison any less apt. In one way or another, the goal is to get rid of an entire set of people and institutions in the service of a radical ideology.

And what is rising in its place is also recognizable from history. From the Covid contrarians running the National Institutes of Health and the Food and Drug Administration to the anti-vaxxers down at HHS headquarters, we have our 21st-century Lysenkos propped up not by the strength of their ideas but by their political patrons in the White House.

While the short-term effects of the administration's policies have

*been well-articulated, the long-term ones are just as chilling. In
less than 100 days, President Trump has created a lasting legacy:
We have lost a generation of expertise, of systems built up to care
for our nation and provide for our collective future in terms of
scientific advances.*[154]

Of course, these attacks on medicine and science can't be separated
from the larger assault on competence, decency, honesty, and the rule of
law that characterizes the Trump administration. All are parts of the same
cruel, destructive process led by cruel, destructive people.

**I'm gonna let him go wild on health. I'm gonna let him go wild on the
food. I'm gonna let him go wild on medicines.**
— Donald Trump

None of this should come as a surprise. Kennedy and his ilk loudly
announced their intentions, and this is not the first dance between Trump
and Kennedy. In 2017, they discussed Kennedy's chairing a "commission on vaccine safety and scientific integrity."[155] Trump spread nonsense
about vaccines long before he was first elected president in 2016,[156] and
he reiterated his beliefs during a phone call with Kennedy in July 2024:

*A vaccination that is like 38 different vaccines and it looks like
it's meant for a horse, not a, you know, 10-pound or 20-pound
baby […] then you see the baby all of a sudden starting to
change radically. I've seen it too many times. And then you hear
that it doesn't have an impact, right?*[157]

The only time Trump received jeers from his followers was when
he suggested they get the COVID vaccine.[158] Having learned to hide
the greatest success of his first term in office, Trump earned applause

by repeatedly vowing not to give "one penny" to schools with vaccine mandates.[159] In one interview, he touted his relationship with Kennedy, saying:

> We're working with Kennedy and we'll take on corruption at the FDA, the CDC, World Health Organization AND other institutions of "Public Health" that are dominated by corporate power and dominated really by China.[160]

Days before the 2024 election, Trump told podcaster Joe Rogan:

> I'm gonna let him go wild on health. I'm gonna let him go wild on the food. I'm gonna let him go wild on medicines.[161]

Unsurprisingly, undermining confidence in vaccines has been one of Kennedy's top priorities. In October 2024, he posted on social media:

> I'm not going to take anyone's vaccines away from them. I just want to be sure every American knows the safety profile, the risk profile, and the efficacy of each vaccine. That's it.[162]

That same day, his organization, Children's Health Defense, posted about a scientist who reportedly used a "4000x microscope to examine the blood of vaccinated and unvaccinated people, alive and deceased." According to the tweet:

> This is easily one of the most disturbing things we have ever had the misfortune to post. **There are blinking lights in peoples' blood.**[163]

The CDC may soon be publishing this kind of material. Kennedy has tapped David Geier, an anti-vaccine activist with no medical training, to "study" the relationship between vaccines and autism.[164] One article about Geier stated:

> Geier, who is not a doctor, and his father co-authored papers claiming that vaccines cause autism. They also worked together

*at a Maryland clinic that treated autistic children with Lupron, a
drug used for the chemical castration of rapists. In 2012, Geier's father lost his medical license for prescribing the treatment
and Geier was fined $10,000 for practicing medicine without a
license.*[165]

There is no doubt what Geier's study will "discover," and again, the
next steps aren't a secret. Just days before the election, journalists reported these conversations with Trump:

*REPORTER: You said you would like RFK Jr do whatever he
wants with healthcare-*

TRUMP: Oh, he's gonna have a big role in healthcare

REPORTER: You're comfortable with his views on vaccines?

*TRUMP: We'll be talking about a lot of things but he's gonna
have a very big role on healthcare.*[166]

On Kennedy and vaccines:

*REPORTER: Do you think banning certain vaccines might be
on the table?*

*TRUMP: Well I'm going to talk to him and talk to other people,
and I'll make a decision, but he's a very talented guy and has
strong views.*[167]

Vaccines may be banned or litigated out of existence in the near
future. Kennedy has profited from suing vaccine makers, prompting Senator Elizabeth Warren to comment:

*His finances will still be tied to the outcomes of anti-vaccine
lawsuits — even as he'd be tasked with regulating them as health
secretary. These are outrageous conflicts of interest that endan-
ger public health.*[168]

I'm gonna say to NIH scientists, God bless you all. Thank you for public service. We're going to give infectious disease a break for about eight years.
— *Robert F. Kennedy Jr.*

Kennedy didn't hide his plans to purge scientists either. In 2023, during his presidential campaign, he said:

> *I'm gonna say to NIH scientists, God bless you all. Thank you for public service. We're going to give infectious disease a break for about eight years.*[169]

Kennedy also outlined his plans during his Make America Healthy Again (MAHA) campaign. According to one news report:

> *HHS oversees 13 separate agencies, and Kennedy has long argued they are in desperate need of reform. In campaign speeches, news interviews, podcasts and other public forums, he has described wanting to gut the scientific agencies in charge of science and health policy, such as the NIH, FDA and Centers for Disease Control and Prevention. He told NBC News last year that the agencies have become "sock puppets" for the industries they regulate, and he wants to replace the scientists and government officials with people who align with his views and aren't burdened by conflicts of interest.*[170]

Another article reported:

> *Former independent presidential candidate and antivaccine advocate Robert F. Kennedy Jr. said that former President Trump wants him to choose leaders for key public health agencies if he wins the election in November.*

> *Kennedy told conservative commentator Tucker Carlson that under a second Trump term, he would be responsible for eliminating "corrupt influences" from agencies, Mediaite first reported. "President Trump has asked me specifically to do two things. One, to help unravel the capture of the agencies by corrupt influence. In other words, to drain the swamp. And, you know, I had to say something about President Trump," Kennedy told Carlson. Kennedy named the Centers for Disease Control and Prevention (CDC), the Food and Drug Administration (FDA) and the National Institutes of Health (NIH) as potential agencies during a Tuesday stop in Wisconsin on Carlson's live tour.[171]*

Kennedy wanted to "*gut the scientific agencies in charge of science and health policy,*"[170] and with the help of Elon Musk and his Department of Government Efficiency (DOGE), that's exactly what he's doing.

Unfortunately, Kennedy has won many converts to his anti-science agenda. Another article, just days before the election, quoted the co-chair of the Trump-Vance transition team as saying:

> *He (Mr. Kennedy) says, 'If you give me the data, all I want is the data, and I'll take on the data and show that it's not safe.' And then if you pull the product liability (protections), the companies will yank these vaccines right off, off of the market.[172]*

Shortly before the election, an article appeared about Vice President JD Vance and his interview with Joe Rogan. It said:

> *Vance, who said he's had COVID-19 five times, claimed on the show he was "red-pilled" after he had side effects following taking an unidentified vaccine.*
>
> *"We're not even allowed to talk about the fact that I was as sick as I've ever been for two days, and the worst COVID experience*

I had was like a sinus infection. I'm not really willing to trade that," Vance claimed.

Vance also said he's worried that there may be a "conflict" in 30 to 40 years with developing countries because they have a negative perception of Westerners for "giving them health care that isn't actually health care," referring to vaccines.[173]

Republican legislators announced their plans to incapacitate public health and scientific agencies. The article "Republicans Have a Post-Pandemic Plan for the Scientific Establishment" confirms this, stating:

House and Senate Republicans are plotting a new battlefront in the Covid wars. They seek to rein in the sprawling National Institutes of Health by bringing to heel its civil servants and the leading scientists awarded the agency's biggest research grants. Republicans plan to do that, if they win control of Congress in November, by demanding to know more about what the NIH is funding, assigning more political appointees to keep tabs on the agency, significantly downsizing it and by spreading the wealth to a bigger group of grantees. Democrats in the Senate majority are blocking changes for now. The fight shows how politicized public health has become since the pandemic.

"You have the NIH in the sights of people who think there were big failures during the pandemic and that we have to change the way things operate," said Joel Zinberg, who worked on health policy on the Council of Economic Advisers during Donald Trump's presidency and is now a senior fellow at the libertarian Competitive Enterprise Institute.

Trump, who clashed with NIH leadership during his term, could make some of the changes Republicans want even if Democrats are able to block legislation. At stake: nearly $50 billion in research funding.[174]

The federal government's public health apparatus has lost the public's trust.
— *Project 2025*

Their blueprint was plainly available before the election. The Heritage Foundation's "Project 2025" has 54 pages devoted to neutering the HHS.[175] The CDC is described as "perhaps the most incompetent and arrogant agency in the federal government." The Project goes on to say:

> ***Goal #4: Preparing for the Next Health Emergency.*** *The COVID-19 pandemic demonstrated how catastrophic a micromanaging, misinformed, centralized, and politicized federal government can be. Basic human rights, medical choice, and the doctor–patient relationship were trampled without scientific justification and for extended periods of time. Excess deaths, not due to COVID-19, skyrocketed because of forced lockdowns, isolation, vaccine-related mass firings, and colossal disruptions of the economy and daily rhythms of life. The federal government's public health apparatus has lost the public's trust. Before the next national public health emergency, this apparatus must be fundamentally restructured to ensure a transparent, scientifically grounded, and more nimble, efficient, transparent, and targeted response that respects the unique needs and input of patient populations and providers.*
>
> *Every one of the overreaching policies during the pandemic—from lockdowns and school closures to mask and vaccine mandates or passports—received its supposed legal justification from the state of emergency declared (and renewed) by the HHS Secretary. Tellingly, however, the threshold for what constitutes*

a public health emergency—how many cases, hospitalizations, deaths, etc.—was never defined. For the sake of democratic accountability, we must know with clarity what will trigger the next emergency declaration and, just as important, what will trigger its end. Unaccountable bureaucrats like Anthony Fauci should never again have such broad, unchecked power to issue health "guidelines" that will certainly be the basis for federal and state mandates. Never again should public health bureaucrats be allowed to hide information, ignore information, or mislead the public concerning the efficacy or dangers associated with any recommended health interventions because they believe it may lead to hesitancy on the part of the public. The only way to restore public trust in HHS as an institution capable of acting responsibly during a health emergency is through the best of disinfectants—light.

Read that again:

> *Excess deaths, not due to COVID-19, skyrocketed because of forced lockdowns, isolation, vaccine-related mass firings, and colossal disruptions of the economy and daily rhythms of life. The federal government's public health apparatus has lost the public's trust.*

You'll see that message repeatedly throughout this book. The revisionist history of "Project 2025" absolves SARS-CoV-2 of all responsibility and blames those who tried to contain it for its consequences. That's the message coming from the White House today, though they also blame a lab leak for this virus.[176] Similarly, you'll read suggestions about how to *"restore public trust"* from doctors who deliberately spread mistrust in public health because they want to destroy it.

Why Doctors Should Learn to Stop Worrying and Love MAHA.
— Dr. Joseph Marine

These drastic events have divided doctors featured in this book. Although any one of the headlines above is enough to disqualify Kennedy as leader of the HHS, many doctors absurdly depicted him as the savior of American medicine. It's no coincidence that the same doctors who spread absurdities about COVID also claimed that the man behind *Vaxxed III: Authorized to Kill*[177] was the perfect guy to save vaccines and science in general. They wrote glowing homages to him, such as:

- "RFK Jr Will Disrupt the US Medical Establishment" by Dr. Jay Bhattacharya and Kevin Bardosh[178]
- "RFK Jr. is Saying Things People Know are True but Don't Want to Hear: Dr. Makary"[179]
- "Why Doctors Should Learn to Stop Worrying and Love MAHA" by Dr. Joseph Marine[180]
- "Donald Trump Has a Plan to Make America's Children Healthy Again. It's a Good One" by Dr. Robert Redfield[181]
- "Sabotaging RFK Jr's Confirmation Will Increase Vaccine Hesitancy" by Dr. Vinay Prasad[182]
- "The Cure for Vaccine Skepticism" by Dr. Martin Kulldorff[183]
- "The Nomination of Robert F. Kennedy Jr. as Secretary of the Department of Health and Human Services: A New Beginning?" by Dr. Frederik Schaltz-Buchholzer[184]

That last article, by a Danish epidemiologist and published on the monetized disinformation Substack *Sensible Medicine*, said:

> *RFK Jr. will be a net positive for public health in the US. The mainstream media – who were the most important enablers of the destructive COVID-19 policies - are falling over themselves and screaming wolf, oblivious to the fact that current US public health is a complete failure.* [...]

While I have not read all of RFK's statements closely, my general impression is that he focuses on topics that are potentially important/relevant, and then unfortunately often exaggerates or distorts the facts.

That's pure propaganda. Kennedy's belief that AIDS is caused by a "gay lifestyle,"[185]not HIV, is not "potentially important/relevant," and saying that Kennedy "exaggerates or distorts the facts" is like saying the Titanic was an unpleasant boat ride. As people who have actually bothered to closely read Kennedy's statements know, he is a paranoid, angry crank who is utterly disconnected from reality and wants to burn it all down.

Dr. Frederik Schaltz-Buchholzer would later try to absolve Kennedy of any responsibility for the 2025 measles outbreaks, saying to me on social media:

A measles outbreak now, 2 months after his nomination, can hardly be his fault, though, could it? Falling vaccine coverage over the years is a problem that likely increased due to the failed COVID-19 policies that you championed.[186]

According to Dr. Schaltz-Buchholzer, Kennedy's 20-year history of anti-vax disinformation was erased the moment he was sworn into office, and he is not to blame for vaccine clinics closing in Texas. In contrast, my articles arguing that COVID vaccine side effects aren't as bad as literal death caused Mennonite parents in Texas to refuse vaccinating their children against measles. Apparently, I have great influence in that community, and it's my fault that a 6-year-old and an 8-year-old,[187] both of whom should have been vaccinated *before* the pandemic, died of measles. While Kennedy is blameless, my words can travel back in time.

> "I think that it's also reasonable to ask questions about the particulars of the vaccines that are on the schedule one at a time,"
> — *Dr. Jay Bhattacharya*

Several doctors—namely Drs. Marty Makary and Jay Bhattacharya—have been rewarded for their willingness to spread COVID disinformation with prominent positions in the Trump administration as heads of the FDA and NIH, respectively. Dr. Tracy Beth Høeg, a sports medicine physician, was also named a "special assistant"[188] to Dr. Makary at the FDA, where one of her first acts was to halt the approval of the Novavax COVID vaccine, demanding that they conduct a new clinical trial.[189] Despite the complete failure of the plan to get rid of SARS-CoV-2 by spreading it, these doctors are not chastened or humbled. They are embittered and emboldened.

They are also powerful and influential. After absurdly railing against the "medical establishment" as if they were outsiders, these doctors are now the epitome of the medical establishment, and reaching these heights required them to legitimize Kennedy's anti-vaccine disinformation.

In his article "Trump Pick for NIH Director: Vaccines May Cause Autism, Alternative Schedules Okay," Walker Bragman reported:

> *On the Dad Saves podcast, Bhattacharya claimed the COVID shots only marginally reduced the risk of death from the virus, and only for a limited time. He argued the boosters lacked adequate evidence of benefit and said the vaccines should be reserved for older populations.*
>
> *Beyond casting doubt on COVID shots, the professor, who has never practiced medicine himself, endorsed alternate vaccine schedules—a popular idea among anti-vaxxers—and suggested*

that pediatricians ought to be respectful and open to concerns about inoculations from parents.

"I think that it's also reasonable to ask questions about the particulars of the vaccines that are on the schedule one at a time,"
he added. "I don't see how, in this post-COVID era, you can just simply say 'trust the experts.'"

When host Papola told him that he and his wife had spaced the vaccines out for their children and asked for a reason not to do that, Bhattacharya responded that "there's not great randomized trial evidence to like, answer that question, so why not just have that?"

"Especially since measles isn't really circulating at very, very high levels in the community at large, right? So you're not actually exposing your child to a risk if you delay by a couple of months," he said. "If it is circulating, then of course you probably want to do it earlier, right?"

Measles cases are currently surging in the U.S. prompting concern from experts. The disease can kill and cause lasting health consequences.

Bhattacharya said that if he had a young child, he would give them "many" of the vaccines on the schedule, but added that "there's uncertainties about all of them." He also noted, "There are ones where I'd be more skeptical."

" 'HPV is generally sexually transmitted. Why give it to a baby?' Someone could easily ask that," Bhattacharya said. "Do I need to give it to my son who's not ever going to get cervical cancer? Hepatitis B is another virus that babies, unless they're exposed from the mother in utero, are not going to get the disease until

they're an adult. Could we wait? I personally would do it, but I could totally understand a parent saying 'no, let's wait on this.'"[190]

In reality, children do not receive the HPV vaccine until they are at least 9 years old, it also protects boys from cancer, and there are important reasons why the hepatitis B vaccine is given to newborns.

During his confirmation hearing to become the NIH director, Dr. Bhattacharya refused to rule out vaccines as a cause of autism, saying "My inclination is to give people good data."[191] However, Dr. Bhattacharya provided bad data throughout the pandemic, and reams of data refuting the link between vaccines and autism already exist.

Despite Kennedy's awful start, Dr. Bhattacharya recently said he "admires" him and:

He wakes up in the morning asking, "How can I make the lives of children better? How can we address the chronic health needs of the American people?" He has ideas about what causes autism. But from a scientific point of view, there's been a tremendous increase in autism diagnoses. [...] And we don't know why. The answer in that situation is to do excellent science so that we can find out what causes it—and then we can address it in an informed way.[192]

That's going to age nearly as well as Dr. Bhattacharya's prediction that COVID would only kill about 20,000–40,000 Americans.[193]

Similarly, during his confirmation hearing, Dr. Makary refused to commit to restarting canceled vaccine meetings and cast doubt on the independence of federal advisors, saying:

We need to review the ethics policy. [...] I want life sciences com-

panies to thrive, but we need to call balls and strikes and to keep
that independent scientific review process free of any conflicts.[194]

Effective pandemic preparedness. Step 1: Fire all the people current-
ly responsible for pandemic preparedness.
— Dr. Jay Bhattacharya

Achieving these lofty positions required Drs. Bhattacharya and Makary to accept Kennedy's purges, and they began their tenures by presid-
ing over mass firings that unsurprisingly targeted women and minority
scientists.

April Fools' Day 2025 perfectly encapsulated the tenures of Drs.
Bhattacharya and Makary so far. On that day, the article "'One of the
Darkest Days': NIH Purges Agency Leadership Amid Mass Lay-offs"
was published. It said:

> *On health economist Jay Bhattacharya's first day as the head of*
> *the US National Institutes of Health (NIH), the chiefs of 4 of the*
> *27 institutes and centres that make up the agency — including*
> *the country's top infectious-diseases official — were removed*
> *from their posts. The unprecedented move comes amid massive*
> *cuts to research funding at the NIH.*
>
> *The directors of the National Institute of Allergy and Infectious*
> *Diseases (NIAID), the National Institute of Child Health and*
> *Human Development (NICHD), the National Institute on Mi-*
> *nority Health and Health Disparities (NIMHD) and the National*
> *Institute of Nursing Research (NINR) were informed late on 31*
> *March that they were being placed on administrative leave.*[84]

Another article that day reported that Dr. Bhattacharya pledged to "implement new policies humanely."[195] Those "new policies" meant firing people, and to his credit, Dr. Bhattacharya acknowledged that the layoffs were entirely political in nature. "Many of our valued colleagues are losing their jobs, which is in no way a reflection of the quality of their work," he said.

He's right. Scientists weren't fired because they were incompetent. They were fired because of their beliefs, and they weren't fired "humanely." According to the article "'A Cruel April Fool's Joke': HHS Layoffs Characterized by Confusion, Errors":

> As NIH workers were digesting the loss of their jobs, they received an introductory email from Jay Bhattacharya, the newly confirmed director of the medical research agency.
> One NIH staffer described Bhattacharya's note as a "thank you and can't wait to work with you email ... in the middle of the massacre."[196]

That same day, contrarian podcaster Bari Weiss posted an interview with Dr. Bhattacharya where he lamented that Dr. Francis Collins, the former NIH director, had called him "fringe" in a private email over four years ago.[197] He said the insult was intended to "destroy" him, and it "really hurt." Dr. Bhattacharya spoke about how meaningful it was that Dr. Collins had apologized to him privately and urged Dr. Collins to make a public apology as well. At that moment, when many of his valued colleagues were "losing their jobs," Dr. Bhattacharya, the current NIH director, was feeling sorry for himself because he had been called a mean name in 2020.

As scientists were closing their labs and cleaning out their desks, he gave another interview on Fox News that day where he said:

> We'll never use this agency to censor scientists who disagree. If scientists are censored, we actually can't have excellent science.[198]

Dr. Bhattacharya also said:

> *The healthcare system ought to be focused on preventing disease*
> *in the first place. The chronic disease problems that we have,*
> *many of them could be prevented. We have all these incentives*
> *to take care of people after they are sick. Let's make incentives*
> *to make people healthier so that they don't get sick in the first*
> *place.*[199]

Again, that sounds compassionate and reasonable. However, Dr. Bhattacharya rose to fame for his proposal to mass-infect unvaccinated people aged 60 and under to reach herd immunity in three to six months, and Kennedy, his boss, has devoted his career to promoting disease in the first place.

Moreover, although Dr. Bhattacharya extolled the virtues of preventing chronic disease, many experts *in* chronic disease were victims of the purge. According to one article published that day:

> *Several top scientists charged with overseeing research into*
> *disease prevention and cures at the National Institutes of Health*
> *(NIH) were notified that they were subject to a reduction in force*
> *on Tuesday as part of a devastating purge of federal employees*
> *carried out by US Health and Human Services Secretary Robert*
> *Kennedy Jr., WIRED has learned.*
>
> *Multiple sources at the NIH, granted anonymity because they*
> *were not authorized to talk to the media, confirmed Tuesday*
> *afternoon that at least 10 principal investigators who were*
> *leading and directing medical research at the agency had been*
> *fired. Among them is Dr. Richard Youle, a leading researcher*
> *in the field of neurodegenerative disorders previously awarded*
> *the Breakthrough Prize in Life Sciences for his groundbreaking*
> *research identifying mechanisms behind Parkinson's disease.*[85]

This April Fools' Day gaslighting was simply a repetition of what happened regarding COVID, where contrarian doctors treated trivialities and persecution fantasies with more importance than unwanted calamities in hospitals. No matter what disaster was happening on the ground with COVID, Dr. Bhattacharya was on Fox News to say that everything was just fine, except for how *he* had been treated. Now, as people are being fired at the NIH, he is on Fox News promoting a new age of tolerance for dissent.

Dr. Bhattacharya's willingness to cut funding for medical research and purge scientists was no surprise. He had previously fantasized about being able to take revenge on scientists this way. In October 2023, he tweeted:

> *Once, I would have lamented funding cuts for the @NIH. Now, I view them as an appropriate response to an out of control agency that funded dangerous research, conducted devastated* [sic] *takedowns of scientists, and hid unclassified documents from public scrutiny.*[200]

Then in January 2024, he posted:

> *Effective pandemic preparedness. Step 1: Fire all the people currently responsible for pandemic preparedness. They likely caused the pandemic, locked you down, kept your kids out of school, demolished economies, and want more power to do it again.*[201]

Dr. Makary similarly purged scientists at the FDA. Though he had recorded a podcast in 2022 titled "Cancel Culture Isn't Good for Science,"[202] headlines from his start read, "FDA's New Commissioner Marty Makary Signed Off on Peter Marks Ouster"[203] and "FDA Commissioner Marty Makary Gets Off to a Bruising Start as Agency Is Wracked by Layoffs,"[204] among others.

According to one article:

> *U.S. public-health agencies on Tuesday morning, and the im-*
> *pact on the Food and Drug Administration so far has been dire,*
> *according to current and former employees.*
>
> *"The FDA as we've known it is finished, with most of the leaders*
> *with institutional knowledge and a deep understanding of prod-*
> *uct development and safety no longer employed," former FDA*
> *Commissioner Dr. Robert Califf wrote in a LinkedIn post.*[142]

Appropriately, these articles were also published on April Fools' Day.

Along with their COVID disinformation, the fate of these agencies will be the permanent legacy of Drs. Bhattacharya and Makary. They became famous during the pandemic for listing the amazing things they *would have* done, but now they have significant real-world responsibility for the first time. It's very early, but things are going terribly so far. Both of them seem to be at the mercy of forces they didn't anticipate and can't control. It turns out that actually running the FDA and NIH is a lot harder than complaining about it on Fox News and Twitter, especially when your boss is Kennedy and DOGE arrived with a chainsaw.

According to the article "RFK Jr. Vowed to Upend American Health Care. It's Happening Faster Than Expected":

> *Many of those people had expressed cautious optimism at the*
> *outset of Kennedy's tenure, encouraged by his focus on chronic*
> *disease and promises to leave hard-edged activism behind in*
> *favor of a "mutual intention to work toward what we all care*
> *about: the health of the American people."*
>
> *Yet that goodwill has run dry, they said, amid Kennedy's deci-*
> *sions to downsize the department while devoting resources to*
> *investigating the debunked theory linking vaccines and autism,*
> *and muddling messaging on a measles outbreak that has now*

killed two children.

"This has set us back dramatically," said Michael Osterholm, an epidemiologist and director of the University of Minnesota's Center for Infectious Disease Research and Policy. "We are nowhere near as safe now as we were even 10 weeks ago." […]

Several officials characterized FDA Commissioner Marty Makary, who signed off on the ouster of Marks and other senior regulators in his first days, as an instant pariah among many of his own employees. Despite Kennedy's insistence that the firings sought only to eliminate redundancies, current and former employees said many offices are effectively nonfunctional as supervisors spend their days figuring out who was cut and what programs are affected.

Alex Saint, a communications official laid off as part of a gutting of the FDA's public affairs operation, told POLITICO that only about a quarter of the staff remains in the communications shop for the division that oversees prescription drugs, which last year handled roughly 42,000 inquiries alone — most of them from the general public. That office also issued the critical alerts FDA sends to doctors and patients when there are new safety concerns with a medicine or medical device.

"There's no one left to write a drug safety communication," Saint said.[108]

According to another article, "RFK Jr. Says Deep State 'Is Real,' Called FDA Employees 'Sock Puppet' of Industry":

HHS Secretary Robert F. Kennedy Jr.'s visit to the FDA Friday was supposed to introduce him as a trusted leader to agency employees. It did anything but.

Over the course of 40 minutes, Kennedy, in largely off-the-cuff remarks, asserted that the "Deep State" is real, referenced past CIA experiments on human mind control and accused the employees he was speaking to of becoming a "sock puppet" of the industries they regulate. [...]

By the end of the event, billed as a welcome from the new commissioner, Marty Makary, several FDA staffers had walked out of the rooms where the speech was being broadcast.[205]

Dr. Makary has used his power and influence to warn about talc, seed oils, and COVID vaccines. He feels that keeping Americans safe from these dangers is a top priority.

Things aren't better at the NIH with Dr. Bhattacharya at the helm. According to one article titled "What Is the Actual Point of Treating the N.I.H. Like This?":

By the time their spending accounts were reactivated on Thursday, some scientists at the National Institutes of Health said they were running on fumes.

They had spent weeks scrambling to keep their labs running amid spending freezes, firing rampages and the chaos and confusion brought on by both. They were reusing latex gloves in an effort to conserve supplies. They were borrowing, donating and sharing a long roster of crucial but dwindling reagents with one another, in email threads that had morphed into virtual bazaars. In interviews, several of them said they would have to close up shop in as little as two or three weeks if something didn't change drastically, and soon. [...]

As if none of that were bad enough, people in the agency said the N.I.H. is also set to lose a majority of staff members who work on contracts on June 2, when the 60-day notice period (legally required for firings related to force reduction) concludes; the scientists I spoke with said all of those working for the scientific institutes had been fired.

After a lifetime spent asking big, complicated questions, what the scientists most want to know now is this: Why? What, truly, is the goal of so much cruel and clumsy destruction?

Efficiency is not being enhanced, nor is waste being eliminated. (If anything, it's increasing.) American interests are not being protected. And the quest to cure diseases or improve human health is not being advanced.

So when it's all over, if the crown jewel of biomedical research — the enterprise that gave us the human genome sequence, Covid vaccines and treatments for cancer and H.I.V. and obesity — has been destroyed, what will have been the point?[206]

Although Drs. Makary and Bhattacharya bemoaned "cancel culture" and "censorship" when it came to their social media content, fear permeates the agencies they now lead. Articles about the FDA and NIH today universally include statements from "employees granted anonymity for fear of retaliation."[205] Understandably, scientists don't want to be caught up in the next round of purges if they say the wrong thing or criticize the wrong people. Dedicated scientists are resigning from the NIH, citing censorship and political interference into their research as the chief reasons.

Currently, Drs. Makary and Bhattacharya are flailing and in over their heads. They are distrusted and reviled by many people at the agencies they lead and struggle to answer *basic* questions from journalists. The public doesn't trust them either. Vaccine advocates are upset at their attempts to limit vaccines, while anti-vaxxers are enraged that they approved them for vulnerable populations. Unaccountable DOGE employees with no medical background seem to be calling the shots. We need the FDA and NIH to function and function well. I hope Drs. Makary and Bhattacharya can turn things around at the agencies they supposedly lead. Meanwhile, over at the CDC, no one is in charge. There is no director.

I have no sympathy for academic researchers and their staff who do shit science and live off NIH grants. I am sorry. Never have. Never will.
— Dr. Vinay Prasad

Other doctors in this book aren't involved in a direct way but have minimized the assault on science from the sidelines exactly as they did with COVID. Dr. John Mandrola, who relentlessly sought to numb people to COVID with articles such as "No, Young Adults Should Not Live in Fear from Coronavirus,"[207] implied that the NIH funded useless "coffee and blueberries studies [...] nonrandom retrospective comparisons" and said, "If NIH-supported studies like this decreased b/c of cuts, medical research would be just fine."[208]

Dr. Mandrola's false assurances were wrong on both counts. COVID became a leading killer of young adults after he told them not to fear this outcome—though death is not COVID's only bad outcome—and the cuts to the NIH affected more than coffee and blueberry studies.

His colleague Dr. Prasad used similar language to belittle massive cuts to funding and staffing. In an article titled "Pausing NIH Study Sections Is Going to Be Fine," he said that "The government cannot be a welfare program for everybody doing low quality, low credibility, irreproducible, low value of information research [sic]."[209]

A White House press release quoted Dr. Prasad as saying:

Cutting indirects might even mean more science. Less money spent on the administration is more money to give out to actual scientists.[210]

When he was not busy spreading Orwellian doublespeak, saying less money is more money, Dr. Prasad gleefully applauded the decimation of our scientific infrastructure. Dr. Prasad spent much of the pandemic spreading doubt about COVID mitigation measures, claiming that only those proven via an RCT were of value. However, now that his ideological allies are in charge, he's stopped demanding RCTs from public health officials. Dr. Prasad bemoaned "censorship" and speculated that mitigation measures might lead to Nazism with COVID, but he's now cheering and justifying every act of sabotage. They can do whatever they want; no RCTs required.

Dr. Prasad was furious at COVID "tyrants" and enjoyed seeing careers and research go up in flames. He felt fired scientists got what they deserved. He was eager to justify every budget cut, every firing, every attack on universities, and every attempt to censor research under the current medical establishment. According to Dr. Prasad, scientists were wrong about the threats to their research, which were merely a fantasy of the dishonest media. His articles reflect this mindset:

- Is More Science Better than Less Science?[211]
- First Defund Bad Science; Then Invest in Good Science[212]
- The Same Media that Lied About All Things COVID is Lying About Peter Marks' Departure from FDA[213]
- Yes, mRNA Vaccine Science Should be Deprioritized by the NIH for 5 Reasons[214]
- Trump Cuts NIH Grants and the Media Screams; VP Pulls up the NIH Grant Funded Papers and Reviews Them- Whoa, They are Useless, and Should be Cut![215]
- Easy Come, Easy Go. DEI Buzzwords Helped You Get a Grant

and Now They Will Cost You One[216]

- Questions the Media Should Ask About Reductions in Work Force[217]
- 3 Ways the Media Coverage of Health Care is Dishonest[218]
- Public Health's Stupidity Will Lead to More Damage & More Measles Outbreaks[219]

In that last article, which does not mention Kennedy, Dr. Prasad said that public health officials are the "dumbest people in the country." Like Dr. Schaltz-Buchholzer, Dr. Prasad blames them for measles outbreaks, saying, "The greatest anti-vax tool ever created was allowing public health to be run by idiots." Dr. Prasad remains a big fan of Mr. Kennedy and is unbothered by his anti-vaccine disinformation.

Dr. Prasad openly fantasized about taking part in the mass purges himself, saying, "I would fire at least ~10000 people (1/4) in the CDC,"[220] and, in his typical profane and childish manner, said:

I have no sympathy for academic researchers and their staff who do shit science and live off NIH grants. I am sorry. Never have. Never will. They do work that cannot be reproduced, just say the same empty slogans that are in vogue. During the pandemic they failed society and lied about the impact of school closure and the viral origins. I can't believe we tax plumbers and bus drivers who do real work to fund this bullshit. It's a welfare program for upper middle class kids. Recently they were saying even a single drink of wine kills you. They should be completely defunded for using low quality science to insert themselves in debates they don't understand, or appreciate. It's not even science. It's propaganda that's government-funded masquerading as science.[221]

Dr. Prasad's willingness to be a cheerleader for the new medical establishment was rewarded with an appointment to head the Center for Biologics Evaluation and Research (CBER)—the FDA division that oversees vaccines and biologic medicines. According to the article "An Anti-Science MAHA Extremist Is Playing a Major Role at the FDA," staff at the FDA

> *Were alarmed by the decision to hire Prasad, who lacks regulatory experience and has more explicitly political views than center directors in the past. "It's very bad," one employee said. "Another completely unqualified person who has no idea what regulation is running an important center."*[222]

Though he was conciliatory on his first day in office, previously Dr. Prasad hurled childish insults and invectives at FDA employees and fantasized about firing the people who now work for him. To pick one example among many, in November 2024, Dr. Prasad complained about the FDA's authorization of the pediatric COVID vaccine and said, "Good News. These idiots will be fired soon."[223] One of his first actions in office was to make the COVID vaccine unavailable to healthy people under age 65.[224]

There's just so much we would have lost, and that we could still lose.
— Dr. Monica Gandhi

Other doctors in this book appear to have woken up to the dangers of disinformation, after it was too late. They are appalled at the forces they helped unleash, though none of them have acknowledged their role in it. Yet it wasn't until after the election, once the consequences of disinformation struck them personally for the first time, affecting their grants and institutions, that they suddenly started to care about it. In their view, it was fine for doctors to spread fake statistics about COVID, but it's wrong to threaten their funding.

Dr. Jeffrey Flier, the former dean of Harvard Medical School, promoted and amplified people like Dr. Prasad during the pandemic. Now he is writing articles such as "I Led Harvard's Medical School, and I Fear for What's to Come"[225] and "The Case Against RFK Jr."[226] These were perfectly adequate, but Dr. Flier promoted pro-Kennedy doctors and their COVID disinformation while personally attacking me and others for correcting their factual errors and exposing their specious reasoning.

Similarly, an article titled "'Devastating': Trump Research Funding Cuts Could Cost Bay Area Billions" said:

> *After news came of the NIH drawdown, Dr. Monica Gandhi, head of the UCSF-Bay Area Center for AIDS Research, spent the weekend worrying about having to shut down labs, lay off scores of people, and grind research to a halt. She and others at the university helped put together long briefs for attorneys detailing their research and spending in an effort to save themselves.*
>
> *"People are acting like these schools are building palaces, but they're supporting direct research by giving us the infrastructure," Gandhi said. "There's just so much we would have lost, and that we could still lose."*
>
> *The Center for AIDS Research is supported almost entirely by indirect rates from the $38 million in NIH grants steered toward Gandhi's research over the past decade. The funding covers electricity, water, janitorial staff, and salaries, among other infrastructure for the 750 researchers under her purview.*
>
> *It also supports efforts well beyond the campus, undertaken via partnerships with public and private entities across the U.S. and in South Africa and India.*

"The degree of anxiety this caused, it's just an incredible waste of time," Gandhi said. "And I have a feeling we're going to go through this again and again over the next four years as the [Trump] administration attacks science in a very chaotic, sudden way."[227]

Another article titled "UCSF 'Borders on Panic' Facing Potential Trump Funding Slash" also featured Dr. Monica Gandhi. It said:

As the lead of the Center for AIDS Research at the University of California, San Francisco, Dr. Monica Gandhi is spending the month in a world of devastating "what-ifs."

What would have happened if a federal judge had not, on Feb. 10, blocked the Trump administration's order to slash billions in biomedical research funding from the National Institutes of Health? Monitoring the health of study participants in biomedical research funded by NIH would be gone. Clinical trials on patients would be stopped. Key services, like maintaining the lab equipment and keeping research data safe, would also vanish.

"All of that, as of Friday, is massively threatened," Gandhi said.[153]

She's absolutely right, and I feel horrible for her and her team. However, I can't help but wonder, "what if" prominent people like Drs. Flier and Gandhi had spoken with a unified voice to oppose disinformation and guard against its threat? Instead, they and other doctors in this book spread disinformation, and, when warned about its dangers, either ignored the alarms or lashed out with juvenile insults against those who tried to warn them.

The anti-vaxxers haven't won yet, but they are in power and on the offensive. I have been studying and battling anti-vaccine disinformation since 2010. What I observe is that, while most parents still want to vaccinate their children, not only are vaccine rates dipping thanks to disinformation spread during COVID,[228] but we are also much less prepared to handle a pandemic than we were in 2020. Unfortunately, the problem of disinformation and the resulting distrust in public health has gotten much worse since March 2020.

Everything that's happening now is just a continuation of a process that's been brewing for decades; it was just supercharged when COVID arrived five years ago. A collective failure to forcefully reject disinformation at that time directly led us to this moment. What's changed is who is in charge. The same doctors who intentionally and relentlessly spread COVID disinformation are featured today in articles about "purges" and "firings." This is not a coincidence.

These doctors are now the medical establishment, and they own everything that's happening. Their harm will reverberate for decades, and many people will be hurt along the way.

How did all of this happen? How could someone like Kennedy even be considered for such a position? How has half the country become indifferent to or even excited by the possibility of an anti-vax disinformation agent gaining power? Why, after a virus killed 1.2 million Americans, are so many people only upset because we tried to contain it for a year? How did the anti-vaccine movement, which sent so many people to early graves, emerge from the pandemic empowered, emboldened, and legitimized? Why were so many "leaders" blind to the threat? How did doctors who spread blatant disinformation and purposely aimed to infect unvaccinated people gain power and influence? How did front-line healthcare workers, who risked their lives to save lives, go from heroes to villains in the eyes of so many people in such a short time?

This book seeks to answer these questions and examine the crucial role doctors and institutions played in bringing us to this sad, dangerous moment. In the prequel to this book, *We Want Them Infected*, I wrote that I underestimated the anti-vaccine movement and threats to science. Once again, I underestimated the danger. I didn't imagine that things would get so bad so fast, and we are just getting started. But at least I and many others left a clear record of how we got here. We tried to warn people that it was dangerous to tolerate and normalize disinformation.

Chapter 2: Public Health is Undervalued, Underfunded, Neglected, Mistreated

Numerous groups, such as the tobacco industry, have deliberately altered and misrepresented knowable facts and empirical evidence to promote an agenda.
— *Rebecca F. Goldberg and Dr. Laura N. Vandenberg*

You may have heard the expression, "The first thing a cult does is to convince you that everyone else is lying to you." Whether or not this is true of cults, the message reinforced repeatedly by the doctors I will discuss in this book is this: *Everyone else is lying to you.*

A small number of prestigious doctors from prestigious universities, in conjunction with right-wing politicians, tech moguls, and business interests, are waging an open war on the very concept of public health as well as the idea that words have specific meanings and that objective facts are real and knowable. Their primary weapon is doubt. As Garry Kasparov said, "The point of modern propaganda isn't only to misinform or push an agenda. It is to exhaust your critical thinking, to annihilate truth."[1]

Drs. David Gorski and Gavin Yamey rightly called these doctors the "the new merchants of doubt"[2]—a reference to the book by Naomi Oreskes and Erik M. Conway about scientists who denied climate change and the dangers of tobacco use.[3] "Doubt is our product," said one tobacco executive. These new merchants of doubt didn't hide their intentions. They are openly hostile to our nation's public health agencies and have called for their destruction. They produced podcasts such as "Stop Trusting the Public Health Establishment"[4] only to turn around to give lectures titled "Why No One Trusts Scientists Anymore."[5]

None of their techniques were new or unusual. In their article, "The Science of Spin: Targeted Strategies to Manufacture Doubt with Detrimental Effects on Environmental and Public Health," Rebecca F. Goldberg and Dr. Laura N. Vandenberg discussed how tobacco, coal, and sugar industries "deliberately altered and misrepresented knowable facts and empirical evidence to promote an agenda, often for monetary benefit, with consequences for environmental and public health."[6]

Goldberg and Vandenberg presented 28 strategies and 10 logical fallacies these groups used to manufacture doubt, and these are featured on every page of this book.

In the lists below, "A" refers to scientific evidence and facts, while "B" refers to information generated to promote narratives that are favorable to the industry.

List 1: Strategies Used to Spread Doubt

- **Attack Study Design:** To emphasize study design flaws in A that have only minimal effects on outcomes. Flaws include issues related to bias, confounding, or sample size
- **Gain Support from Reputable Individuals:** Recruit experts or influential people in certain fields (politicians, industry, journals, doctors, scientists, health officials) to defend B in order to gain broader support.
- **Misrepresent Data:** Cherry-pick data, design studies to fail, or conduct meta-analyses to dilute the work of A.
- **Suppress Incriminating Information:** Hide information that runs counter to B.
- **Contribute Misleading Literature:** Use literature published in journals or the media to deliberately misinform, either pro-B, anti-A, or to distract with peripheral topics.
- **Host Conferences or Seminars:** Organize conferences for scientists or relevant stakeholders to provide a space for

dissemination of only pro-B information.

- **Avoid/Abuse Peer-Review:** Avoid the peer-review process to publish poor literature, publish without revealing funding sources, use the journal name to add weight to claims, or minimize need for peer-review among lay audiences.
- **Employ Hyperbolic or Absolutist Language:** Discuss scientific findings in absolutist terms or with hyperbole, use buzzwords to differentiate between "strong" and "poor" science (i.e. sound science, junk science, etc.).
- **Blame Other Causes:** Find related, alternative causes for negative effects that are reported or observed.
- **Invoke Liberties/Censorship/Overregulation:** Invoke laws to emphasize equality and rights for expression of B, despite differences in evidence quality.
- **Define How to Measure Outcome/Exposure:** Attempt to set guidelines for 'proper' measurement of exposures or outcomes, while undermining guidelines used in A.
- **Take Advantage of Scientific Illiteracy (media/individuals):** Emphasize scientific obscurity to confuse lay audiences, or deliberately disseminate unscientific or false but digestible information.
- **Pose as a Defender of Health or Truth:** Represent the goals of B as health-conscious or dedicated to truth.
- **Obscure involvement:** Ghostwrite, create shell companies, use attorney client privilege to hide association.
- **Develop a PR Strategy:** Devise methods for specifically reaching public audiences to spread B messages.
- **Appeal to Mass Media:** Appealing to journalistic balance, developing relationships with media personnel, preparing information for media personnel, invoking the Fairness Doctrine.
- **Take Advantage of Victim's Lack of Money/Influence:** Silence or abuse individuals by out-spending or exploiting a power imbalance.

- **Normalize Negative Outcomes:** Normalize the presence of negative effects to reduce importance and make them seem inevitable.

- **Impede Government Regulation:** Overwhelm governmental regulatory agencies to slow or stop their function.

- **Alter Product to Seem Healthier:** Make modifications to harmful product to reduce ostensible negative effects.

- **Influence Government/Laws:** Gain inappropriate proximity to regulatory bodies and encourage pro-B policy.

- **Attack Opponents (scientifically/personally):** Conduct targeted attacks on opponents by undermining their professional or personal reputations.

- **Appeal to Emotion:** Manipulate an audience's emotions to draw support for claims in the absence of facts.

- **Inappropriately Question Causality:** Argue that correlation does not equal causation despite the presence of strong evidence.

- **Make Straw Man Arguments:** Publicly refute an argument that was not made by the opposition.

- **Abuse Credentials:** Use qualifications in one discipline to assume authority in another discipline.

- **Abuse Data Access Requests:** Requesting access to data in order to misrepresent and attack, employing Shelby Amendment, Freedom of Information Act, etc.

- **Claim Slippery Slope:** Illogically or falsely claiming that there will be disastrous consequences if B ideology is not supported.

List 2: Fallacies Used to Spread Doubt

- **Gain Support from Reputable Individuals:** Appeal to authority (*ad vercundiam*): saying that because an "authority" believes something, it must be true.

- **Misrepresent Data:** Texas Sharpshooter: utilizing a subset of evidence that supports a theory but ignoring the full picture.

- **Blame Other Causes:** Questionable Cause (*cum hoc ergo propter hoc*): confusing correlation with causation.

- **Define How to Measure Outcome/Exposure:** Definist Fallacy:

redefine a term to make a position easier to argue.

- **Pose as a Defender of Health or Truth:** Righteousness Fallacy: using evidence of good intentions to support other claims.
- **Attack Opponents:** *Ad hominem*: by attacking the arguer instead of the argument, the argument can be dismissed.
- **Appeal to Emotion:** Appealing to emotion: manipulating an emotional response in place of a valid, factual, compelling argument.
- **Make Straw Man Arguments:** Strawman argument: misrepresenting an argument to make it easier to attack.
- **Abuse Credentials:** Use of false authority: using an expert with dubious or unrelated credentials to promote the industry's position.
- **Claim Slippery Slope:** Slippery Slope: avoiding the main argument by using extreme hypotheticals as distractions.

The biggest danger to my kids isn't the measles, but the thought process that leads people to reject the vaccine in the first place.
— Dr. Jonathan Howard

I have been interested in the anti-vaccine movement, and anti-vaccine doctors in particular, since 2010, when a doctor I trained with, Dr. Kelly Brogan, morphed into one of the country's most prominent anti-vaccine celebrities. As such, I was very familiar with these targeted strategies to manufacture doubt when the pandemic started. In 2018, I co-wrote a book chapter with law professor Dorit Reiss titled "The Anti-Vaccine Movement: A Litany of Fallacy and Errors,"[7] which examined how anti-vaccine advocates spread doubt. That chapter concluded with this observation:

> *Anti-vaccine activists draw on different strands of thoughts and*
> *may have differing motives when they promote misinformation*

that may scare people from vaccinating. However, many common
themes run through the movement, all of which reinforce the ba-
sic reality that anti-vaccine claims have little basis in fact. They
appeal to the way people think and can mislead even rational,
well-intentioned people into putting their children at risk.

That same year, there was a measles outbreak in New York City,
where I live. According to one article, "Consequences of Undervaccina-
tion—Measles Outbreak, New York City, 2018–2019" there were 649
measles cases. It further reported:

The median age was 3 years; 81.2% of the patients were 18 years
of age or younger, and 85.8% of the patients with a known vacci-
nation history were unvaccinated. Serious complications includ-
ed pneumonia (in 37 patients [5.7%]) and hospitalization (in 49
patients [7.6%]); among the patients who were hospitalized, 20
(40.8%) were admitted to an intensive care unit.[8]

Fortunately, no children died but this was all preventable. Children
suffered needlessly because their parents had been told not to trust experts, particularly doctors who warned them measles could be dangerous,
while the MMR was safe and effective.

At the time, I posted, "The biggest danger to my kids isn't the measles, but the thought process that leads people to reject the vaccine in the
first place,"[9] on Twitter (now X).

The bedrock underlying that thought process is anger and doubt.
There is overwhelming evidence that vaccines are safe and effective, and
while most anti-vaxxers know these studies exist, they don't trust them.
They believe doctors, scientists, pharmaceutical companies, and medical
institutions from around the world are corrupt and dishonest to the core.
A dozen more studies showing that the MMR vaccine doesn't cause au-

tism won't move the needle an inch.

Before the pandemic, anti-vaccine doctors like Dr. Brogan nurtured this doubt. They extolled the "benefits" of "natural immunity" and fear-mongered about vaccines. In her article, "Vaccination: Your Body. Your Baby. Their Flu," Dr. Brogan wrote:

> *This better way embraces periodic sickness as part of comprehensive wellness. The only way to truly protect ourselves and our infants is through natural immunity bolstered by wild-type exposure in the community. Once you have a particular flu strain, when it comes around again, you will be uniquely protected, and you will pass on this protection to your newborn. There is no replacement for this. We cannot outsource our health to pharmaceutical companies. They just don't know what health is.*[10]

Dr. Sherri Tenpenny, another anti-vaccine doctor, said:

> *We've got to stop calling chickenpox and measles diseases, because they're not. They're infections, and infections come and go in a week to ten days, and leave behind a lifetime of immunity. A disease is something that comes and stays, and frequently can't be cured. So when you vaccinate to avoid an infection, what you potentially are doing is causing a disease.*[11]

In her article, "The Benefits of Having a Natural Measles Infection," Dr. Suzanne Humphries claimed that measles treats kidney disease and cancer:

> *Why not just let wild measles circulate and do the job nature intended at the time of life it was intended, which leads to 65 years of immunity and no need for life-span vaccination?*[12]

Anti-vaccine doctors abused their credentials to speak directly to parents. According to an article about Dr. Larry Palevsky, a "holistic pediatrician," who publicly urged parents not to vaccinate their children:

> *"Hundreds of thousands, if not millions, of mothers… have*
> *witnessed children regressing after they get the MMR," Palev-*
> *sky told the crowd, largely composed of members of Rockland's*
> *Orthodox Jewish community, according to a Gothamist reporter*
> *who attended the event. […] He reportedly added: "Children*
> *stop talking, they don't look at you, they start flapping their arms,*
> *they start banging their head."*[13]

What bothered me so much about these doctors was not only that their disinformation hurt children—though this was obviously the worst part—but that they were entirely sheltered from the consequences. Their casual ability to dismiss dangerous viruses wouldn't have been possible if they had real world responsibility for children who were hospitalized due to those viruses. However, sick children were just an abstraction for these doctors, and they used vaccines to build a brand, gain social media followers, and attract paying customers. They were intentionally provocative to draw attention to themselves, and they vilified doctors who had real-world responsibility, saying they were beholden to Big Pharma and had financial incentives to vaccinate children.

Measles and COVID are not the same. Until recently, measles last killed American children in 1990–1991, when nine unvaccinated children died in Philadelphia.[14] In contrast, COVID killed nearly 200 American children in the first two months of 2022,[15] though death is not the only harm from either virus. The MMR vaccine is better than the COVID vaccine. Two doses of the MMR offer near-perfect, lifelong protection against measles. The COVID vaccine is not nearly this effective, though it greatly limits COVID's gravest harms. While measles and COVID are different, the underlying philosophy behind their vaccines is identical. Though most children fully recover, both viruses can hurt them, and vaccination blunts those harms.

Measles and COVID share another similarity: Anti-vaccine doctors used the same strategies to manufacture doubt, undermining not only vaccines but also doctors, public health officials, and everyone and everything else—except for them.

However, there are some significant differences between doctors who spread disinformation about measles in 2019 and doctors who spread disinformation about COVID. Before the pandemic, anti-vaccine doctors were pariahs in the medical community, rightfully treated with scorn and contempt. Pre-pandemic anti-vaccine doctors also weren't particularly influential with regard to COVID. They didn't advise powerful politicians, and they weren't given space to write editorials in major newspapers.

Unfortunately, other doctors replaced them, and today's anti-vaccine doctors get glowing profiles in mainstream newspapers and are celebrated by their university leadership. Their obvious disinformation is either deliberately ignored or, even worse, absurdly reframed as "differing viewpoints."

In this book, I will toggle back and forth between an imaginary world, where the pandemic ended many times, and the real world.
— Dr. Jonathan Howard

My first book on this topic, *We Want Them Infected*, discussed disinformation spread by doctors and the purposeful movement to infect unvaccinated young people with SARS-CoV-2 in the failed quest for herd immunity. In the introduction to that book, I described two pandemic narratives; the real one that occurred in hospitals and an imaginary one that occurred in university faculty offices and podcast booths. I wrote:

> *In this book, I will toggle back and forth between an imaginary world, where the pandemic ended many times, and the real*

world, where COVID remains the third leading cause of death
in the U.S. In the imaginary world, COVID only threatened the
old and infirm. In the real world, tens of thousands of children
and young adults were seriously harmed or killed by COVID.
In the imaginary world, pediatric vaccines were dangerous
and useless. In the real world, the vaccines are imperfect but
much safer than the virus for children. In the imaginary world,
all it took to protect nursing homes and open schools was to
say "protect nursing homes" and "open schools." In the real
world, this was impossible when the virus was allowed to
spread freely. In the imaginary world, contrarian doctors were
silenced and suppressed. In the real world, they were loud and
influential.[16]

This book will return to the mirror world, where advocates of herd
immunity through mass infection now claim to have been vindicated
and that only America's leading anti-vaxxer, Robert F. Kennedy Jr., can
restore confidence in vaccines.

I will use the phrase "WWTI doctors" to describe a group of doctors
who were either overt advocates of herd immunity through mass infection or who spread blatant disinformation, always minimizing the risk of
the virus and maximizing the risk of the vaccine. Their desire to infect
unvaccinated children hasn't waned, and several of them have the power
to enact their agenda. This book will discuss the same doctors as *We Want
Them Infected*, and it will follow the same format: namely, it will be full
of accurate quotes from sheltered doctors in the mirror world, paired with
news headlines and quotes from doctors who treated COVID patients in
the real world.

In *We Want Them Infected*, seeking to give people the benefit of the doubt, I used the term "misinformation," which refers to the unintentional spread of false information. In this book, I will primarily use the term "disinformation," which implies intentionality. While I am not a mind reader, I no longer see the need to sugarcoat things or to pretend these doctors' errors were all mere accidents.

In many ways, I am a collector and curator more than an author, and my books are reference books. My goal is to keep a record of how we got to this moment and to preserve WWTI doctors' words. They may want their false declarations of herd immunity and bogus statistics to be forgotten, but I do not. Twenty-five pages of *We Want Them Infected* were nothing more than direct quotes of doctors declaring the pandemic over. This book will have similar lists, and all information will be referenced so that my work can be fact-checked. Like *We Want Them Infected*, it will be hard to challenge for that reason. However, unlike Kennedy's "MAHA Report: Make Our Children Healthy Again," which includes Drs. Jay Bhattacharya and Marty Makary as authors, none of my references are fake, AI-generated hallucinations.[17]

Neither book is about doctors who said some silly things in a couple of hastily written social media posts. There are a few stupid tweets of my own lurking out there. Rather, the material that I present reflects a steady stream of consistent, coordinated communication. WWTI doctors had a message, and they repeated it relentlessly in blogs, podcasts, social media posts, documentaries, TV interviews, and editorials in mainstream newspapers and the "heterodox" media. I strongly encourage you to view the material yourself, especially their YouTube videos. Many WWTI doctors are polished speakers who are very charismatic and comfortable in front of cameras.

I will be able to share only a small fraction of their disinformation here. However, I will present lists of articles and collections of quotes to show how seemingly credible doctors repeatedly drilled certain messages into the public consciousness to minimize COVID, promote their political agenda, and elevate their public profile. Thanks to their efforts, many people are convinced that we greatly overreacted to COVID and that everything would have been perfectly fine had we made only a minimal effort to contain it.

I view this book as a sequel to *We Want Them Infected*, though I also intend for it to stand on its own and tell a different story. *We Want Them Infected* was about *why* these doctors were wrong. Unlike in *We Want Them Infected*, I will not present exhaustive data about rare, mild, temporary vaccine side effects but, instead, expect readers to agree with me that they are not as bad as death from COVID. However, I will repeat some material again when appropriate.

For example, it's important to repeat that I have no personal animosity towards any doctors in this book. I have not met with nor spoken to any of them. In fact, I even admired several of them very much prior to the pandemic, favorably quoting them in my book on cognitive biases in medicine.[18]

I write about these doctors because they have impeccable credentials, can speak in scientific jargon, and were highly influential in our pandemic response. They were omnipresent in the media and advised powerful politicians. They were clear that COVID threatened the elderly and infirm, but they said that it was just a cold for everyone else. They mixed good advice with bad advice, making it impossible for many people to recognize that they were spreading disinformation. They spoke with great certainty when they falsely reassured the public that COVID was nothing to worry about and it was all going away.

I will not skimp on discussing the disinformation spread by WWTI doctors. It remains disturbing and relevant. It's important to review the trustworthiness of doctors who told us to distrust everyone else and who will wield great power and influence moving forward. Previously, anti-vaxxers distrusted the medical establishment and heads of institutions such as the NIH and FDA. Those roles are now reversed.

Many people found it hard to get through *We Want Them Infected* without throwing it against the wall. I hope and expect this will trigger a similar reaction. However, while *We Want Them Infected* was the refutation of these doctors' disinformation, my aim here is to zoom out and reveal the techniques they used to undermine trust, the threat they pose to the entire concept of public health, and the failure of institutions to respond.

Public health is undervalued, underfunded, neglected, mistreated.
— *Dr. Vinay Prasad*

Public health officials had a near-impossible job during the pandemic. They were going to be raked over the coals no matter what. This was their first pandemic too, and the virus changed rapidly and unpredictably, upending everything we thought we knew about it. Prominent forces opposed every attempt to control the virus, and public health officials were not nearly as powerful as people imagined them to be. In April 2020, Dr. Vinay Prasad gave the following warning:

> *Public health is undervalued, underfunded, neglected, mistreated, and it is easy to get away with that for years, decades, but someday that ends up biting you in the ass.*[19]

He was right about all of this. Researchers who think seriously about this stuff wrote reports such as "The Impact of Chronic Underfunding on America's Public Health System: Trends, Risks, and Recommendations" that examined the conditions contributing to COVID's rapid spread:

> *Lack of funding in core public health programs slowed the response to the COVID-19 pandemic and exacerbated its impact, particularly in low-income communities, communities of color, and for older Americans – populations that experience higher rates of chronic disease and have fewer resources to recover from an emergency.*[20]

However, while making YouTube videos from the safety of their offices, WWTI doctors lambasted "undervalued, underfunded, and neglected" public health officials because they couldn't do *everything*. WWTI doctors tasked them with protecting the vulnerable, keeping everything open, and running endless randomized controlled trials—all this in addition to their regular duties. Yet instead of helping public health officials with these crucial tasks, WWTI doctors purposefully undermined them.

When the next history of the CDC is written, 2020 will emerge as perhaps the darkest chapter in its 74 years.
— *James Bandler, Patricia Callahan, Sebastian Rotella, and Kirsten Berg*

Certainly, the purpose of this book is not to say everything is just fine and that public health leaders and institutions are beyond reproach. It's vital to have well-intentioned discussions of the proper role and scope of public health, as well as their performance. Even some of the "good guys" gave numerous reasons for the public to be skeptical of them. We overreacted in some ways and underreacted in many ways, though the harms of these errors were not equal. Surfers should not have gotten tickets for violating quarantine orders in 2020, but they are better off than many thousands of young people who died because they were told they didn't need a vaccine.

Some errors were honest mistakes, obvious only in hindsight. Others were more intentional, and these sowed doubt. To pick one example, according to news reports, Dr. Jay Varma, the COVID czar in New York City, confessed to having participated in drug-fueled sex parties during the height of the pandemic, a violation of the COVID policies he helped write.[21] His transgressions will make it harder for future public health leaders to respond to the next pandemic. WWTI doctors know this and used the personal failings of some public health leaders to spread doubt about the science of public health. Dr. Prasad, for example, wrote an article titled "Dr Jay Varma's Sex Parties Are a Metaphor for Public Health: Do as I Say, Not as I Do." He said, "Public health is a broken field,"[22] as if every public health official were just like Dr. Varma. This sort of hypocrisy damages the public trust in a significant way.

So does incompetence. One of my first articles on *Science-Based Medicine*, a blog devoted to exposing medical disinformation, was titled "The CDC Should Do Better." In it I said:

> The CDC's failure to report clear and accurate data about how COVID-19 is affecting children has opened the door to those who wish to minimize its impact by spreading fear, uncertainty, and doubt.[23]

That's exactly what happened. Many WWTI doctors took advantage of the CDC's failure to report clear and accurate data. Several of them devoted great effort to spreading doubt about the data regarding pediatric COVID. They always claimed that the numbers were inflated, of course, though COVID seriously hurt a non-trivial number of children regardless of the *exact* numbers.

A ProPublica investigation from December 2020, "Inside the Fall of the CDC," [24] was even more unsparing in its criticism:

> *When the next history of the CDC is written, 2020 will*
> *emerge as perhaps the darkest chapter in its 74 years,*
> *rivaled only by its involvement in the infamous Tuskegee*
> *experiment, in which federal doctors withheld medicine*
> *from poor Black men with syphilis, then tracked their*
> *descent into blindness, insanity and death.*
>
> *With more than 216,000 people dead this year, most*
> *Americans know the low points of the current chapter*
> *already. A vaunted agency that was once the global gold*
> *standard of public health has, with breathtaking speed,*
> *become a target of anger, scorn and even pity, [...]*
>
> *Senior CDC staff describe waging battles that are as*
> *much about protecting science from the White House as*
> *protecting the public from COVID-19. It is a war that*
> *they have, more often than not, lost.*
>
> *Employees spoke openly about their "hill to die on"*
> *— the political interference that would prompt them to*
> *leave. Yet again and again, they surrendered and did as*
> *they were told. It wasn't just worries over paying mort-*
> *gages or forfeiting the prestige of the job. Many feared*
> *that if they left and spoke out, the White House would*
> *stop consulting the CDC at all, and would push through*
> *even more dangerous policies.*
>
> *To some veteran scientists, this acquiescence was the*
> *real sign that the CDC had lost its way. One scientist*
> *swore repeatedly in an interview and said, "The coward-*

ice and the caving are disgusting to me." […]

Now, 10 months into the crisis, many fear the CDC has lost the most important currency of public health: trust, the confidence in experts that persuades people to wear masks for the public good, to refrain from close-packed gatherings, to take a vaccine.

Dr. Martin Cetron, the agency's veteran director of global migration and quarantine, coined a phrase years ago for what can happen when people lose confidence in the government and denial and falsehoods spread faster than disease. He called it the "bankruptcy of trust." He'd seen it during the Ebola outbreak in Liberia in 2014, when soldiers cordoned off the frightened and angry residents of the West Point neighborhood in Monrovia, the capital. Control of a pandemic depended not just on technical expertise, he told colleagues then, but on faith in public institutions.

Today, some CDC veterans worry that it could take a generation or longer to regain that trust. "Most of us who saw this could be retired or dead by the time that's fully fixed," one CDC official said.

This was important journalism, and it's fine for anyone to criticize the NIH, CDC, and FDA, as well as Dr. Fauci and anyone else—so long as they do so in good faith. However, while skepticism of institutions and authorities is healthy, mistrust solely for the sake of mistrust is not. The avalanche of spurious criticisms of these agencies prevented needed improvement from taking place. They are in much worse shape now than they were in 2020. Doubt was used as a weapon to drive policy.

I have one wish, it would be that lockdown becomes a dirty word, that whenever someone mentions lockdown, people shudder in horror.
— *Dr. Jay Bhattacharya*

Though WWTI doctors claimed that "natural immunity" was a "triumph," in reality, it killed and disabled millions of people. It's not over yet. Although I will use the phrase "during the pandemic" in this book, SARS-CoV-2 is still infecting and hurting people every day. It remains more deadly than the flu,[25] and it hasn't become any less severe for babies who are born without immunity to it. One study from England reported that babies make up 64% of all pediatric COVID hospitalizations.[26] We'll be learning about the consequences of repeated COVID infections for the rest of our lives. Fewer infections are better than more infections, but if someone can't avoid the virus, it's best they encounter it with up-to-date vaccines.

While accurately remembering the history of the pandemic would be of value in its own right, we must also learn from our mistakes. A sage commenter at *Science-Based Medicine* discussed the importance of remembering the past to help prepare for the future:

> *To step back just a bit in perspective, I think there is an unspoken narrative here. Something along the lines of, "why is Doctor Howard still writing all these articles about these same people? Isn't that old news now?"*
>
> *And I think the first is that there is an ongoing, competitive process of writing the history of the pandemic. What happened? How did it go? What did we do right? What went wrong? What should we do the next time? Some of this is happening in the usual scientific channels, where researchers continue to study the*

virus, how it affects the body and the vaccines and drugs we developed to prevent or treat it. But much of it is now happening in non-traditional channels, like Substack articles, YouTube videos, Congressional hearings and even this blog.

And many of the same people whom Dr Howard wrote about in his book are major participants in that process. So it's important to look at what are they saying now? Does it make sense? How does it mesh with what they said previously?

The second element is the aspect of self-assessment that should happen when things get really messed up. Did I make any mistakes? Was there something I overlooked in my thinking or choices? What should I change to do better next time? ... But these articles show that practically everyone on his list is doubling down on their positions, or at best trying to ignore them, while continuing to argue against public health measures.[27]

Everything about that is right. There is an ongoing, competitive process of writing the history of the pandemic, and my exploration of that process ventures into non-traditional channels, including social media, Substack articles, YouTube videos, and Congressional hearings. This book is as much about the future as the past. Indeed, there is a connection between these two questions. *What went wrong? What should we do next time?*

When the next pandemic arrives, we are in big trouble. WWTI doctors bluntly told the public to "stop trusting public health" and to trust anti-vaccine disinformation agents like Kennedy instead.[3] Predictably, many people now believe that measures to contain a deadly virus are useless at best and a sign of impending Nazism at worst.[28] WWTI doctors also instructed the public to forget COVID's carnage and to remember only the worst aspects of the measures needed to contain it. In a pandemic where 1.2 million Americans died, Dr. Bhattacharya only regretted these measures. He wrote, "I have one wish, it would be that lockdown becomes a dirty word, that whenever someone mentions lockdown, people shudder in horror."[29]

He likely got his wish. If COVID-26 arrives, there's virtually no chance public health officials would be able to employ mitigation measures as they did in 2020. Not only would much of the public not comply, but our current medical establishment would also stand in the way. You'll be on your own.

> **A key theme emerging in analysis of the COVID pandemic globally is public trust – or lack thereof – in governments, public institutions and science.**
> — *Shauna Hurley and Rebecca Ryan*

Indeed, one of the key lessons of the pandemic is that messages of doubt are both effective and dangerous. In 2023, the Pew Research Center issued a report, "Americans' Trust in Scientists, Positive Views of Science Continue to Decline,"[30] with the following key findings:

Impact of science on society

Overall, 57% of Americans say science has had a mostly positive effect on society. This share is down 8 percentage points since November 2021 and down 16 points since before the start of the coronavirus outbreak.

About a third (34%) now say the impact of science on society has been equally positive as negative. A small share (8%) think science has had a mostly negative impact on society.

Trust in scientists

When it comes to the standing of scientists, 73% of U.S. adults have a great deal or fair amount of confidence in scientists to act in the public's best interests. But trust in scientists is 14 points lower than it was at the early stages of the pandemic.

The share expressing the strongest level of trust in scientists – saying they have a great deal of confidence in them – has fallen from 39% in 2020 to 23% today.

As trust in scientists has fallen, distrust has grown: Roughly a quarter of Americans (27%) now say they have not too much or no confidence in scientists to act in the public's best interests, up from 12% in April 2020.

Ratings of medical scientists mirror the trend seen in ratings of scientists generally.

We should never forget that there were real-world consequences when doctors told the public that those who suggested getting vaccinated for COVID were dishonest and untrustworthy. According to one study:

Trust in physicians and hospitals decreased substantially over the course of the pandemic, from 71.5% in April 2020 to 40.1% in January 2024. Individuals with lower levels of trust were less likely to have been vaccinated or received boosters for COVID-19.[31]

If "doubt & mistrust" could be listed as an underlying cause of death, it would be on countless death certificates.

None of this bodes well for the future. As Shauna Hurley and Rebecca Ryan wrote in their article, "How Can We Improve Public Health Communication for the Next Pandemic? Tackling Distrust and Misinformation is Key":

A key theme emerging in analysis of the COVID pandemic

globally is public trust – or lack thereof – in governments, public institutions and science.

Mounting evidence suggests levels of trust in government were directly proportional to fewer COVID infections and higher vaccination rates across the world. It was a crucial factor in people's willingness to follow public health directives, and is now a key focus for future pandemic preparedness.[32]

They also said:

Misinformation is not a new problem, but has been supercharged by the advent of social media. […] The Lancet Commission on lessons from the COVID pandemic has called for a coordinated international response to countering misinformation.

This encouraged mistrust in science is going to extend well beyond the pandemic and impact much more than COVID. According to the article "Trust in Physicians and Hospitals During the COVID-19 Pandemic in a 50-State Survey of US Adults":

Among more than half a million survey responses from US adults between April 2020 and January 2024, we found that trust in physicians and hospitals decreased throughout the COVID-19 pandemic across all sociodemographic groups. A lower level of trust was associated with decreased likelihood of vaccination against SARS-CoV-2 as well as influenza.[31]

Indeed, this encouraged mistrust in science is also going to impact much more than medicine. In our current environment, anyone who reports unwanted news is blamed for it. Meteorologists get blamed for hurricanes the same way virologists get blamed for pandemics and doctors get blamed for the deaths of COVID patients. In his article, "I'm Running Out of Ways to Explain How Bad This Is," journalist Charlie Warzel said:

The pandemic saw Americans, distrustful of authority, trying to discredit effective vaccines, spreading conspiracy theories, and attacking public-health officials. But what feels novel in the aftermath of this month's hurricanes is how the people doing the lying aren't even trying to hide the provenance of their bullshit. [...] What is clear is that a new framework is needed to describe this fracturing. Misinformation is too technical, too freighted, and, after almost a decade of Trump, too political. Nor does it explain what is really happening, which is nothing less than a cultural assault on any person or institution that operates in reality. If you are a weatherperson, you're a target. The same goes for journalists, election workers, scientists, doctors, and first responders. These jobs are different, but the thing they share is that they all must attend to and describe the world as it is. This makes them dangerous to people who cannot abide by the agonizing constraints of reality, as well as those who have financial and political interests in keeping up the charade.[33]

He's right. In the mirror world, people do more than dismiss unwanted reality; they blame anyone who accurately reports it. This is the inevitable result of seemingly credible, influential doctors deluging the public with the message—*everyone else is lying to you.*

Chapter 3: Trust in Scientists Should Be Down, Rationally

*In the final analysis, public health officials actively propagated
misinformation that ruined lives and forever damaged public trust
in the medical profession.*
— *Dr. Marty Makary*

In 2023, Dr. Marty Makary published an article titled "10 Myths Told
by COVID Experts — And Now Debunked." In it, Dr. Makary enumerat-
ed ways he felt Americans had been misled by public health officials:

*In the past few weeks, a series of analyses published by highly
respected researchers have exposed a truth about public health
officials during COVID:*

Much of the time, they were wrong.

*To be clear, public health officials were not wrong for making
recommendations based on what was known at the time. That's
understandable. You go with the data you have. No, they were
wrong because they refused to change their directives in the face
of new evidence.*

*When a study did not support their policies, they dismissed it and
censored opposing opinions. At the same time, the Centers for
Disease Control and Prevention weaponized research itself by
putting out its own flawed studies in its own non-peer-reviewed
medical journal, MMWR. In the final analysis, public health
officials actively propagated misinformation that ruined lives and
forever damaged public trust in the medical profession.*

Here are 10 ways they misled Americans:

-     ***Misinformation #1****: Natural immunity offers little pro-*

tection compared to vaccinated immunity

- **Misinformation #2**: *Masks prevent COVID transmission*
- **Misinformation #3**: *School closures reduce COVID transmission*
- **Misinformation #4**: *Myocarditis from the vaccine is less common than from the infection*
- **Misinformation #5**: *Young people benefit from a vaccine booster*
- **Misinformation #6**: *Vaccine mandates increased vaccination rates*
- **Misinformation #7**: *COVID originating from the Wuhan lab is a conspiracy theory*
- **Misinformation #8**: *It was important to get the second vaccine dose three or four weeks after the first dose*
- **Misinformation #9**: *Data on the bivalent vaccine is 'crystal clear'*
- **Misinformation #10**: *One in five people get long COVID*[1]

There's a lot to unpack there, and WWTI doctors produced an overwhelming amount of material like this. I'll revisit this article several times, but following Dr. Makary's lead, I've created a list of 16 themes I want you to notice throughout this book.

#1: Most of These "Myths" Aren't Myths, and They Were Chosen to Spread Mistrust

Many of these "*myths spread by COVID experts*" were not actually myths, and Dr. Makary's criticisms were not made in good faith, but rather to spread mistrust. His first complaint about public health was this:

**Misinformation #1: Natural immunity offers little protection
compared to vaccinated immunity**

*A Lancet study looked at 65 major studies in 19 countries on nat-
ural immunity. The researchers concluded that natural immunity
was at least as effective as the primary COVID vaccine series.*
[...]

*Since the Athenian plague of 430 BC, it has been observed that
those who recovered after infection were protected against severe
disease if reinfected.*

*That was also the observation of nearly every practicing physi-
cian during the first 18 months of the COVID pandemic. Most
Americans who were fired for not having the COVID vaccine
already had antibodies that effectively neutralized the virus, but
they were antibodies that the government did not recognize.*

Even though unvaccinated people died at much higher rates than
vaccinated people,[2] Dr. Makary felt it was vital for the public to know
that "natural immunity was at least as effective as the primary COVID
vaccine series."[1] Elsewhere, he alleged a grand conspiracy to hide the
wonderful news about "natural immunity." He said that public health
officials refused to "recognize" it because, "It would undermine the
indiscriminate vaccine vaccination policy for every single human being,
including extremely low-risk people."[3]

It's certainly true that immunity from the virus is at least as strong as
immunity from the vaccine,[4] though neither triggers durable immunity,
unfortunately. Indeed, the study Dr. Makary cited to support his claim
showed that, while "natural immunity" was decent at the start of the
pandemic, the study's authors noted, "Protection was substantially lower
for the omicron BA.1 variant and declined more rapidly over time than

protection against previous variants."[5]

An unvaccinated person who contracted COVID in March 2020 isn't protected today, while someone who has had zero COVID infections but is 100% up to date on their vaccines has superior, though imperfect, protection.[6] Considering the pandemic lasted longer than 18 months, it is entirely true that *natural immunity offers little protection compared to vaccinated immunity*. Moreover, one study, which was published before Dr. Makary wrote his article, revealed more favorable outcomes in vaccinated individuals when compared to those with "natural immunity." It reported:

> *Significantly, the all-cause death and hospital admission rates for vaccinated individuals were 37 percent lower than the rates for those with natural immunity acquired from previous COVID infection. The rate of ED visits for all causes was 24 percent lower for vaccinated individuals than for the previously infected.*[7]

Dr. Makary didn't share this information with his readers.

Is this "myth" consequential? Would it have been a disaster if people believed "*natural immunity offers little protection compared to vaccinated immunity?*" While public health officials should always strive to be 100% honest, Dr. Makary didn't even attempt to explain why it would be so catastrophic if people believed this "myth," especially considering there is evidence that vaccination after infection is beneficial.[8] Dr. Makary implied it would be a disaster for someone to get the vaccine after getting COVID, yet he expressed no concern about someone getting COVID before they were vaccinated. In fact, he tacitly encouraged it by frequently describing "natural immunity" as "powerful" and "27 times more effective"[3] than vaccine immunity.

Finally, who specifically spread this "myth?" Who strenuously asserted that the main reason to get vaccinated was because *"natural immunity offers little protection compared to vaccinated immunity?"* Perhaps someone somewhere said this, but Dr. Makary provided no examples. *He didn't quote anyone.*

In reality, public health officials said it was wiser to get vaccinated instead of infected, because gaining immunity via the vaccine is infinitely *safer* than gaining immunity via the virus. After all, "natural immunity" killed over a million Americans, and using a virus to protect yourself against that virus is like fireproofing your home by burning it down.

In contrast, the vaccine protected millions of Americans against grave outcomes without killing them in the process. This was the *obvious* case public health officials made, and while Dr. Makary refused to quote them, I will. Here's what the CDC said on this topic:

> **Getting a COVID-19 vaccine is a safer and more dependable way to build immunity to COVID-19 than getting sick with COVID-19.** *COVID-19 vaccination causes a more predictable immune response than an infection with the virus that causes COVID-19. COVID-19 can cause severe illness or death. You can also continue to have long-term health issues after COVID-19 infection. Getting sick with COVID-19 offers protection from future illness. This protection is sometimes called "natural immunity". The level of protection people get from a COVID-19 infection may vary depending on how mild or severe their illness was, the time since their infection, and their age.*[9]

Dr. Makary doesn't want anyone to trust the doctors and CDC officials behind this message.

But notice how he didn't engage with the argument they actually made—*getting a COVID-19 vaccine is safer*. Instead, he created a strawman to misrepresent their arguments and declare victory over his invented caricature of dastardly public health officials. Thankfully, public health officials refused Dr. Makary's advice and didn't repeatedly glorify "natural immunity."

Several of Dr. Makary's other "myths" contained factual errors. For example, his "Misinformation #4" was that "myocarditis from the vaccine is less common than from the infection." In reality, myocarditis *from* COVID is both *more common* and *more severe* than myocarditis from the vaccine. Prior to Dr. Makary's article, the American Heart Association had published articles titled "COVID-19 Infection Poses Higher Risk for Myocarditis Than Vaccines,"[10] "Young People Recover Quickly from Rare Myocarditis Side Effect of Covid-19 Vaccine,"[11] and "Post-Vaccine Myocarditis in Young People is Rare and Usually Mild, Study Confirms."[12]

In contrast, COVID-myocarditis killed some young people. The article "'Wrecked Our Lives': Families of 3 Young Adults Who Died From COVID-19 Share Heartbreaking Stories" quoted the grieving mother of Michael Lang as saying, "Eighteen years old and his future ahead of him. That part of it is hard to wrap our brains around — that he won't be with us any longer."[13]

Michael, who died of COVID-myocarditis, "had no preexisting conditions and had never been in the hospital prior to COVID-19." Of course, COVID's harms are not limited to myocarditis, and the vaccine has benefits, while COVID does not. Therefore, the question of which causes more myocarditis—the virus or the vaccine—isn't even the proper comparison.

There were real consequences when doctors treated vaccine side effects as a fate worse than death. The article "'A Devastating Shock':

UNCW Student Dies Due to Covid-19 Complications, Funeral Arrange-
ments in Place," reported on Tyler Gilreath, a 20-year-old university
student who died of COVID in September 2021. It said:

> *"I cajoled, encouraged, threatened, and nagged for him to get
> vaccinated," Tyler's mother, Tamra Demello, told WECT. "I did
> everything I could possibly think. I think he did some research
> where he was thinking that it was going to hurt his heart long-
> term or something... I'm not even sure where he was getting his
> information which is super frustrating. Sometimes, I felt like the
> harder I pushed the more — he basically said to me, 'mom, leave
> me alone. I can take care of myself.'"[14]*

Refuting such disinformation was the goal of *We Want Them Infected*, which revealed the truth of Brandolini's law, an adage that states the
amount of energy needed to refute bullshit is an order of magnitude bigger than that needed to produce it.[15] WWTI doctors created false and misleading claims much faster than anyone could correct them. Dr. Makary's
article was a written version of a Gish Gallop, a debating technique that
uses "a rapid series of specious arguments, half-truths, misrepresentations
and outright lies, making it impossible for the opponent to refute all of
them within the format of the debate."[16]

As political propagandist Steve Bannon famously said, the goal was
"to flood the zone with shit,"[17] which is exactly what WWTI doctors did.

#2: All Of These "Myths" Are Trivial Compared to COVID's Toll

COVID was the greatest mass death event in American history. The
virus killed 1.2 million Americans and injured millions more. It was going to be bad no matter what, but it didn't have to be this bad. One study

estimated that 232,000 deaths could have been prevented in unvaccinated adults from May 30, 2021, to September 3, 2022, had they been vaccinated with at least the primary series.[18]

That should matter. It's worth remembering there were real lives behind these grim statistics. According to one article:

> *Daniel Macias wanted to wait until he and his wife, Davy Macias, recovered from the coronavirus before naming their newborn daughter. But about a week after giving birth, the mother died of Covid-19 complications. And nearly two weeks after she died, so did her husband.*
>
> *Davy Macias was 37, and Daniel Macias was 39, Terri Serey, Davy Macias' sister-in-law, told NBC News on Monday. The couple, both of Yucaipa, California, left behind five children, ages 7, 5, 3, 2 and 3 weeks.*
>
> *"They were the kindest, most amazing people," Serey said.*
>
> *"They were the ones who got everyone together — for every birthday, every holiday."*
>
> *Davy Macias was unvaccinated because she was pregnant, Serey said, but it was unclear if Daniel was vaccinated.[19]*

Yet these preventable tragedies never seemed to bother WWTI doctors. COVID's victims never appeared on their list of "10 Myths Told by Covid Experts." They showed no compassion for the children who appeared in the article, "Parents Mourn Teens Who Refused to Get Covid Vaccine,"[20] and they mocked those who showed concern for children affected by COVID. Dr. Vinay Prasad called them "idiots,"[21] for example.

Instead of caring about COVID's victims, WWTI doctors worried deeply about issues that were significantly less consequential, and they berated public health officials for not sharing their warped priorities.

Dr. Makary, for example, bemoaned the fate of people who lost their jobs because they refused a vaccine. Indeed, that happened, and it's not inconsequential. Reasonable people can disagree about vaccine mandates, especially for a vaccine with a limited impact on transmission, and I never advocated for or against them. However, WWTI doctors often acted as if mandates were the pandemic's greatest tragedy. They spent valuable time arguing against them on social media and writing papers such as "COVID-19 Vaccine Boosters for Young Adults: A Risk Benefit Assessment and Ethical Analysis of Mandate Policies at Universities."[22] While WWTI doctors casually brushed aside anything COVID could do, they went to great lengths to stand up for anyone who didn't want a COVID vaccine. Now they have power, several of them are taking away people's right to have one. Their belief in bodily autonomy and medical freedom was unidirectional, applying only to anti-vaxxers.

They worried more about sore arms from potentially unneeded vaccine doses than about cold bodies due to missed vaccine doses. Even though Dr. Makary didn't mention them, hundreds of thousands, if not millions, of Americans lost their jobs because COVID killed or disabled them. Moreover, some people who are presently upset about vaccine mandates are alive because of them. One paper from *JAMA* reported:

> *Mask requirements and vaccine mandates were negatively associated with excess deaths, prohibitions on vaccine or mask mandates were positively associated with death rates. […] Using the primary specifications, the estimates suggested that if all states had weak restrictions, there would have been 1.3 million to 1.4 million excess deaths from July 2020 to June 2022, that is, 271 000 to 447 000 more than estimated with universal strong restrictions, a 25% to 48% difference.*[23]

WWTI doctors worried *deeply* about trivialities. Dr. Prasad wrote articles such as "Let Djokovic Play"[24] and "Aaron Rodgers and the Absurdity of Media Coverage of Covid Policy."[25] The fate of anti-vaccine millionaire athletes *really* mattered to them.

Conversely, WWTI doctors never criticized public health officials for failing to protect young people. The only things that bothered them about SARS-CoV-2 were that public health officials tried to contain it and didn't say enough positive things about it. For example, Dr. Martin Kulldorff authored an article named "The Triumph of Natural Immunity"[26] and posted on social media that, "The denial of natural immunity after Covid disease is the worst unscientific folly in the past 75 years."[27]

In actuality, the only people who denied the "power" of "natural immunity" were those who claimed COVID only hurt old, vulnerable people.

#3: Most WWTI Doctors Never Treated COVID Patients

Obviously, being a frontline healthcare worker was just one of thousands of ways that people made crucial pandemic contributions. It was not a requirement to comment on COVID or a guarantee that the person had anything valuable to say.

However, most WWTI doctors never treated COVID patients, and their ignorance and inexperience were obvious in nearly everything they said. The phrase *"no one who worked on a COVID unit would have said anything like that"* could appear after most quotations in this book. For example, on January 14, 2021, Dr. François Balloux, an infectious disease epidemiologist and microbial geneticist at University College London, said:

> The pandemic has unleashed a vision of an apocalypse bordering on the religious at times. Once it will become clear this is not the end times, I expect the addiction to pandemic doom and gloom will recede, with people resuming more meaningful lifes [sic].[28]

Indeed, no one who worked on a COVID unit would have said anything like that, especially at that moment. We knew COVID was the *end times* for many people, and the middle of January 2021 was the peak of the deadliest month of the entire pandemic in both the U.K. and U.S. A February 1, 2021, article titled "Pandemic's Deadliest Month in US Ends with Signs of Progress," reported the death toll in the U.S. climbing past 440,000, with over 95,000 lives lost in January alone. Deaths averaged 3,150 per day at that point of the pandemic.[29]

The toll would have been *much* worse if more people had the attitude that "doom and gloom" was worse than the virus. However, according to Dr. Balloux, who treated zero COVID patients, anyone who was more cautious than he wasn't credible. He said they were "grifters and ghouls"[30] who had an "addiction to pandemic doom and gloom."[28] Even when 3,000 Americans were dying of COVID every day, Dr. Balloux was offended and upset that people weren't cheerful enough. As those of us who worked in hospitals know, graveyards are full of people who resisted "doom and gloom."

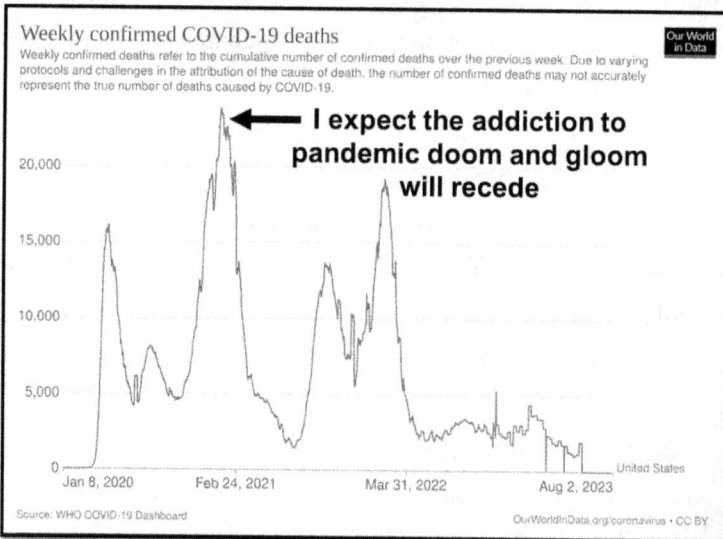

Source: OurWorldInData.org. Customization by author.

Not only did WWTI doctors lack an essential perspective, they were also entirely incurious about it. They completely disregarded frontline workers and had no interest about what happened in hospitals. They never paused to listen to what doctors who treated COVID patients had to say or consider that frontline doctors had an important perspective they lacked.

Had WWTI doctors been willing to listen, they would have learned valuable lessons. Most deaths occurred in older, sick people, but we all saw some young people die. Although death was the only negative consequence recognized by WWTI doctors, it was not the only bad outcome from COVID. Many people survived COVID but were seriously injured by it. No one who worked on a COVID unit casually brushed aside what the virus could do with banal claims that the "old have a thousand-fold higher mortality risk than the young,"[31] as Drs. Kulldorff and Jay Bhattacharya put it in their article "The Ill-Advised Push to Vaccinate the Young," written right before Delta spiked.

Mostly, WWTI doctors would have learned that SARS-CoV-2 was hard to contain. The virus invariably found people to infect when it was left to spread unchecked in the community. No one who saw what it could do was under any illusion that vulnerable people could have been sealed in a magic bubble, as WWTI doctors claimed.

We saw COVID spread widely within the hospital. Countless healthcare workers contracted the virus, and the World Health Organization (WHO) estimated that 115,000 healthcare workers died from COVID by May 2021.[32] Dr. James Mahoney was one of them. He was on the verge of retirement when the pandemic hit but refused to abandon his community as recounted in the article "A Legend at a Brooklyn Hospital Dies of Covid-19":

> *Mahoney was well-trained to treat Covid-19 patients. And public hospitals, already stretched thin, were bracing for an influx of*

*patients. So he went "running into the fire," Melvin said. Brooklyn
has had 40,000 Covid-19 cases, and the virus hit black and Latino
communities the hardest.*

*"The last time I saw him was at the beginning of the pandemic,"
Cavanagh said. "I said, are we going to get through this? And he
said, oh yeah, we're going to get through this."*

*But in early April, Mahoney started coughing and running a fever.
On Easter Sunday, after Chisolm [Dr. Mahoney's sister] recovered, Mahoney's family noticed on a video chat that he didn't look
well. The next day, he was admitted to his own hospital, SUNY
Downstate.*

*At first, Mahoney seemed to be improving – he gave his family a
thumbs up on FaceTime. Then his health deteriorated and he was
transferred to NYU Langone for a higher level of care. He died on
27 April.*

*Physicians at SUNY Downstate said Mahoney's death has left a
hole in the institution after his three decades there. "He was what
we call a 'lifer'" at the hospital, said colleague Alex Hieu Ly.*[33]

Dr. James Mahoney was 62 and had worked at his hospital for 30
years. WWTI doctors never mentioned people like him.

Their lack of real-world responsibility also meant that WWTI doctors
were sheltered from the consequences of their words. Although they told
people not to "live in fear," they never saw what happened to the people
who listened to them. They never met people like Christian Cabrera.
According to the article, "Father Dying of Covid Regrets Not Getting
Vaccine in Heartbreaking Texts":

*Shortly before dying of Covid-19, a father in Los Angeles
texted family members to express his regret over not getting*

vaccinated.

Christian Cabrera, 40, tested positive for the coronavirus around Christmas. Not long afterward, he was in an emergency room with pneumonia in both lungs.

"I can't breathe again," he texted his brother, according to KTLA. "I really regret not getting my vaccine. If I can do it all over again I would do it in a heartbeat to save my life. I'm fighting for my life here and I wish I [had] gotten vaccinated."[34]

This happened to many thousands of young people, and Dr. Abraar Karan, an infectious disease expert at Stanford, explained why no one who witnessed this would minimize the virus. He said:

One thing I guarantee you will notice if you pay attention, doctors who have cared for #COVID19 patients will never underestimate what this virus is capable of. The antivaxx, antimask pundits who have been tweeting from the safety of their home for the past two years often will.

I have yet to meet a fellow physician who has spent the majority of their time caring for these cases who would claim to know exactly what to expect from #SARSCoV2 — because we continue to be surprised. Surprised by people who die that shouldn't. People who suffer for longer than we would expect. People who seem to get better & then suddenly turn for the worse. People who are doing poorly & who end up surviving.

Medicine humbles us as clinicians; this virus has too. Hearing non-clinicians downplay it after long days/weeks/months where we are working hard to try & save people's lives Honestly-eventually you can't help but feel like half of the people on here

who claim to know what the right answer is or what's "safe
enough" are full of BS.

Because if you get sick, they won't be responsible for it. They
won't be accountable to you, your family, your loved ones.
Your doctors will be at your bedside. Your antimask, antivaxx
saviors will not. A common response I hear from sick patients
once it's too late — I wish I had listened.[35]

Instead of being curious and willing to learn from people like Dr.
Karan, WWTI doctors mocked and excoriated doctors who intruded on
their fantasy mirror world with facts about what was actually happening
in the real world. For example, Dr. Scott Atlas blamed doctors who treated patients for the loss of trust in medicine. He said in an interview:

Dr. Scott Atlas: *I mean, the medical community really failed*
and we see the results of their failure. First of all, you know that
they're trusted. You know [...] we're doctors. People are intim-
idated by doctors, but also we occupy a special position of trust
in society, almost blind trust. People depend on you. You have
to take that role very seriously. Now how do what do I mean
by that? That means. When somebody comes in and asks you a
question, you don't just spit out a memorized guideline, you, you
explain what the data is, if they want to know. You don't, you
don't persuade by coercion and pressure, you persuade by show-
ing people the facts. I mean, your role is to be the information
giver, not to coerce people. And they really failed. And I have to
say, you know, doctors... it's a disgrace what they did and how
little they know about the data. A disgrace in my opinion. But
you see it in the polling, you know, you realize that pre-pandem-
ic, the trust, "high trust in doctors" - 71%. Now January 2024,

from 71% have plummeted to "trust doctors a lot." - Now that
answer is 40%. It's very disheartening.

Dr. Drew Pinsky: *It may be continuing to drop.*[36]

While Dr. Atlas was on TV and podcasts speculating that COVID would only kill approximately 10,000 Americans[37] and that "natural immunity" would lead to herd immunity, other doctors were dealing with consequences of his disinformation in ERs and ICUs. Later, Dr. Atlas, a radiologist who never treated COVID patients, berated these doctors for reporting their experience and trying to limit COVID's harms—"*it's a disgrace what they did.*"

#4: WWTI Doctors' Expressed Concern About Social Justice Issues, But Only With Regards to COVID Mitigations

Although WWTI doctors openly opposed COVID mitigation efforts, they sought to obscure their motives. They woke-washed the pandemic and waged their battle under the guise of being "inherently left-wing,"[38] "progressive doctors,"[39] and "a far-left democrat."[40] WWTI doctors temporarily and selectively co-opted social justice issues, claiming they were only concerned about the plight of the global poor, the vulnerable, and the working class.

Despite their professed concern about these groups, WWTI doctors mentioned them only in relation to their opposition to mitigation measures. For example, Dr. Kulldorff said, "Lockdowns harmed children, the poor and the middle class,"[41] and an article about Dr. Sunetra Gupta portrayed her as a leftist. It said:

She rejected being bracketed with libertarian lockdown sceptics, saying her opposition came from the left. "I personally think that only thinking along the lines of eliminating coronavirus, without giving heed to the consequences on the disadvantaged young and globally, is a dereliction of our duties as global citizens.[42]

Dr. Bhattacharya, who co-authored the Great Barrington Declaration (GBD) with Drs. Kulldorff and Gupta, reported similar motives. He said:

Some culturally influential people regret that a few places kept schools open. The study cites doesn't evaluate the effect closed schools on disease spread. Nor does it evaluate the harms to kids (especially poor & minority kids) from such draconian restrictions on their lives.[43]

Dr. Bhattacharya often claimed that mitigation measures were merely a luxury of the "laptop class," as if COVID's victims would have been better off if only more bankers and lawyers had died next to them. Some examples are below:

- *Unfortunately for the global poor, the vulnerable, and the working class, the pandemic ends when the **laptop class** decides it ends, and not a moment sooner.*[44]
- *Lockdown were a luxury of the **laptop class**.*[45]
- *Lockdowns were focused protection of the **laptop class**. Undiluted trickle down epidemiology.*[46]
- *The lockdowns were neither necessary nor sufficient to protect vulnerable people from covid, and were destructive to human life in so many other ways. They were a policy by, of, and for the **laptop class**.*[47]
- *The brutal reality of lockdown in the poorest parts of the world was police power crushing the poor. The **laptop class** conceit of "stay home, stay safe" was a cruel joke to the world's poor.*[48]
- *The public health establishment pretends it cares about the well being of the poor and vulnerable. But when the test came, it adopted a policy of trickle down epidemiology and focused*

*protection of the **laptop class**.*[49]

- *Public health, the way it is currently constituted, will never do anything other give lip service to protecting anyone outside the **laptop class**. The lockdown orders were designed to protect the laptop class, though they ultimately failed at that.*[50]

Of course, Dr. Bhattacharya and nearly all WWTI doctors are exemplars of the laptop class, and they never polled the "global poor, the vulnerable, and the working class"[44] before claiming to speak on their behalf.

Instead of listening to the people they claimed to represent, wealthy academics declared themselves as champions of the working class. Laptop-class doctors claimed to represent all doctors and White doctors anointed themselves as spokespersons for "minority children." For example, during her testimony before the U.S. Select Subcommittee on the Coronavirus Pandemic, Dr. Tracy Beth Høeg said, "School closures were a regressive policy that disproportionately affected minority children and children of lower socioeconomic status."[51]

No one deputized Dr. Høeg to speak on behalf of these "minority children," and her "advocacy" was largely in opposition to the wishes of their parents. An article titled "Why Is This Group of Doctors So Intent on Unmasking Kids?" written about Dr. Høeg's group, Urgency of Normal, reported that wealthier, White parents like her were less likely to support mitigation measures. It said:

In one poll conducted in January, 65 percent of parents with household income of less than $75,000 a year said they were either "very worried" or "somewhat worried" about their kid getting seriously sick from Covid-19, and 45 percent said they were "very worried." Wealthier parents were far less concerned, with only 10 percent saying they were "very worried." In the *same survey, 49 percent of Black or Hispanic parents said they were very worried, as compared to 12 percent of white parents. This isn't the first poll to point to divides by class and race. In an August poll, 75 percent of Black parents wanted all kids to wear masks in schools, compared to 54 percent of white parents. Families of color have also been more concerned about the risks of in-person learning, according to some research.*[52]

The same article quoted Dr. Lakshmi Ganapathi, a pediatric infectious diseases physician at Harvard Medical School:

That's precisely because these are the communities that have been disproportionately impacted. This is fundamentally a pandemic of inequity. African American, Latino, and Indigenous children have significantly higher rates of hospitalizations and death.

She's right, but Dr. Høeg did not care that COVID disproportionately affected "minority children and children of lower socioeconomic status."

At times, WWTI doctors spread blatant disinformation to oppose mitigation measures while pretending to stand up for the downtrodden. For example, Dr. Bhattacharya blamed "lockdown-induced solitary confinement" for the suicide of an Air Force cadet,[53] when, in reality, she was a distraught rape victim.[54]

Despite their professed concern about *minority children and children of lower socioeconomic status,* many WWTI doctors were stars of the right-wing media and partnered with anti-public education billionaires and overt pro-tobacco, child-labor advocates. Their "concern" about *minority children and children of lower socioeconomic status* didn't extend that far.

#5: Outside of Nursing Homes, WWTI Doctors Blasted Public Health Officials for Anything They Did to Limit the Virus

Aside from protecting nursing homes, WWTI doctors labeled public health officials as extremists and unscientific fearmongers for any attempt they took to limit the virus. WWTI doctors claimed *any* mitigation measure was too much, useless, dangerous, and an indication of massive government overreach. They opposed masks, ventilation, testing, vaccines, and anything else to prevent young people from getting COVID.

WWTI doctors talked about the potential harms of mitigation measures in histrionic, overwrought language. Dr. Bhattacharya, for example, routinely called lockdowns "the worst avoidable peacetime public catastrophe in history,"[55] "absolutely catastrophic,"[56] and the "biggest public health mistake we've ever made. [...] The harm to people is catastrophic."[57] In another interview, he said it would "take a generation" to reverse the harms of lockdowns, adding:

> It's absolutely devastating the amount of damage that it's done worldwide, especially to the poor.[58]

However, WWTI doctors didn't just want mitigation measures to be gone on a societal level; they wanted individuals to embrace the virus. They sought to numb individuals to COVID by describing infections as "mild" for the vast majority of people, even before anyone was vaccinated. They portrayed viral avoidance as "panic," or a sign of mental illness. As the pandemic progressed, several of them mercilessly shamed the few non-conformists who still tried to avoid COVID. They laughed at anyone who wanted a booster vaccine and even took pictures of strangers on the street to mock them for wearing masks.

Conversely, at least after the first half of 2021, WWTI doctors were

livid whenever anyone said anything positive about vaccines. They treated *theoretical* harms from them—even a mere abnormal lab value—much
more seriously than *actual* harms from COVID. Dr. Prasad, for example,
fretted mightily about "subclinical myocarditis" from the vaccine but
casually blew off literal death from COVID, saying such concerns were
"breathless."

This is how badly they wanted them infected.

#6: WWTI Doctors Claim to Have Been Vindicated, But They Refuse to Acknowledge Their Own Errors or Even Their Own Words

In April 2020, Dr. John Ioannidis said:

> *I would say that covid-19 will result in fewer than 40,000 deaths this season in the USA.*[59]

Dr. Atlas estimated that COVID "would cause about 10,000 deaths"[60]
at the start of the pandemic, while Dr. Bhattacharya postulated that
COVID had "one-tenth of the flu mortality rate of 0.1%,"[61] writing in
March 2020 that a "20,000- or 40,000-death epidemic is a far less severe
problem than one that kills two million."

These doctors never deviated from this erroneous perspective. Nothing the virus did led them to alter their opinion, formed in spring 2020,
that COVID was overblown, and that it was all going away.

Today, 1.2 million deaths later, they've left their 2020 predictions in
the rearview mirror. While WWTI doctors seek to reinforce unpleasant
lockdown memories from 2020, they act as if their absurd predictions
from that time never happened at all.

If I predicted in major newspapers that COVID would kill 40,000
Americans, I would count that as my biggest mistake. WWTI doctors did

not. In 2022, Dr. Ioannidis starred in a movie about himself, *Out to See*, where he reflected on his "biggest mistake" by saying:

> *And I think my biggest mistake, and I think that others can probably think about their mistakes, is that I underestimated how much power politics and media and powers outside of science could have on science. I think that I had no clue and no preparation for this invasion of science.*[62]

Dr. Bhattacharya also reflected on his "biggest mistake," stating:

> *The biggest mistake I made was that I thought in March that it would be impossible to get a vaccine so quickly, and so I hadn't thought through the implications of what that meant—that we could get one so quickly, right.*[63]

More than this, WWTI doctors now claim that time has vindicated their pandemic visions. In 2022, Dr. Ioannidis had the following exchange with Dr. Prasad:

> ***Dr. Prasad****: Early in the pandemic you were viciously attacked for expressing a policy viewpoint and intuition that is different from others. In a number of ways your core thesis was: in an effort—well intentioned—to control the coronavirus, we may inflict great damage on ourselves. That lesson appears to be borne out in a number of historical and recent events. How do you judge you original intuition?*
>
> ***Dr. Ioannidis****: I wish I had been wrong on this point. Unfortunately, I am afraid I might have been correct.*[64]

Dr. Atlas is similarly convinced that he was totally right about everything. A typical example of this was a social media post that said:

> *Scott Atlas or Anthony Fauci?*
> *One man: 100% right on lockdowns, masks, schools; honest; da-*

ta-driven; ethical outsider

Other man: 100% wrong on lockdowns, masks, schools; dishonest;
no data; conflict-of-interest-filled lying insider

Who is who? #TruthPrevails @Stanford[65]

Dr. Atlas lamented that other doctors could not admit error. He posted:

> *We now have a frightening crisis of both competence and integrity. Lockdowners will never admit they were wrong—and I and others here were right—that would take integrity.*[66]

Similarly, in an interview from 2021 titled "I Stand by the Great Barrington Declaration," Dr. Bhattacharya said:

> *I do think I've been, we've been vindicated. I think the focus practice was [the] right strategy. I think the lockdowns were, I call the single biggest mistake in public health history.*[67]

He authored an article, "Anti-Lockdown Great Barrington Declaration Vindicated, But Much Too Late," in 2023, which said future public health leaders "must embrace the principles of the GBD [...] if we are to avoid a repeat of [...] history during the next pandemic."[55]

Instead of reflecting on their own poor predictions, WWTI doctors are engaged in a deliberate amnesia project. Not only do they seek to memory hole the hellish scenes of 2020, they also actively deny their own words and their plan to reach herd immunity via mass infection, despite this discourse dominating the first 1.5 years of the pandemic. The reality of the WWTI movement has been replaced with a fiction where doctors who advocated for mass infection in 2020 now claim they *really* only cared about the education of poor, minority children. WWTI doctors actively seek to vilify and discredit anyone who *remembers* their pro-infection advocacy as well as its tragic real-world consequences.

#7: WWTI Doctors Seek to Reinforce Negative Memories of Mitigation Measures that Ended Long Ago

Most people hated lockdowns. Our lives were turned upside down in an instant, all for a virus we couldn't even see. Lockdowns were a brutal solution to a brutal problem, and we shouldn't minimize their harms. People lost their incomes, education environments, and social networks, and those of us who were mostly spared this should recognize our privilege. However, as bad as they were, the lockdowns were temporary and ended years ago. Most people have moved on.

Not WWTI doctors. They discuss mitigation measures constantly and blame them for nearly every societal ill. In the 2023 interview, "The Man Who Talked Back: Jay Bhattacharya on the Fight Against COVID Lockdowns," Dr. Bhattacharya said, "We're in a situation where the harms of the lockdowns have become and are becoming clearer and clearer every day, and the benefits, in terms of protecting people from COVID, it's becoming clearer that they did none of that."[68]

WWTI doctors have been complaining about lockdowns for longer than lockdowns lasted, and they don't want anyone to forget their harms, both real and imagined. WWTI doctors particularly seek to reinforce memories of unpopular mitigation measures that haven't existed for years. For instance, in September 2023, Dr. Kulldorff tweeted:

> One of the most disturbing images of the Covid-19 pandemic was when a teacher .. forced a mask on a crying toddler.[69]

As recently as October 2024, Dr. Prasad complained about "the harms of lockdowns, school closures and masking toddlers,"[70] while Dr. Bhattacharya posed the following question:

> Why won't the conventional media ask about the school closures,

masking toddlers, and vax mandates?[71]

Dr. Atlas similarly lamented school closures in November 2024:

They closed schools & kept them closed; isolated our kids, caus-
ing suicides, psych harms, drug abuse; forced toddlers to wear
masks; coerced/mandated experimental drug injections… It takes
a damaged person lacking self-respect to now vote for people
who did that.[72]

While WWTI doctors seek to memory hole COVID's carnage and their own farcical forecasts, they'll be talking about "masking toddlers" for the foreseeable future. Although children wore masks during the 1918 flu pandemic and turned out fine, WWTI doctors don't want this to happen ever again.

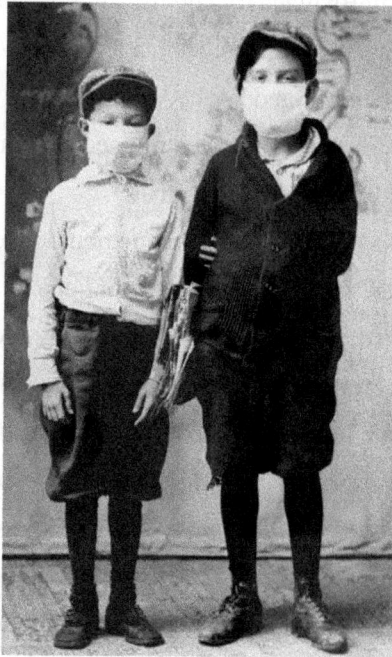

Children in masks during 1918 flu
epidemic. Source: Wikimedia Commons

#8: WWTI Doctors Portrayed Mitigation Measures as an Avoidable Choice

WWTI doctors always blamed people, never the virus. While every country implemented drastic mitigation measures at some point, WWTI doctors portrayed them as an avoidable choice. In their mirror world fantasy, so long as vulnerable people were hermetically sealed in a bubble, then schools, hospitals, businesses, and everything else could have continued normally. Sure, some kids would have gotten the sniffles, but beyond that, no one would have even noticed the innocent, harmless virus. WWTI doctors claim that if we had just listened to them, everything would have been perfectly fine.

For example, Dr. Atlas said:

> *Remember—lockdowns weren't caused by the virus. Human beings decided to do lockdowns—they own the results. Their lockdowns were implemented. Their policies killed and destroyed millions. That's fact. That's the data.*[73]

Another article about a speech by Dr. Atlas said:

> *Atlas broadened his polemic to the academic sphere, making the clear distinction that the significant decline in students' educational performance owed largely to "the shutdowns, not the virus."*[74]

Similarly, the GBD claimed life could go on as normal if only mitigation measures were removed. It said:

> *Current lockdown policies are producing devastating effects on short and long-term public health. The results (to name a few) include lower childhood vaccination rates, worsening cardiovas-*

cular disease outcomes, fewer cancer screenings and deteriorating mental health – leading to greater excess mortality in years to come, with the working class and younger members of society carrying the heaviest burden. Keeping students out of school is a grave injustice. Keeping these measures in place until a vaccine is available will cause irreparable damage, with the underprivileged disproportionately harmed.[75]

This was a fantasy spun by insulated doctors who never saw what the virus could do. Had WWTI doctors worked in hospitals, they would have known that cancer screenings were impossible during COVID surges. Even if elderly people had been willing to get a colonoscopy while forklifts were moving the corpses of their relatives and neighbors into refrigerated trucks, there was no space and no personnel.

Schools were no different. There too, the virus *forced* people with actual responsibility to make hard, often unpopular choices. An article from 2021 titled "Four Kansas School Districts Temporarily Close as Covid-19 Outbreaks Hit 31 Schools" reported:

With the rise in Covid numbers in our staff and student population, as well as in our county, the board was forced to make adjustments," the district said in a Facebook post Tuesday. "One of those adjustments includes the requirement to wear masks while case numbers are high."[76]

These local officials didn't want to "make adjustments." They didn't want to close schools or require masks, but the virus left them with no choice. As a result, they faced furious backlash and outright threats from the public. According to one survey:

Sixty percent of principals and district leaders responding to the survey said at least one of their staff members has faced threats from people who are dissatisfied with their district's approach for dealing with COVID-19.[77]

However, by framing every mitigation measure as an avoidable choice, WWTI doctors aimed not just to absolve SARS-CoV-2 of any responsibility but to displace its consequences onto people who, unlike them, had to deal with it in the real world.

#9: WWTI Doctors Claimed Their Approach Was "Nuanced Middle Ground"

WWTI doctors claimed that their approach represented a nuanced middle ground. Dr. Zubin Damania (ZDoggMD) made podcasts such as "Covidiots vs. Covidians? An Alt-Middle View"[78] and sold shirts that said "nuance: truth is found on all sides." Other examples include:

- ***Great Barrington Declaration:*** *In the Great Barrington Dec-laration, co-signed now by many thousand medical scientists and practitioners, we laid out such a middle-ground alterna-tive, with greatly improved focused protection of older people and other high-risk groups.*[79]
- ***Dr. Sunetra Gupta:*** *There is this middle ground between letting it rip and letting it drip where lockdowns extend the problem to a point where more vulnerable people will eventu-ally die.*[80]
- ***Dr. François Balloux:*** *So I kind of captured the market for corona centrism – not to be systematically optimistic or pessi-mistic and to make it clear there are major uncertainties. And this is empowering, because understanding things is.*[81]
- ***Dr. Jay Bhattacharya:*** *The GBD & focused protection of the vulnerable is a middle ground between lockdown.*[82]
- ***Dr. Vinay Prasad:*** *I'm no fan of anti-vax forces pushing propaganda for decades, but I see now that the anti-anti-vax*

side is also often irrational & unscientific. In the middle is
nuance.[83]

• **Dr. John Mandrola**: *You can love the vaccine (I do) but also*
accept nuance in the decision for the young.[84]

WWTI doctors also asserted that they were the only ones who considered the harm of COVID mitigations. For example, Dr. Bhattacharya
said:

Dr. Fauci is utterly blind to the collateral damage from a lockdown, including our liberty but also our other health needs.[85]

In reality, WWTI doctors never discussed trade-offs in a nuanced
way. They only described COVID's risk to children and teachers as
"low" or "zero," for example. Moreover, they exclusively criticized those
who tried to limit COVID. They never complained about anti-vaccine
disinformation or recognized its victims. However, by falsely portraying
themselves as the reasonable middle, WWTI doctors depicted anyone
who was more cautious than they as extreme and histrionic.

#10: Although They Portrayed Themselves as Outsiders, WWTI Doc-tors Were the Establishment

WWTI doctors attacked the "medical establishment" as if they were
neutral watchdogs and outsiders. They often said things like:

• **Dr. Scott Atlas**: *The public health establishment - journal*
editors & govt advisers - the Faucis and Deborah Birxes of the
world – don't want us to look back.[86]

• **Dr. Vinay Prasad**: *It doesn't help that many establishment*
positions were wrong or lies. Fauci lied about cloth masking
(psst it was the second time when he said it worked). Views on
transmission and possibility of lab leak were also lies.[87]

• **Dr. Vinay Prasad**: *One of the reasons there is massive loss*

of trust in elites/ establishment is when people (falsely) claim
that unproven or dubious interventions are 100% backed by
science, when it just isn't.[88]

- **Dr. Martin Kulldorff**: *Covid restrictions: The worst as-*
  sault on children, workers and the third world poor in many
  decades. The Great Barrington Declaration aims to protect
  them, so predictably, it is slandered and mischaracterized by
  establishment servants.[89]

- **Dr. Marty Makary**: *Just amazing. The establishment group-*
  think bypassed the scientific method of using data and instead
  arrogantly used political absolutism as they decreed medical
  dogma and censored respected physicians with different opin-
  ions (who ended up being correct). The science is now clear.[90]

- **Dr. John Mandrola**: *Are there not "bullshitters" within the*
  anointed establishment?[91]

- **Dr. Monica Gandh**i: *Well done studies should be the ones to*
  make determinations of how to combat a pandemic; otherwise,
  the public health establishment loses trust & that has conse-
  quences on uptake of other health-related recommendations.[92]

By portraying themselves as outsiders, WWTI permitted themselves
to make absurd demands of public health officials while absolving themselves of any responsibility. WWTI doctors then claimed that the "establishment" failed us and that they were heroes because they "called for"
things to be done.

However, WWTI doctors were not just random doctors spouting off
on social media and podcasts. They had prominent academic positions
and enormous media footprints. They were everywhere, except hospitals. They were loud, famous, and influential pandemic celebrities who
advised world leaders. It's impossible to get more elite and establishment
than this. Like essentially all doctors, I don't have a fraction of their
clout, influence, and connections.

Several of them have since been appointed to high positions in the Trump administration. If they weren't "the establishment" before, they are now. Every COVID death will be under their watch, and they'll own every measles and pertussis outbreak in the U.S. for the next four years, at least.

#11: WWTI Doctors Often Blended Medicine with Politics and Business

WWTI doctors claimed to be neutral, objective scientists, and they wielded this as a shield to fend off potential criticism. Yet many of them openly blended politics and medicine. They testified before Congress and in courts; they partnered with presidents and governors. All of their "scientific" communication aligned perfectly with their political beliefs, and there is no mystery what these beliefs were. They only objected to the "*lockdowns and school closures to mask and vaccine mandates or passports,*"[93] which were mentioned by the Heritage Foundation's "Project 2025."

Many WWTI doctors were very well connected politically. Their philosophy was indistinguishable from right-wing legislators, such as the GOP Doctors Caucus, which put out statements like the following:

> *It is un-American for the federal government to mandate what personal health Choices private businesses must require of their employees. Some have correctly perceived federal mandates as tyrannical.*[94]

Several WWTI doctors blended business interests and medicine as well. In fact, some of them *became* businesses, monetizing their social media content, like X, YouTube, and Substack.

Despite this, WWTI doctors claimed that anyone who tried to limit the virus was blinded by "tribalism" and "politics." In their telling, only they saw the world clearly, free of bias.

#12: WWTI Doctors Normalized Quackery

In *We Want Them Infected*, I made a distinction between "contrarian" doctors and pre-pandemic anti-vaccine doctors, such as Drs. Sherri Tenpenny and Kelly Brogan. For many WWTI doctors, that distinction no longer exists. Several of them teamed up with stars of the anti-vax movement in order to achieve political power.

#13: Institutions Were Silent or Enabled WWTI Doctors

WWTI doctors have set up a parallel, insulated world inside academia, with conferences and a media ecosystem that is closed to outsiders who might remind them of their disinformation. They interview each other on podcasts and write blogs and papers together. As Dr. Gregg Gonsalves put it in his article, "Some of Our Top Schools are Embarrassing Themselves Over Covid":

> *But just as the Federalist Society has established influence over law schools and the judiciary, the Covid contrarians and their supporters would like to do the same for medicine and public health, by mainstreaming their views—both in academic settings and then in public policy—by sheer brute force. They won't give up, and they have the money and resources to continue their campaigns.*[95]

Indeed, Leonard Leo, the co-chairman of the Federalist Society's board of directors, featured Dr. Bhattacharya in a promotional video for an organization he founded, the Teneo Network, which aims to "crush liberal dominance."[96]

Universities, meanwhile, have signaled that, for the sake of "academic freedom," WWTI doctors can spread blatantly false statistics without the slightest hint of disapproval. Not only does their disinformation often go unchallenged, it often gets amplified and rewarded. At certain institutions, facts no longer matter, and the most important thing is not to hurt anyone's feelings.

#14: WWTI Doctors Centered Themselves and Considered Themselves Victims

Many WWTI doctors developed main character syndrome. They felt that all of society should have aligned with their personal standards with regard to COVID. They centered themselves and lamented that they didn't get enough attention and respect. They wrote volumes because someone called them "fringe" in an email, and they treated their social media content more seriously than COVID's victims. YouTube removing one of their hundreds of videos was a seminal moment of the pandemic for them.

#15: WWTI Doctors Attacked Their Critics in Bad Faith

WWTI doctors vigorously defended themselves in the war for public opinion. They claimed to value civil debate, and indeed they demanded courtesy and civility when they were criticized. However, they never engaged with their critics in good faith, and several of them launched a deluge of bad faith attacks against anyone who corrected their disinformation.

Whenever anyone used evidence and science to criticize WWTI doctors, they responded with grievance and emotion. They blatantly misrepresented their critics' arguments and reflexively claimed all criticism was "slanderous attacks"[97] and "harassment."[98] It was impossible to write an article criticizing them without it being labeled a "hit piece"—even before it was written. They hurled a tsunami of childish insults against their critics, seeking to intimidate and discredit anyone who might correct their factual errors and pro-infection advocacy.

Of course, it's also true that vile slurs were directed towards many WWTI doctors, which is unacceptable.

#16: WWTI Doctors Portrayed Themselves as Truth-Telling Scientists, While Using Emotional Language and Accusations to Spread Doubt

The key line in Dr. Makary's article "10 Myths Told by COVID Experts — And Now Debunked" was this:

> *In the final analysis, public health officials actively propagated misinformation that ruined lives and forever damaged public trust in the medical profession.*[1]

This was the central message of WWTI doctors, and their statements of anger and mistrust permeate this book. As the pandemic progressed, doctors who claimed in 2020 that COVID would kill 40,000 Americans also claimed they had been right about everything. To make their case that they hadn't underestimated COVID, they began to cast doubt on its death toll, casually claiming that even the pandemic's most basic numbers were distorted and elevated. They claimed that death certificates couldn't be trusted and that doctors killed patients through premature intubations.

WWTI doctors were epistemological warriors who wanted the public to doubt even the most basic facts and to trust no one—except for them.

One of the most important qualities of a physician is humility, knowing your limits, and having the self-awareness that you could be wrong.
— *Dr. Marty Makary*

Indeed, WWTI doctors wanted the public to trust them alone. For this reason, they flaunted their credentials and portrayed themselves as humble scientists driven by data and evidence alone. Dr. Joseph Ladapo wrote about his commitment to "transparency and scientific integrity,"[99] while Dr. John Mandrola boasted of his skills in evaluating science and data. "Appraisal of medical evidence is just like a procedure or surgery. It takes practice, effort, desire and mentors. No shortcuts," [100] he said.

Dr. Atlas bragged of his dedication to truth while under great adversity:

- *No matter how difficult it may seem to speak truth against a tidal wave of hostility, character assassination, death threats, backstabbing from my employer, it was never even a remote consideration to stop. Why not? Because people were dying & I know right from wrong.*[101]

- *I don't care what people think of me—right is right. People were dying, I had to say the truth. One of the things that comes with becoming a public figure [is] there's a burden of responsibility. You're speaking for millions of people, and they depend on you to say it.*[102]

- *We're an ethical society. The truth matters. My children matter to me. I don't want them to inherit a country that ignores facts. We have to persevere.*[103]

During one interview, Dr. Atlas advised young people:

> *Be bold, be empowered, & know it's liberating to say the truth. Once you stand firm in that truth—bc there is only one truth—and you don't have to adhere to the coercion, the lies and the silencing, it feels like a weight is off your shoulders.*[104]

In a podcast titled "Reforming Medicine: Uncovering Blind Spots, Challenging the Norm, and Embracing Innovation," Dr. Makary said:

> *One of the most important qualities of a physician is humility, knowing your limits, and having the self-awareness that you could be wrong.*[105]

In his article, "Why Was My Talk at a Medical Conference Canceled?" Dr. Prasad wrote:

> *As a physician and medical scholar who has published over 450 academic articles and two books, my research team and I base our opinions on a sober assessment of available evidence.*[106]

Similarly, in another article, Dr. Bhattacharya spoke of his commitment to truth. He said:

> *The COVID era has been difficult for scientists whose ideas run against the grain of powerful scientific and government bureaucracies. Even for university scientists with unblemished reputations in the before times, the price of speaking up has been vilification by social media companies, the media, and, unfortunately, even scientific journals and our fellow scientists. It is a wonder that any scientists dared to speak out, with only their commitment to the truth as a reason to do so.*[97]

Dr. Ioannidis said, "Science is the best thing that can happen to humans,"[107] and in an interview from 2021 called "The Quest for Better Science," he spoke of the importance of trust:

Trust in science is at two different levels: between scientists on the one hand and between scientists and the general public on the other. For the first level, I believe that transparency and the sharing of knowledge and know-how enable the best possible understanding of the study and thus give confidence in the work done. For the second level, being able to say "we don't know" seems essential to me. We should be able to separate the scientific environment from the political and cultural environment, to leave science as impartial as possible.[108]

WWTI doctors portrayed themselves as neutral, unbiased scientists who were able to admit to errors.

This is also how they were presented to the public. For instance, in an interview on Fox News in April 2020, the host Mark Levin introduced Dr. Ioannidis by saying:

You are co-director of the Meta Research Innovation Center at Stanford University, the Rehnborg Chair In Disease Prevention chair of disease prevention, professor of medicine and health research policy of biomedical data science and statistics. You are one of the most cited medical scientists ever, a professor of statistics at Stanford University. You are a member of the US National Academy of Medicine.[109]

All of that is true, and this was an entirely appropriate way to introduce Dr. Ioannidis, and his impressive credentials understandably made many people trust him. After this introduction, Mr. Levin then quoted Dr. Ioannidis as saying:

The risk of dying from the coronavirus for a person 65 years old is equivalent to the risk of dying driving a distance of 9 to 450 miles by car per day.

Even though the headlines from that time read "New York City Deploys 45 Mobile Morgues as Virus Strains Funeral Homes,"[110] Dr. Ioannidis told viewers to *doubt* everything they'd heard so far. He said that "the evidence we had early in the pandemic was utterly unreliable."[109] He called mathematical models of mass death "completely off; it is just an astronomical error." He had good news to share—most people with COVID didn't even know they had it. He said:

> There are far more people who are infected with this virus. The vast majority of them don't even realize that they have been infected. They are asymptomatic, they have no symptoms, or they have very mild symptoms that they would not even bother to do anything about. The best data that we have now suggest that it's not one out of 30 or one out of 100 people who get infected who will die. It's probably in the range of one in 1,000.

This low death rate was mathematically impossible at the time given how many people had already died in New York City. Yet, despite the great confidence he projected early in the pandemic, Dr. Ioannidis later portrayed himself as a humble scientist who said, "*Being able to say 'We don't know' seems essential to me.*"

Public health wasn't always a dystopian hellscape intent on using police and military power to maximize compliance with interventions that are based on 0 RCTs. But it is now!
— *Dr. Vinay Prasad*

Although WWTI doctors demanded that they be treated as *sober, impartial medical scholars*, they did not extend this courtesy to anyone else. WWTI doctors didn't feel those who disagreed with their plans for "natural immunity" were well-intentioned, though mistaken. They said that public health officials engaged in "lies and propaganda,"[111] and they spread this message relentlessly, drilling it into the public's consciousness daily for years.

According to WWTI doctors, public health officials weren't people just doing their best in tough times; they were corrupt, authoritarian tyrants with a body count who deserved to be exposed and punished. Many WWTI doctors spoke in scornful terms, full of mockery and insults, about public health officials and anyone who acknowledged COVID's toll. They blamed them for starting the pandemic and everything that went wrong with it after that.

WWTI doctors called for mass firings and shared their revenge fantasies against beleaguered public health officials. Dr. Kulldorff, for example, posted a picture of a guillotine[112] along with an article by the right-wing provocateur Jeffery Tucker titled "Who Will Be Held Responsible for this Devastation?" That article said:

> The response relied on compulsion imposed by all levels of government. The policies in turn energized a populist movement, Covid Red Guard that became a civilian enforcement arm. They policed the grocery aisles to upbraid the maskless. Drones swarmed the skies looking for parties to rat out and shut down. A blood lust against non compliers came to be unleashed at all levels of society.[113]

Dr. Bhattacharya similarly raged about *covidian cruelty, covidian tyranny, and covidian authoritarian overreach*, and Dr. Atlas said:

> Lockdowners killed and destroyed millions. That's fact. That's the data. They did that. Never forget.[114]

Dr. Prasad said public health officials were part of a "*totalitarian regime"* that *"used the power of the police state,"*[115] and he routinely said things like, "Public health wasn't always a dystopian hellscape intent on using police and military power to maximize compliance with interventions that are based on 0 RCTs. But it is now!"[116]

Dr. Prasad called for prosecutions and mass purges of government scientists. On social media, he posted a picture of a mask along with the following message:

> *I saw a 4 year old wearing this outside today. The makers of this should be prosecuted. There is no evidence it is certified to this standard in children of this age. The use of this in a child is disgusting. An adult mental illness that hurts kids. CDC and AAP failed.*[117]

After the election, Dr. Prasad complained about masking children and posted the following on X:

> *I would fire at least ~10000 people (1/4) in the CDC and everyone who touched this decision or didn't stop it. Anyone working from home should go, as well.*[118]

In one video, Dr. Prasad said doctors who advocated for COVID vaccines were "motherfuckers" and "fucking morons."[119] He stated they "don't know anything about evidence-based medicine" and were as "stupid as the people shooting ivermectin up their ass." Dr. Prasad also had this conversation with Dr. Damania in 2024:

> ***Dr. Damania:*** *What do you think should be done, Vinay, because there's this… there's two camps on this, like, "Let's forgive and have a reconciliation about all this and move on and forget it. Why are we beating the dead horse?" and others who say, "But if we do that when the next, you know, Marburg pandemic or whatever comes or bird flu the same shit's gonna happen."*

> ***Dr. Prasad:*** *Yeah, I don't believe in forgiveness because, in my opinion, these pieces of shit are still lying. I mean like, if you want forgiveness, the first thing you have to say is what you actually did wrong and they're still fucking like this well based on the best information we had that the time cloth masking two-year-olds was a sensible... no, it wasn't you fucking liar.*[120]

All this from a doctor who described himself as a "physician and medical scholar"[106] who based his "opinions on a sober assessment of available evidence."

These appeals to raw emotion were successful. Many people were enraged at anyone who tried to limit COVID in 2020, and they could be found in the comments section of many WWTI doctors. Here are some of the replies that Dr. Prasad received for his call to fire 10,000 CDC employees:

- *I hope you can contribute in an official role to Make Science Great Again!*[121]

- *Closing schools... injecting experimental products in children.. They need to be arrested first. Then, you can fire them.*[122]

- *My presumption based on these agencies' decisions so far is that they are filled top to bottom with politically possessed, self righteous, Quacks. I'd love at least 2/3 of them gone! I bet 90% of the real work is probably done by 10% of the employees there.*[123]

- *Masking toddlers was state sanctioned child abuse. The risk benefit analysis is obvious risk, implausible benefit.*[124]

- *Only 1/4?? I'd close the place down & rehire based on their progress during COVID..ie did they challenge/speak out, if so then yes you're on track to having smart people in situ who also have integrity. You can't put a price on that!*[125]

- *I agree . . . we need a decisive leader at CDC who is willing to hold the institution, and its people, accountable for that colos-*

sal failure in judgment.[126]

- *Fire anyone who obscured the reality of Antigenic Sin, innate/
adaptive immunity, risk stratification and mRNA safety signals.
Reinstate everyone with backpay who were fired due to the
unethical, unconstitutional injection mandate.*[127]

These furious calls for revenge were a normal, everyday occurrence on the social media feeds of WWTI doctors. These were the emotions they were hoping to trigger and the responses they were hoping to generate. These people agreed with Dr. Prasad and his calls for purges and prosecutions. They won't cooperate when the next pandemic hits.

#NeverAgain

— *Dr. Scott Atlas*

However, by depicting themselves as *sober medical scholars,* WWTI doctors seemed much more credible when they turned around and depicted public health officials as tyrants attacking honest citizens with needles. Indeed, some WWTI doctors spoke about their pro-infection mission in grandiose ways, invoking the language of the Civil Rights movement.

In September 2023, at a time when there were essentially no remaining mitigation measures, Dr. Prasad wrote an essay titled "Do Not Report Covid Cases to Schools & Do Not Test Yourself If You Feel Ill" that said, "Only non-violent resistance can halt irrational public health actors."[128] Drs. Kulldorff, Gupta, and Bhattacharya routinely described lockdowns as "the worst assault on workers and the working class since segregation and the Vietnam War."[129] In his essay titled "Why I Spoke Out Against Lockdowns," Dr. Kulldorff wrote:

When writing the declaration, we knew we were exposing ourselves to attacks. That can be scary, but as Rosa Parks said: 'I

have learned over the years that when one's mind is made up,
this diminishes fear; knowing what must be done does away with
fear. '130

In one social media post, Dr. Atlas even co-opted language from the
Holocaust to describe attempts to limit the virus. He said:

Why did the public accept illogical, draconian policies? [Be-
cause of] lies—propaganda reminiscent of the most heinous lies
used to sway the public in modern history." #NeverAgain[131]

None of this was new. Since the days of Edward Jenner, doubt and
mistrust have been the jet fuel of the anti-vaccine movement. So has a
sense of victimization. Anti-vaxxers compared themselves to Holocaust
victims before the pandemic, and spooky drawings of tyrannical doctors and cops attacking people with needles have long been a staple of
anti-vaccine propaganda. I was *very familiar* with these images and this
way of thinking prior to the pandemic.

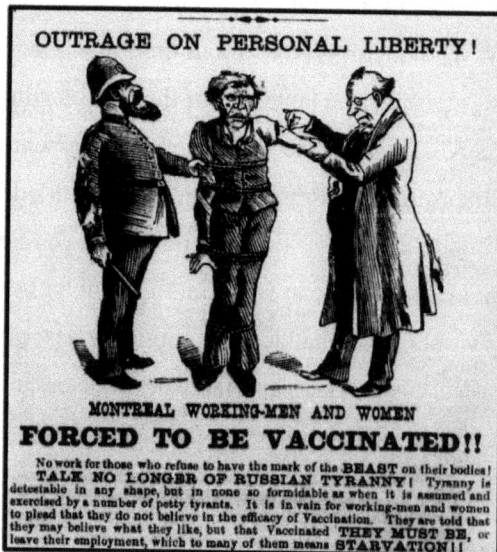

Source: HathiTrust Digital Library

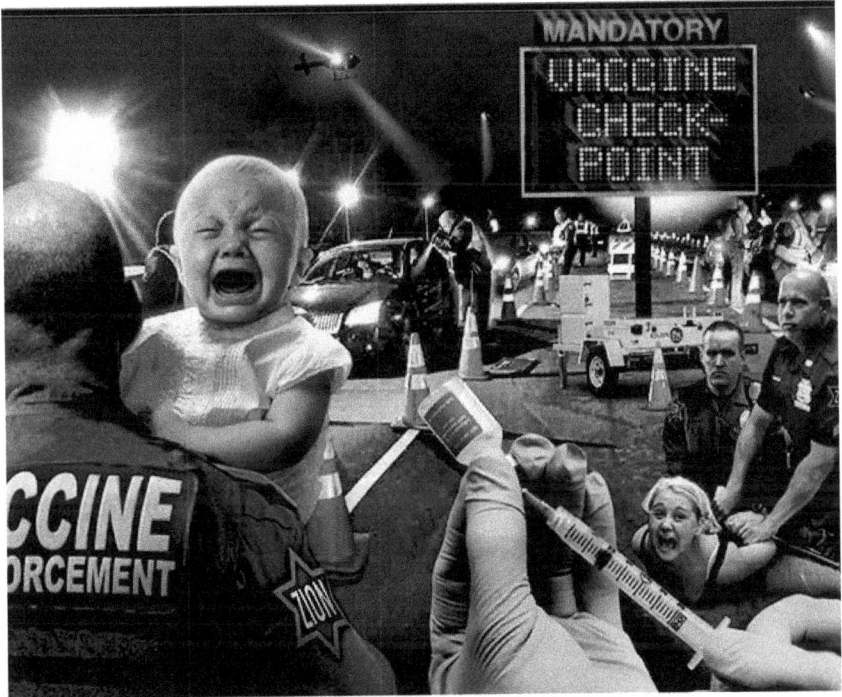

Source: DDees.com

Like the illustrators who created those anti-vax images, the goal of WWTI doctors wasn't to communicate science in a sober way but rather to enrage and provoke people under the pretense of sober science communication. The last chapter of this book is devoted to the linguistics of WWTI doctors, but until then, pay attention to the inflammatory language they used. Though they mindlessly accused everyone else of "groupthink" and "tribalism," they repeated the same phrases and buzzwords in unison to signal in-group identity and to trigger anger and mistrust. For the most part, their arguments weren't scientific, they were emotional.

Dr. Prasad revealed the core goal when he complained once again about masks, lockdowns, and vaccines, and said:

> *Trust in scientists should be down, rationally.*[132]

Lowering trust in scientists to advance their political agenda was the primary aim of WWTI doctors.

Chapter 4: Distrust in Public Health is Good

Trust is the glue in patient care.
— Dr. Lucy McBride

WWTI doctors were right about one thing: at both an individual and societal level, medicine depends on trust. Yet despite repeatedly botching basic facts and making erroneous predictions, WWTI doctors had a clear message for the public—they were highly qualified, brave truth-tellers, while those who tried to limit COVID were lying manipulators. They relentlessly reinforced this message, only to turn around and bemoan the lack of trust in medicine.

One of those WWTI doctors is Dr. Lucy McBride. A concierge primary care physician, she did not hide her impressive credentials or media appearances. According to her webpage:

Dr. Lucy McBride is a native Washingtonian. She attended the National Cathedral School, Princeton University, and Harvard Medical School, where she graduated with honors. She earned a Master's Degree in Pharmacology as a 1996 Fulbright scholar at the University of Cambridge, U.K. Dr. McBride completed her internship and residency in Internal Medicine at the Johns Hopkins Hospital. She then spent several years in the Emergency Medicine faculty at Hopkins.

Dr. McBride has been practicing internal medicine in private practice for nearly two decades. She is passionate about evidence-based, patient-centered primary care. She believes in treating the whole patient and empowering patients with tools and evidence-based guidance to navigate mental and physical health in tandem. She considers her patients her best teachers, and the relationship with them the foundation for patients' sense of agency over their health.

Dr. McBride has become a nationally recognized voice in addressing mental and physical health. She is the author of the popular medical newsletter, "Are You Okay?" now reaching over 27 thousand people a week and is the author of a forthcoming book about whole-person health with Simon & Schuster (due in March 2025).

She hosts a top-rated podcast called Beyond the Prescription, *where she interviews guests like she does her patients, pulling the curtain back on what it means to be healthy. She has been published in* The Atlantic, The Washington Post, *and* USA Today. *She has appeared on NPR, CNN, MSNBC, and PBS NewsHour, providing evidence-based medical advice, advocating for a holistic approach to health care, and helping redefine health as more than our cholesterol and weight. Health, she argues, is a process, not an outcome.*[1]

While it's not clear if Dr. McBride ever treated a hospitalized COVID patient, she was a vocal media commentator during the pandemic. In addition to the media appearances in her biography, she recorded many podcasts and has a large social media presence. In March 2022, she testified in front of the House Committee on Science, Space, and Technology Subcommittee on Investigations and Oversight. Dr. McBride's core message then was "Trust is the *glue* in patient care."[2] She testified:

Trust is the glue in patient care. Being human carries occupational risk; our job in primary care is to help people navigate it. Trust is born when doctors first acknowledge uncertainty—and then lean into things that are certain.

Dr. McBride was absolutely right about this. I've been a doctor for over 20 years and studied the anti-vaccine movement and medical disinformation for 15 years. I fully agree that trust matters more than raw knowledge. Dr. Marty Makary was also correct when he stated in January 2020:

> *We can do more to rebuild the public trust in American medicine. After all, aren't anti-vaxers people who have lost that trust?*[3]

Tragically, trust in medicine has deteriorated since then, and the medical profession bears much of the blame. Not only did WWTI doctors deceive the public about COVID's risks, those same doctors also repeatedly told the public not to trust anyone who corrected their disinformation.

I'll return to Dr. McBride's testimony and pandemic record at the end of this chapter, but first, let's meet some other doctors who—like Dr. McBride—have impressive credentials, were pandemic influencers, and spread copious COVID disinformation. They relentlessly minimized COVID's risk for young people, mocked concerns about variants, and prematurely declared the pandemic over. They greatly oversold the vaccine in early 2021, only to later deny its benefits and treat its side effects as a fate worse than death.

Instead of reflecting on their own mistakes, they instead called on public health officials to admit to errors and apologize. They said that anyone who tried to stop the virus outside of nursing homes was wrong, incompetent, and, most of all, dishonest. The presentations below are just a small sample of their disinformation and accusations.

Immunity is built through illness.
— Dr. Vinay Prasad

Dr. Vinay Prasad has impressive credentials and accomplishments.

According to his webpage:

> *Vinay Prasad MD MPH is a hematologist-oncologist and Profes-*
> *sor in the Department of Epidemiology and Biostatistics at the*
> *University of California San Francisco. He runs the VKPrasad*
> *lab at UCSF, which studies cancer drugs, health policy, clini-*
> *cal trials and better decision making. He is author of over 500*
> *academic articles, and the books Ending Medical Reversal, and*
> *Malignant. He hosts the oncology podcast Plenary Session, the*
> *general medicine podcast the VPZD show is active on Substack*
> *and runs a YouTube Channel VinayPrasadMDMPH. He runs The*
> *Drug Development Letter, a must read for industry insights. He*
> *tweets @VPrasadMDMPH.*[4]

Dr. Prasad was a prominent influencer during the pandemic. He has a popular Substack, podcast, YouTube channel, and social media presence. He was a guest on multiple other podcasts and wrote articles for *The Atlantic, The Washington Post*, STAT News, and MedPage Today. Dr. Prasad's pandemic output might help explain "the erosion of trust in medicine and in public health."[2]

In the first half of 2021, immediately after vaccination campaigns began, Dr. Prasad overhyped them well beyond what the evidence showed. He claimed they offered perfect protection against severe COVID (which was false at the time[5]), that they blocked transmission, and they would end the pandemic. Some of his assertions from that time are below:

- **January 2021**: *Because vaccination primes the body to fight off SARS-CoV-2, you are massively less likely to get sick and less likely to infect others. Some ask about the new variants, but data out from Moderna are reassuring.*[6]
- **February 2021**: *We know the vaccine is 100% effective against protecting against bad outcomes for grandparent.*[7]
- **February 2021**: *This NYTimes story of Jan 24th, "Vaccines*

Alone Won't End Pandemic" Did not age well (as of Feb 18).
It was completely off, and just another squeeze of fear. Enough
with these models. They have often been erroneous.[8]

- **February 2021:** *Vaccines reduce transmission and will lead us back to normal life.*[9]

- **April 2021:** *Media coverage that will backfire, I bet Jan - Feb Bizarre pessimism vaccines will not reduce transmission- Remember that long list of vaccines that don't slow transmission?*[10]

He recorded a podcast in March 2021 titled "Monica Gandhi on The End of the Pandemic."[11] In an interview titled "What We Got Wrong (and Right) About COVID-19" from July 2021, just before Delta ripped through much of the country, he said:

> *I think the worst is over. The better way to judge how much of a*
> *public health threat is happening is the number of people who*
> *are hospitalized, the number of people who are dying. And maybe*
> *cases won't be the best metric going forward, because many peo-*
> *ple might have mild, very mild infections.*[12]

After saying the pandemic had mostly ended in the first half of 2021, Dr. Prasad began casting doubt on all measures to limit COVID, including vaccines, masks, boosters, testing, and ventilation, as well as anyone who supported those measures. He wrote articles such as "Covid Vaccines Shouldn't Be 'Routine' for Kids,"[13] "Covid Vaccines for Children Should Not Get Emergency Use Authorization,"[14] "The Downsides of Masking Young Students Are Real,"[15] and "The Case Against Masks at School."[16]

Though Dr. Prasad initially claimed that vaccines would end the pandemic, he devoted most of his subsequent pandemic energy towards discouraging them. Dr. Prasad's YouTube videos exposed his anti-vaccine agenda:

- Most People Should Not Get a Fall 2023 Covid19 Booster | An Analysis of the Evidence[17]
- No One Wants the Covid19 Booster | CDC Reports 3% Uptake | CDC And FDA Have Failed America[18]
- 11 Reasons an Annual Covid-19 Booster Is Not Like an Annual Flu Shot[19]
- Singapore Study on Kids' Vax Only Included Kids W/O COVID| Does It Apply to US? | A Doctor Reflects[20]
- The Fall Covid19 Booster Is A PUBLIC HEALTH FIASCO - It Has No Clinical Evidence| Total Scam[21]
- The CDC's Changing Vaccine Story (Vinay Prasad Analyzes Walensky Statements)[22]
- Concerning Vaccine Safety Signals Documented by FDA[23]
- Boosters Do Not Work If You Have Had Covid19[24]
- The White House Former Covid Czar Spreads Misinformation to Sell Fall Booster[25]
- Kids Vaccine Efficacy Requirement is GONE![26]
- FDA's Marks Demoted Krause, so Biden Could Ram COVID Vax Approval & Mandate It[27]

While Dr. Prasad claimed to be driven by evidence and data, this was not the case. In December 2021, for example, Dr. Prasad mocked people who wanted the first booster dose in a podcast titled "Omicron Panic"[28] with Drs. Makary and Zubin Damania (ZDoggMD). While laughing uproariously, they said:

> **Dr. Makary:** *Are you guys boosted being that close or is this an unboosted contact?*
>
> **Dr. Damania:** *We're unmasked, unboosted and unrepentant, Marty.*
>
> **Dr. Makary:** *Well, I'm an unboosted male. That's my preferred pronoun, by the way.*
>
> **Dr. Damania:** *Oh, is that your pronoun? An unboosted male? Yes, my pronouns are it, they, those and currently unboosted*

because I got Moderna, which apparently kicks ass.

[…]

Dr. Prasad: […] *I haven't gotten my booster yet and-*

Dr. Makary: *You mean this week you haven't gotten, 'cause you do weekly boosters, I'm sure.*

Dr. Prasad: *Well, eventually, we're all gonna have to keep boosting.*

Dr. Makary: *Yeah, boosting.*

Dr. Damania: *You know, my vaccine card looks like one of those like frequent flyer like coffee cards where they punch the hole, like I boosted here and boosted here and boosted here and when I get 10 boosters, Fauci sends me a Fauci bobblehead that says I am the science.*

Dr. Makary: *I'm getting my booster sent with the GNC nutrition vitamins.*

Dr. Prasad: *They had the same evidence, you know.*

None of this was true. By December 2021, there was already clear evidence a third vaccine dose was beneficial. Though the results were only available as a press release, a randomized controlled trial (RCT) of 10,000 people showed that a booster was safe and 95% effective at preventing COVID.[29] The results were published in the *NEJM* several months later,[30] and it doesn't take a genius to imagine a vaccine that prevented COVID infections would also lessen severe COVID. The results from a large observational study were also available at the time.[31] It estimated the booster to be 93% effective for hospital admission, 92% effective for severe disease, and 81% effective for COVID-related death. None of this mattered to these doctors. As Omicron loomed, they couldn't stop making jokes.

The Omicron wave hit with force in January 2022, just a month after the podcast. According to the article "During the Omicron Wave, Death Rates Soared for Older People":

> *Despite strong levels of vaccination among older people, Covid killed them at vastly higher rates during this winter's Omicron wave than it did last year, preying on long delays since their last shots and the variant's ability to skirt immune defenses.*
>
> *This winter's wave of deaths in older people belied the Omicron variant's relative mildness. Almost as many Americans 65 and older died in four months of the Omicron surge as did in six months of the Delta wave, even though the Delta variant, for any one person, tended to cause more severe illness.*
>
> *While overall per capita Covid death rates have fallen, older people still account for an overwhelming share of them.*
>
> *"This is not simply a pandemic of the unvaccinated," said Andrew Stokes, an assistant professor in global health at Boston University who studies age patterns of Covid deaths. "There's still exceptionally high risk among older adults, even those with primary vaccine series."*[32]

Though Dr. Prasad discouraged it, a single vaccine dose could have prevented much of this.

Similarly, Dr. Prasad's opposition to the pediatric COVID vaccine was not supported by data and evidence. In fact, he began his campaign against it months before there was any data or evidence about it. The first data about the pediatric COVID vaccine—an RCT showing it was safe and 100% effective against COVID[33]—was published in May 2021. However, in January 2021, Dr. Prasad had already speculated that children wouldn't need it as the pandemic seemed to be "abating." He wrote:

Let me be perfectly clear: children DO NOT NEED a sars-cov-2 vaccine before they are permitted to return to normal activities, such as school and visiting loved ones. […] If the epidemic is abating, how can you justify giving 100 kids those AEs (adverse events), so that perhaps 1 or 2 or even 3 will be spared a case of covid that might be as mild as the AEs themselves? […] Once adults, particularly older adults are vaccinated, and if *god willing* there is not vaccine escape, covid19 is over. We are going back to normal.[34]

He formalized his thoughts in an essay the next month in which he gave "five reasons why schools can and should open at 100% capacity before a vaccine for those under age 16 is available."[35] Dr. Prasad fearmongered about mundane vaccine side effects such as fevers, and used obviously erroneous statistics—*"the vaccine might save one life for every 1 million kids who get it"*—a death rate that was mathematically impossible at the time based on the number of children who had already died. Dr. Prasad also repeatedly stated that COVID was "on par with seasonal influenza" for children,[34] another obvious falsehood.

In June 2021, he continued to claim that children didn't need to be vaccinated because they could avoid the virus altogether. He wrote:

Remember cases are FALLING PRECIPITOUSLY […] The fraction of all cases that are adolescents is not the point. The raw number of adolescent cases is the point THAT IS FALLING […] The actual numbers show both COVID and MIS-C is plummeting with adult vaccination.[36]

Shortly after this, Delta arrived, and headlines would soon read, "COVID Hospitalization Rate in Kids Rose 5x as Delta Variant Spread, CDC Says."[37] Unvaccinated teenagers died preventable deaths,[38] and a

CDC report found, "hospitalization rates were 10 times higher among un-vaccinated than among fully vaccinated adolescents."[39] Omicron arrived soon after this, and headlines would read, "COVID Hospitalization for Young Children 5 Times Higher During Omicron Than Delta."[40] During the Omicron wave in New York City, 54% of hospitalized children had no underlying conditions,[41] and once again, unvaccinated children suffered the most.[42]

As the pandemic progressed, Dr. Prasad used contradictory reasons to support his unshakable belief that children should not get the COVID vaccine. In 2021, he opposed vaccinating children, writing that "kids are less likely to acquire SARS-CoV-2."[43] In 2022, he opposed vaccinating children because "Most kids already had COVID-19." He didn't mention that, in between these two statements, the headlines read, "Every Day, Hundreds of Kids Are Getting Hospitalized with Covid-19."[44]

As with the booster vaccine, Dr. Prasad was entirely unmoved by studies of the pediatric COVID vaccine. An RCT showing it perfectly prevented COVID infections in adolescents[33] did not sway him, nor did dozens of observational trials from around the world showing the vaccine limited rare but grave harms in children. In fact, Dr. Prasad managed to find a "flaw" in every study whose conclusion he did not like. He made YouTube videos such as "New Vaccine Study Stays Covid19 Boost-ers Lower Heart Attacks; It Is Flawed; Here Is Why,"[45] "CDC Pushes a Flawed Analysis | Does COVID Cause Diabetes in Kids? | A Doctor Analyzes an MMWR Paper,"[46] and "FLAWED Booster data was used by FDA for Mass Vax Campaign & We PROVE it in our new PAPER."[47]

He later said that it was "good" to report parents who wanted to vac-cinate their child to Children's Protective Services,[48] that vaccine boosters were "crazy, malpractice medicine. An annual vaccine for a 20-year-old man is dangerous."[49]

In addition to minimizing the benefits of the vaccine, Dr. Prasad relentlessly minimized pediatric COVID. After COVID killed 19 children in a single month, he said children didn't need the vaccine because there were 330 million Americans.[50] He repeatedly said that anyone who even discussed pediatric COVID was "breathless." Some examples include:

- *Two++ years of breathless, fear-mongering news coverage of COVID-19 in kids*[51]
- *Breathless coverage of rare anecdotes of MIS-C & death in kids, which sabotaged school reopening?*[52]
- *Media's breathless coverage of MIS-C and variants has been a disservice.*[53]

That last quote was from April 2021, just before the arrival of the Delta and Omicron variants. However, no matter what was happening on the ground, Dr. Prasad continued to minimize pediatric COVID deaths. In February 2022 he wrote:

While the death of any child is a tragedy, Covid-19 is less deadly to children than many other risks we accept as a matter of course, including drowning, vehicle accidents, and even cardio-vascular disease.[54]

That sentence was factually wrong when he wrote it. COVID was a leading killer of children at the time, and we do not accept kids drowning and getting hit by cars "as a matter of course." In May 2022, he wrote an article that said:

A few sadly were hospitalized and very few died.[55]

In reality, around 2,000 children died of COVID, and the American Academy of Pediatrics estimated that 234,000 were hospitalized from Fall 2020 to Spring 2024.[56] Meanwhile, Multisystem Inflammatory Syndrome in Children (MIS-C) is a devastating COVID complication that affects around 10,000 children, killing at least 80 of them.[57] All of this would have been much worse had there been no pediatric COVID vaccine as Dr. Prasad wished.

Dr. Prasad routinely humiliated anyone who tried to avoid COVID and claimed they were mentally ill. In January 2021, the pandemic's deadliest month, he tweeted:

> *I want to write a children's book about a bear who didn't want to leave home till it was perfectly safe. He never left and life passed him by. In the sequel, he stands at the window shouting at anyone outside that they are killing fellow bears and spreading disinformation.*[58]

He wrote articles such as "Legitimizing Irrational Anxiety Is Bad Medicine"[59] and made collages of other doctors wearing masks to shame them on social media.[60] He mocked science journalist Ed Yong for wearing a mask and said, "He did invent long COVID."[61] Nonconformists bothered Dr. Prasad so much, he even took a picture of a stranger on the street and wrote an entire article to mock them for wearing a mask.[62] Dr. Prasad also ridiculed Long COVID patients on social media, joking, "Haha double long covid. Just like double IPA!"[63] Even when COVID was killing 1,000 Americans per week, Dr. Prasad said:

> *Covid is a cold now. Don't take anything. Don't test. Drink OJ. Toughen up.*[64]

Dr. Prasad also minimized COVID's cardiac effects. In the article titled "Setting the Record Straight: There Is No 'COVID Heart,'" he wrote that:

> *Even in the sickest of the sick, Covid-19's effect on the heart appears to be modest. [...] People who have recovered from Covid-19 have no special reason to worry about their hearts.*[65]

However, Dr. Prasad felt *very differently* about rare, mild, temporary vaccine side effects.[66] While Dr. Prasad casually brushed off anything COVID could do, he developed a laser-like focus on vaccine-myocarditis, scolding anyone who didn't treat it as more consequential than death from COVID. In contrast to COVID, he warned about the vaccine that:

> *The problem is that scar tissue created in response to heart inflammation can be the source of the rhythm disturbance. It's one of the reasons we feel that even the slightest bit of inflammation in the heart should be treated seriously.*[67]

While Dr. Prasad said a rate of 21 of 3,000 patients with COVID-myocarditis was "reassuring," he was troubled about the rare occurrences of vaccine-related myocarditis, saying, "That 1/3-5k ballpark is deeply concerning."[68]

Dr. Prasad produced an overwhelming amount of content on this side effect. Some of his YouTube videos are:

- Our New Myocarditis Paper - Shows the Risk Highest in Young Men[69]
- Myocarditis From Moderna 2nd Dose Higher in Men Under 40 Than Covid19[70]
- Myocarditis & Teens: Vaccine Benefit & Risk[71]
- New MMWR CDC Study Compares Covid Myocarditis to Vax Myocarditis | Is It Good Science?[72]
- The Good, The Bad, and The Ugly of the Covid Vaccine[73]
- Thailand Myocarditis After Vaccine Study[74]
- New Study Documents Covid19 Vaccine Harms - Low Platelets, GBS, Myocarditis - I Unpack[75]
- UPDATED DATA: UK Myocarditis Authors Stratify by Sex for Men under 40- Vax vs Virus[76]
- How Are Kids and Young Adults Doing 90 Days After Vaccine Myocarditis?[77]
- Kaiser Northwest Estimate of Myocarditis/Pericarditis Com-

pared to CDC's Estimate[78]
- How CDC's Vaccine Safety Missed Cases of Myocarditis | ID doc Dr. Katie Sharff Discusses New Study[79]
- Myocarditis | Kids Vax | Kids Mask[80]
- Myocarditis Data from Ontario Province: Specific Vaccine & Interval Between Doses[81]
- CDC Director Is Wrong Re Myocarditis Numbers 5-11 & CDC Cannot Count Vaccine Doses - Huge Blunders![82]
- Myocarditis Update - Israeli Data - Sweden - Denmark - So Much More[83]
- Closing Thoughts on Myocarditis and Vaccines[84]
- Myocarditis In The UK: Moderna Vs. The Virus! New Nature Medicine Paper[85]

All this about a rare effect that is universally described as "mild, transient, and self-limiting."[66]

In one video, he even fretted mightily about "subclinical myocarditis,"[86] which is nothing more than an abnormal lab value in a child who feels fine. In contrast to literal death from COVID, Dr. Prasad didn't say concerns about this lab value were "breathless, fear-mongering."[51]

Eventually, Dr. Prasad came to embrace the mass infection of unvaccinated children so they could theoretically serve as human shields for more vulnerable adults. He laid out his pro-infection position in an article written in February 2022, toward the end of the worst wave of the pandemic for children, titled "Should We Let Children Catch Omicron?"[54]

According to the American Academy of Pediatrics, "The largest peak was in winter 2022 during the omicron surge, with 6,527 child hospitalizations the week of Jan. 15."[56] The headlines that month read, "A Record-High Number of Kids are Getting Hospitalized with Covid-19 as Overall Covid-19 Hospitalizations Soar Past the Delta Peak."[87] Furthermore, the youngest children, who are most vulnerable to COVID, were not yet eligible to be vaccinated. COVID killed nearly 200 American children in January and February 2022.[88] When the dust settled, an article quoted Dr. Jason Kane, a pediatric intensivist, as saying, "We saw a massive surge of hospitalized young children during Omicron that we didn't see in the earlier months of the pandemic."[89]

Despite what was happening in pediatric hospitals at that moment, Dr. Prasad spoke of the benefits of infecting children, both to them and society at large:

> *What kids really need, however, is a return to normal. And when it comes to infectious disease, normality means a world where they are routinely exposed to, and overcome, viral illness. For children, getting sick and recovering is part of a natural and healthy life. […]*
>
> *Dropping masks, quarantines, distancing, and all other mitigations will allow children to develop the kind of broad immunity gained by living a normal life. Shielding kids from exposure only increases their future risk. This is partly why the UK does not vaccinate against chickenpox. Serious complications from the disease are rare among children, and the circulating virus allows adults to be naturally boosted against reactivation-driven shingles. By rebuilding population immunity among the least at-risk, moreover, we help buffer risk for those most vulnerable. […]*
>
> *The epidemiologist and researcher Francois Balloux puts it this way:*
>
> > *I'm not sure how to convey this message in a half-acceptable way. But, if the objective were to send SARCoV2 into endemicity, then healthy kids have to be exposed to the virus, ideally earlier than later. This is not 'eu-*

genism'; it is bog-standard infection disease epidemiol-
ogy.

It's time to allow children to resume normal life, not simply be-
cause their exclusion is unfair or hurts them socially and psycho-
logically, but because it is immunologically in their best interest.
Parents must consider that exposures are how we best protect our
children against the variants of the future. In fact, it is reckless to
let children age into a more serious encounter with a disease best
dealt with while younger.

This view is shared by the authors of a May 2021 paper in The
British Journal of Medicine, who wrote: "Once most adults are
vaccinated, circulation of SARS-CoV-2 may in fact be desir-
able, as it is likely to lead to primary infection early in life when
disease is mild, followed by booster re-exposures throughout
adulthood... This would keep reinfections mild and immunity up
to date." […]

Schools are not sterile, nor should they be. Immunity is built
through illness.[54]

None of this is true. Repeated SARS-CoV-2 infections are not beneficial for children, exposures do not protect against "variants of the future,"
immunity can be safely built through vaccines, and pediatric infections
do not "buffer risk for those most vulnerable." In fact, children turned out
to spread the virus quite effectively, with one study reporting that 70% of
outbreaks in US households started with a child.[90]

Dr. Prasad expanded on his pro-virus philosophy in his essay, "I Am
Going to Mask Because I Want to Get Fewer Colds & Other Flawed
Ideas." In it, Dr. Prasad shamed and ridiculed anyone who wanted to stay
healthy and claimed the best way to *avoid* feeling sick was to *get* sick.

"We may even feel worse when we get sick," he warned, "having lost some cross immunity the longer we postpone things."[91]

Dr. Prasad spoke of the dire consequences of stopping viruses, warning that worse variants might arise if we didn't give them opportunities to infect us and mutate. He wrote, "That would only mean we are selecting for fitter viruses. Viruses that can spread with less and less breath."

Parroting old anti-vaccine talking points about measles and smallpox, Dr. Prasad speculated that *preventing* infections could cause cancer and autoimmune disease, even though viruses can cause cancer and autoimmune diseases. He wrote:

> There is the arrogance that avoiding colds and flu is good for us. Of course it is the case that getting sick is unpleasant, but our knowledge of immunology and the body is so primitive we should not conclude that avoiding it is 'good for us.' We have no idea if that is true in the long run.
>
> It is natural to be infected repeatedly with respiratory viruses— if we got fewer infections what would that mean for auto-immunity for cancer? We have no idea if we would actually live longer or healthier lives trying to dodge seasonal runny noses and coughs.

In the real world, SARS-CoV-2 can cause autoimmune diseases.[92] In the mirror world, however, sickness was health.

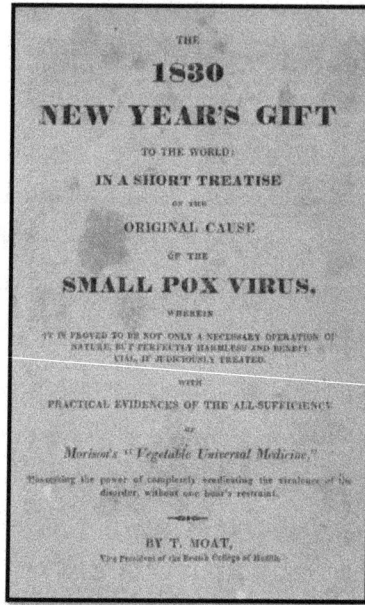

THE
1830
NEW YEAR'S GIFT
TO THE WORLD:
IN A SHORT TREATISE
OF THE
ORIGINAL CAUSE
OF THE
SMALL POX VIRUS,
WHEREIN
IT IS PROVED TO BE NOT ONLY A NECESSARY OPERATION OF
NATURE, BUT PERFECTLY HARMLESS AND BENEFI-
CIAL, IF JUDICIOUSLY TREATED.
WITH
PRACTICAL EVIDENCES OF THE ALL-SUFFICIENCY
OF
Morison's "Vegetable Universal Medicine,"
Possessing the power of completely eradicating the virulence of the
disorder, without one hour's restraint.
BY T. MOAT,
Vice President of the British College of Health.

Smallpox is "perfectly harmless and
beneficial, if judiciously treated."

Distrust In Public Health Is Good
— Dr. Vinay Prasad

Despite that inglorious track record, Dr. Prasad gave an interview to the libertarian publication *Reason* in 2023 titled "Stop Trusting the Public Health Establishment,"[93] which described him as a "progressive doctor." "The truth is, the entire public health apparatus failed," Dr. Prasad said. He added:

> *Yeah, I think this is an article that sort of makes the argument that we should trust institutions in so far as their past perfor-*

mance. And unfortunately, public health, by that I mean the institutions of public health, the CDC, the National Institutes of Allergy and Infectious Disease, NIAID, which Tony Fauci ran, and even some local public health officials should lose your trust because of their poor performance. And I go on to detail, seven domains where I think we can all agree they really underperformed and maybe even in fact told us some falsehoods along the way.

He recorded other podcasts titled "When Trust in Experts Goes Too Far."[94] and "How Politics Corrupted Science: Dr. Vinay Prasad on COVID."[95] Although Dr. Prasad assured his audience that vaccines halted transmission and would end the pandemic, he said:

What I think is most problematic is that we [in the medical field] were a bit dishonest in saying we had more confidence than we really did. The place that I have been most critical of the pandemic response is communication around the certainty of the evidence when it is, in fact, a lot more uncertain.

Dr. Prasad made multiple YouTube videos where he spoke about "lies" and "deception" from public health leaders. Some examples are:

- COVID 19 Recap - I am Interviewed About Covid19 Errors, Particularly Those Made by Government[96]
- Lies and Exaggerations Re: Kids Vax Under 5 Is Bad Public Health[97]
- Why Has Public Health Lost Trust | A Brief Recap of Things We Got Wrong[98]
- Media Was Complicit with Public Health's Lie About Natural Immunity[99]

- Public Health Failures with ID Ethicist Zeb Jamrozik | Mandates, RCTs, Masks, Deception[100]
- Public Health Lied About Natural Immunity[101]

He wrote an article titled "The Fragmented Trust in Public Health," which said:

> Public health, the institution, must own these absurdities and contradictions because the CDC has the scope and authority to correct them with clear guidance. Just as we need trust, public health seems poised to destroy it.[102]

Much of the article lamented the fate of wealthy athletes. Dr. Prasad was very upset that "Kyrie Irving can watch the basketball game from the first row, but not play on the court – and worse, that this rule only applies in New York city."

In another article, Dr. Prasad spoke of "myths from the brave new world of science as political propaganda."[103] He said.

> Throughout this pandemic, the CDC has been a poor steward of that balance, pushing a series of scientific results that are severely deficient. This research is plagued with classic errors and biases, and does not support the press-released conclusions that often follow. In all cases, the papers are uniquely timed to further political goals and objectives; as such, these papers appear more as propaganda than as science. The CDC's use of this technique has severely damaged their reputation and helped lead to a growing divide in trust in science by political party. Science now risks entering a death spiral in which it will increasingly fragment into subsidiary verticals of political parties. As a society, we cannot afford to allow this to occur. Impartial, honest appraisal is needed now more than ever, but it is unclear how we

can achieve it.

Dr. Prasad repeatedly spread this message of doubt to his over 300,000 followers on social media. Some examples include:

- **Misinformation** *like: covid vaccines halt transmission, cloth masking works, vaccine mandates work, school closure has net benefit, paxlovid works in vaccinated people-- so much misinformation these days. Mostly from the federal government.*[104]

- *The most dangerous type of* **misinformation** *is when government officials like Mandy* [CDC Director Dr. Mandy Cohen] *make false statements. There is no evidence that this fall booster will lower the rate of long covid. The CDC has failed to demand randomized studies. Disgraceful conduct.*[105]

- *The idea that public health would force a fit young man to get a vaccine for a disease he already had--- and one that was known to not halt transmission-- is an* **acid poured on society's trust***. It will keep rotting away and the next 25 years will be tumultuous.*[106]

- *It is hardly a question. Why did public health* **lose trust***? Their own actions. Their own errors.*[107]

- *Public health* **lied** *about: Natural immunity Myocarditis Mask evidence School closure Long COVID Ethics of vaccine mandates Ran 0 RCTs of NPIs in US Public health forfeited its own trust and may never earn it back Backlash 100% deserved.*[108]

- *Situation critical. Public health experts* **lied** *about harmful covid policy, and silenced criticism. Conflict of interest is out of control. Public trust in science is going to collapse this decade. Scientists must talk to people where they are. No more high horse.*[109]

- *Why is trust in public health so low? -- says person who has been telling a steady stream of* **lies.**[110]

- *The* **number one cause of loss of trust in public health** *is public health. Random people on the internet is not the problem. If you want a police information, start by getting the CDC to provide accurate counts of death.*[111]

- *The biggest reason for loss of trust are **errors** made by CDC and FDA.*[112]
- ***Misinformation** is the number one cause of distrust in public health. The problem is they forgot it was their own misinformation.*[113]
- *Everything Ashish says here in @npr is a **lie**. No one has ever shown that taking this booster keeps you in school more. No one has ever shown that it slows transmission in any useful way. This is just misinformation. Make Pfizer run a study and measure these end points.*[114]
- *An amazing @CNN clip, posted by @TheEliKlein where an anchor confronts Fauci with Cochrane's report showing no proven benefit to community masking Fauci says it works for individuals not populations Yet, this is also a **lie**.*[115]
- *CDC director is still **lying**. Specifically about what was known on transmission, and on the Cochrane mass review being retracted Good scientist run RCTs Bad scientists **lie**.*[116]
- *It's weird to see the FDA commissioner **lie** about the efficacy of primary vaccination based on his misinterpretation of non randomized data. You don't see this often.*[117]
- *It was one of many **lies** as part of the "audition" package to work for White House. The lie supported White House policy goal (70%), which they invented Very dangerous when scientists become politicians.*[118]
- *Very few faculty have called out @DrCaliff_FDA's false statements including 'Misinfo is leading cause of death,' which is a **lie** he made up and has not provided a ref for Another **lie** is need to EUA bival boosters without RCTs.*[119]

After seeing someone comment that "Trust in doctors and hospitals: 70%+ in 2020, 31.4% now. On its way to zero," Dr. Prasad felt this was still too high, posting:

> *It should be zero Doctors and hospitals created unproven policies, ran zero RCTs, continue those policies, and **lie** about the*

evidence.[120]

Dr. Prasad did not want civil discussion and debate. He wanted heads to roll. He called for mass purges of anyone who tried to limit pediatric COVID. His article, "Entirely Predictable: More Parents Don't Want Routine Vaccination for Their Kids," blamed the CDC for falling vaccination rates. He said that the "CDC recommended unnecessary COVID19 vaccines for kids and lost all credibility."[121] He wrote:

> *In order to regain trust, the CDC needs to be reorganized. First, any employee responsible for masking 2 year olds or adding COVID19 vaccines to the pediatric schedule should be fired. [...] The CDC is failing every day; only drastic action can overcome the public doubt they have created by their own incompetence.*

Though Dr. Prasad still talks about COVID nearly every day, he wrote an article in January 2023 titled "Should We Just Stop Talking About Covid19?" that—again—called for mass firings, not just at the CDC, but also at the American Academy of Pediatrics (AAP). He wrote:

> *It's important to remember that it was likely a lab leak, masks don't work, mandates didn't work, vaccines were not needed in people who had COVID, nor children, closing school was a human rights violation, masking kids didn't work, vaccine mandates were unethical, vaccine passports were useless, boosters don't have good data, paxlovid doesn't have good data, long COVID is overblown, etc.. These are obvious things to those of us who can read. The CDC lied repeatedly, and all the employees at CDC and AAP who told us to cloth mask 2 year olds should be fired for stupidity.*[122]

Dr. Prasad wrote another article titled "AAP (American Academy Of Pediatrics) Is Broken, Failed Organization," which began:

*The American Academy of Pediatrics (AAP) is a failed organi-
zation. For years, they have made mistakes, but the pandemic
elevated their failings to catastrophic errors.*[123]

Dr. Prasad concluded by saying the AAP was motivated only by its
hatred for Trump and calling for its destruction. He said:

*COVID-19 has revealed that no organization in the USA defends
the interests of kids. Kids don't have lobbyists. But, it is vital that
they do. I support the creation of a non-partisan federal agency
whose sole task is to evaluate, in real time, the impact of policies
on children. Just as the CBO scores legislation for fiscal impact,
this group would score the balance of an intervention's impact on
kids.*

*The agency will also be tasked with issuing prospective guidance
to promote the welfare of children. The agency can suggest and
enforce policies to correct the deficiencies of the pandemic. If
money is allocated to schools, and I support this, the agency can
enforce that it be spent on kids, not teachers unions. The fate of
all societies depends on how we treat the next generation.*

*The AAP was happy to sacrifice millions to score a pyrrhic
victory against Trump. We must have a new group empowered to
protect kids interests in the face of incompetence, irrationality
and tribalism. The AAP is not fit for that task. A new group must
be created.*

He wanted the AAP's replacement to be carefully monitored by government overseers to make sure it didn't get out of line.

He wrote an article titled "Public Health's Truth Problem," which
said:

Throughout the pandemic, public-health officials have omitted

uncomfortable truths, made misleading statements, and advanced
demonstrably false assertions. In the information era, where
what one says is easily accessible and anyone may read primary
literature, these falsehoods will be increasingly recognized and
severely damage the field's credibility.[124]

He asked readers to "Consider some messages the field has promoted to the public over the last two years and their shaky relationship with the truth." Dr. Prasad complained about masks and vaccines and concluded:

Falsehoods and half-truths have consequences. Publishing
flawed science to raise irrational fear, making false statements
about the efficacy of treatments, and extrapolating data from
one vaccine to another all constitute bad scientific practice. In
normal times, scientists would not tolerate such behavior. Yet,
repeatedly, federal agencies and respected organizations push
recommendations that are deeply uncertain, rely on fearmonger-
ing, or provide hollow reassurances. The right answer would be
to acknowledge the massive residual uncertainty surrounding
these issues and embark on studies to reduce it.

We need public-health institutions in times of crisis. But if they
won't tell the truth, they don't deserve the public's trust. If we
meet future health threats as a more polarized society, these insti-
tutions will deserve their share of the blame.

In yet another article, "Public Health Should Lose Your Trust," Dr. Prasad wrote:

Trust is justified based on how an organization or system per-
forms. And the truth is, the entire public health apparatus, failed.
In addition to that, leaders at FDA and NIH and CDC engaged
in lies and propaganda. As such, they should lose your trust, and

without serious reforms you should not return the trust of these organizations.[125]

He felt that public health officials tried too hard to limit COVID and were not appropriately deferential to SARS-CoV-2. His complaints about public health included: *"Lack of debates/ smearing scientists who disagreed natural immunity counts for nothing, masking efficacy, vaccine-myocarditis, Paxlovid, and one size fits all booster recs."* His sole concern about the virus was that it didn't get enough praise and respect. Dr. Prasad said:

> *Whether or not having prior COVID-19 means you are less likely to get seriously ill from a repeat bout of COVID-19, is now well accepted as obviously true. And yet, this information was steadily suppressed. A paper out this week in the Lancet shows durable reduction in severe disease after natural infection.*

He accused public health officials of "suppressing" information about "natural immunity," while simultaneously sharing that such information had been published in a leading medical journal. Later research showed that severe infections often follow a severe first infection.[126]

Dr. Prasad depicted himself "as a scientist,"[125] in the article and stated that "it's my duty to call balls and strikes." He again spoke of "lies and errors" and concluded:

> *There is no question going forward, public health is facing an existential crisis. Hundreds of millions of Americans don't trust them. That trust was lost because of lies and errors.*
>
> *Public health has aligned itself with democratic partisan politics, further alienating itself from half of America. If something bad happens, we are doomed. The country will tear itself apart before we ever succumbed to restrictions again.*

The situation is very dire. The only way to regain trust is brutal honesty and accountability. As a scientist, it's my duty to call balls and strikes. This administration struck out a long time ago.

In an article titled "We Need to Strip CDC and Public Health of Powers," Dr. Prasad called for the decimation of the CDC because they took measures to limit COVID.[127] He wrote:

Eventually politicians will strip CDC and other public health agencies of their power, and I won't be able to argue with them. Why? Public health misused and abused its powers with:

- *Closing beaches*
- *Pouring sand into outdoor skateboard parks*
- *Discouraging people from outdoor activities*
- *Lying about the evidence for cloth masks in community settings (to this day)*
- *Lying about the evidence for masking outside*
- *Not running any randomized control trials of masking in high income nations*
- *Pushing masks on 2-year-olds in contrast with world health organization recommendations, evidence, and basic common sense*
- *Culling animals*
- *Using the police state to enforce lockdown*
- *Not letting people hold their father's hand when their father dies*
- *Not letting people visit their mother when she's hospitalized*
- *Restricting visitor access from parents & siblings to their sick, hospitalized, and dying children*
- *Closing schools (but just for poor kids who go to public school, rich kids get to go to school)*
- *Making testing companies rich by recommending unproven*

testing

- *Inventing a 6-ft distance*
- *Enforcing stupid distances to make it hard to run school buses*
- *Lowering the regulatory bar for vaccines*
- *Lying about the myocarditis after the safety signal is found in Israel*
- *Never making drug companies test lower doses in young men*
- *Doing absolutely nothing to mitigate the risk*
- *Lying about natural immunity/ never accepting it*
- *Repeatedly lying about it so you can force boosters on people who've already had Covid, despite no evidence, and lacking biological rationale*
- *Continuing the emergency state long after it's appropriate*
- *Continuing emergency powers when the emergency has passed*
- *Vaccine passports*
- *Discriminating against people by vaccine status*
- *Preventing Novak Djokovic from competing in US Open*
- *Preventing Kyrie Irving from playing but he can watch the game*
- *Making children wear masks to go to the zoo in California in November 2022 to protect the animals who shouldn't be close to the kids anyway, and they're all outside anyway*
- *Firing healthcare workers who got COVID-19 taking care of sick patients, because they didn't want to get a vaccine for the virus they had already had and cleared*
- *Firing healthcare workers to the point that no one wants to work in healthcare anymore, and it is hard to staff*
- *Discouraging people from getting routine health care*
- *Publishing propaganda in MMWR to justify your broken agenda*
- *Funding the ecotrust dude after all the issues about where the virus is coming from*
- *Spending 10 billion on paxlovid without randomized data in*

> *vaccinated people*
> - *Spending billions on remdesivir when it doesn't do s****
> - *Spending so much money on useless tests, that faculty members quit universities to go run testing companies selling said useless tests*
> - *Using useless test to keep kids out of school*
> - *Inventing unproven Quarantine policies to keep kids out of school*
> - *Closing Palo Alto schools, but leasing the space, so parents can drop their kids off in zoom school, wear an instructor who's an underpaid worker opens a laptop so they can take a class with their teacher.*
>
> *If you stand back and consider the million things public health did to combat the pandemic, the ratio of incorrect to correct things might be 100,000 to one. And doing all this without running a single cluster randomized trial to figure out anything. To just do it on a whim without data.*
>
> *So as someone who has long believed in the value of the regulatory state, and long been a champion for increased funding of public health, if the politician asks me should we destroy the CDC, I would have to say 'yes, please and let me help you'. We have to totally destroy it and try to build a new institution that actually uses science to guide policy and realizes that you can never follow the science. Science can just articulate trade-offs, but all trade-offs must be decided by citizens.*

Dr. Prasad expressed no regret that COVID killed tens of thousands of young people and injured many more. He never asked if public health officials could have done more to prevent such tragedies. Instead, he was upset about closed skateboard parks and a zoo that required children to wear masks.

In his YouTube video "Public Health Needs Restrictions | Placed Upon It | Errors in Pandemic Policy," he complained about a museum's booster policy for visitors and said:

> *Public health has been placing restrictions on people for a long time now, but it's time for the shoe to be on the other foot. It's time for a taste of its own medicine. Public health needs to face restrictions. [...]*
>
> *Somebody need to face some restrictions, but it's not people. It's public health itself. It has been misused and abused. Things have been done in its name that it does not stand for. These are things that are scientifically gray, medically gray, and it's okay to do medically gray things, but not to use the brute force, not to use the brute force of government or the brute force of public health to carry those things out. [...]*
>
> *It's time for a taste of its own medicine.*[128]

However, Dr. Prasad's most provocative article was "How Democracy Ends." In it, he concocted an elaborate fantasy where measures to control a virus might one day end democracy and lead to Nazism. He wrote:

> *The pandemic events of 2020-2021 outline a potential pathway for a future democratically elected President of the United States to systematically end democracy. The course of events leading to this outcome need not be a repeat of the direct assault on the Capitol, but a distortion of risk of illness as a justification for military force and suspension of democratic norms. [...]*
>
> *When democratically elected systems transform into totalitarian regimes, the transition is subtle, stepwise, and involves a combination of pre-planned as well as serendipitous events. Indeed,*

this was the case with Germany in the years 1929-1939, where Hitler was given a chance at governing, the president subsequently died, a key general resigned after a scandal and the pathway to the Fuhrer was inevitable.[129]

Anti-vaxxers often wore yellow stars and openly compared their fate to Holocaust victims, and his essay triggered responses such as "Pandemic Essay from Oncologist Criticized for Antisemitism"[130] and "Vinay Prasad's Nazi Analogy is Imbecilic, Ignorant, and Dangerous," in which Dr. Arthur L. Caplan said, "I don't think the public health side of Germany led to Nazism or to a Nazi genocide."[131]

Yet, after overwhelming the public with the message that Nazi-like scientists were constantly lying to them, Dr. Prasad felt entitled to give a lecture called "Why No One Trusts Scientists Anymore." In it, he spoke about the:

Existential question facing scientists who communicate in the public domain, which is this, fewer Americans now say science has had a mostly positive effect on society.[132]

Dr. Prasad said his core responsibility was *"the communication of scientific ideas to the public."* He continued:

The pandemic has unearthed, I think the very sobering fact that trust in science and scientists is plummeting. Routine childhood immunization is plummeting and I think if we do not come to terms with the root reasons why trust in science is plummeting we will have failed in our core responsibility as scientists, which is the communication of scientific ideas to the public.

Trust in science and scientists is plummeting. I wonder who could be blamed for that.

The most compassionate approach that balances the risks and benefits of reaching herd immunity, is to allow those who are at minimal
risk of death to live their lives normally to build up immunity to the
virus through natural infection, while better protecting those who are
at highest risk.

— *Dr. Jay Bhattacharya*

Dr. Jay Bhattacharya is a medical school graduate-turned-health
economist with impressive credentials. According to his biography from
Stanford University:

> *Jay Bhattacharya is a Professor of Health Policy at Stanford
> University and a research associate at the National Bureau of
> Economics Research. He directs Stanford's Center for Demog-
> raphy and Economics of Health and Aging. Dr. Bhattacharya's
> research focuses on the health and well-being of vulnerable pop-
> ulations, with a particular emphasis on the role of government
> programs, biomedical innovation, and economics. Dr. Bhattacha-
> rya's recent research focuses on the epidemiology of COVID-19
> as well as an evaluation of policy responses to the epidemic. His
> broader research interests encompass the implications of popula-
> tion aging for future population health and medical spending in
> developed countries, the measurement of physician performance
> tied to physician payment by insurers, and the role played by
> biomedical innovation on health. He has published 135 articles
> in top peer-reviewed scientific journals in medicine, economics,
> health policy, epidemiology, statistics, law, and public health
> among other fields. He holds an MD and PhD in economics, both
> earned at Stanford University.*[133]

Dr. Bhattacharya became a pandemic celebrity despite never treating
COVID patients. He met with President Trump in August 2020 and HHS

Secretary Alex Azar in October 2020. He also advised Florida Governor Ron DeSantis. He testified before Congress and in courts to oppose mitigation measures. He also has a large social media following and was on countless podcasts.

Dr. Bhattacharya was omnipresent in the media, writing articles in *The Wall Street Journal*, *Newsweek*, and *The Hill*. All of his articles opposed measures to limit COVID. Some examples include, "The Ill-Advised Push to Vaccinate the Young,"[134] "The Case Against Covid Tests for the Young and Healthy,"[135] and "The White House Keeps Stoking Covid Fears: Covid Is 'a Far Greater Threat to Kids Than the Flu Is,' Ashish Jha Claims, Citing a Flawed Study."[136] He appeared 33 times on Fox News in 2021, according to the article "The Dishonest Doctors Who Were Fox News' Most Frequent Medical Guests in 2021."[137]

Dr. Bhattacharya published his first article "Is the Coronavirus as Deadly as They Say?" in March 2020. It said that "current estimates about the Covid-19 fatality rate may be too high by orders of magnitude."[138] He continued:

> *If it's true that the novel coronavirus would kill millions without shelter-in-place orders and quarantines, then the extraordinary measures being carried out in cities and states around the country are surely justified. But there's little evidence to confirm that premise—and projections of the death toll could plausibly be orders of magnitude too high.*
>
> *Fear of COVID-19 is based on its high estimated case fatality rate — 2% to 4% of people with confirmed. COVID-19 have died, according to the World Health Organization and others. So if 100 million Americans ultimately get the disease, 2 million to 4 million could die. We believe that estimate is deeply flawed. […]*

If our surmise of six million cases is accurate, that's a mortality rate of 0.01%, assuming a two week lag between infection and death. This is one-tenth of the flu mortality rate of 0.1%. Such a low death rate would be cause for optimism.

Dr. Bhattacharya noted that "a 20,000- or 40,000-death epidemic is a far less severe problem than one that kills two million." His article concluded:

If we're right about the limited scale of the epidemic, then measures focused on older populations and hospitals are sensible. [...] A universal quarantine may not be worth the costs it imposes on the economy, community and individual mental and physical health. We should undertake immediate steps to evaluate the empirical basis of the current lockdowns.

Dr. Bhattacharya was horribly wrong about "the limited scale of the epidemic," yet *nothing* the virus did changed the opinions he formed in March 2020.

Although he never acknowledged that a dangerous pandemic ever started, he repeatedly declared it over. In July 2020, he spoke about New York and Sweden and said:

"There's some places where I think we've reached herd immunity actually. [...] They've reached herd immunity there."[139]

In October 2020, before anyone was vaccinated, he said:

An infection is a severe problem for older populations, and also for people who have certain chronic conditions. For younger populations under 70, it's much milder.[140]

This was just a few months before the worst wave of the pandemic, when COVID would kill 3,000 Americans every day. Thousands of young Americans had already died of COVID by then, and it would become a leading killer of young adults and middle-aged people in 2021.

Then, in March 2021 Dr. Bhattacharya said:

> *The virus is seasonal and late fall/winter is its season. It is very unlikely, given that this is the case, that the virus will spread very widely during the summer months. It is also the case that a large fraction of the UK population has already been infected or vaccinated and is immune, which will greatly reduce hospitalization and mortality from the virus in coming months.*
>
> *There are tens of thousands of mutations of the SARS-CoV-2 virus. They mutate because the replication mechanisms they induce involve very little error checking. Most of the mutations either do not change the virulence of the virus, or weaken it. There are a few mutations that provide the virus with a selective advantage in infectivity and may increase its lethality very slightly, though the evidence on this latter point is not solid.*
>
> *We should not be particularly concerned about the variants that have arisen to date. First, prior infection with the wild type virus and vaccination provide protection against severe outcomes arising from reinfection with the mutated virus. Second, though the mutants have taken over the few remaining cases, their rise has coincided with a sharp drop in cases and deaths, even in countries where they have come to dominate. Their selective infectivity advantage has not been enough to cause a resurgence in cases.*[141]

He proclaimed COVID "defanged" on at least five occasions: April 14, 2021; May 3, 2021; July 21, 2021; July 28, 2021; and January 6, 2022.[142] During a podcast with Dr. Damania from April 2021, Dr. Bhattacharya stated:

I think that the central problem right now I think is the fear that
people still feel about COVID. […] I think that that, that we are
so used to this fear that we've lived under for a year that we
don't know how to get out of it. There's still this fear, how do we
decondition it?[…]

I think it's partly the fear, right? I think that it's hard to let go of
that. You've lived your, for a full year under it. It's hard to let go.
I'd say it's, I mean in some ways you can understand it, right?
It's like we've been conditioned to be careful. And when the,
when the danger is gone, we're still careful.[143]

The danger was not gone, and the variants proved to be worth worrying about. Delta and Omicron would arrive before the year was out,
though Dr. Bhattacharya brushed them off too. He said, "I don't think the
Delta variant changes the calculus or the evidence in any fundamental
way"[144] and gave interviews, such as "Delta Variant Spread 'Not a Cause
For Fear'"[145] and "Covid Delta Variant 'Does Not Pose a Risk to You If
You're Vaccinated or Recovered.'"[146] In December 2021, he starred in a
podcast titled "Why No One Should Panic About the Omicron Variant,"
in which he said "this is not something to panic about."[147] He then gave
an interview in 2023 titled "Why The New COVID-19 Variant Shouldn't
Scare You."[148]

Dr. Bhattacharya spread copious disinformation about vaccines
despite initially overselling them early in 2021, claiming they eliminated
COVID's risk. During a podcast with Dr. Damania in April 2021 he said
the risk of two vaccinated people spreading the virus was "zero," adding:

There's just good news about the, I mean we can talk about the
Johnson Johnson bit in a bit but like on the whole, the vaccine,
or just it's an incredible achievement. And in many ways has de-

fanged the epidemic, it's taken away the, the specter of death and
hospitalization that comes with the disease for the older popula-
tion to the extent that the older population is vaccinated.[143]

However, he also spread anti-vaccine disinformation with regards
to young people. His article, "The Ill-Advised Push to Vaccinate the
Young," written in June 2021 before Delta peaked, claimed it would be
better to vaccinate no one than everyone:

> *The idea that everyone must be vaccinated against COVID-19 is*
> *as misguided as the anti-vax idea that no one should. The former*
> *is more dangerous for public health.*[134]

Though Dr. Bhattacharya routinely brushed off death from COVID in
young people, he treated vaccine side effects with the utmost seriousness,
calling "myocarditis, a serious side effect of this vaccine."[149]

Dr. Bhattacharya was most famous for being one of three authors of
the Great Barrington Declaration (GBD), which was written in October
2020—just two months before vaccines arrived. The GBD claimed that
we could get rid of the virus in three to six months by spreading the virus.
It said:

> *The most compassionate approach that balances the risks and*
> *benefits of reaching herd immunity, is to allow those who are*
> *at minimal risk of death to live their lives normally to build up*
> *immunity to the virus through natural infection, while better pro-*
> *tecting those who are at highest risk.*[150]

Dr. Bhattacharya claimed herd immunity was inevitable in October
2020:

> *Herd immunity is a fact about most infectious diseases, the*
> *course that they spread through the population. Even if we were*
> *to have an effective vaccine, we would be relying on herd immu-*

nity as the end point of this infectious disease epidemic.[151]

Unfortunately, things didn't work out that way. We do not have herd immunity to COVID, the virus is still hurting and injuring people every day, and the death count is still rising. Much of this is preventable. According to an article published in May 2025 titled "Why Are More Than 300 People in the US Still Dying of COVID Every Week?":

> *The experts said there are a few reasons why people might still be dying from the virus, including low vaccination uptake, waning immunity and not enough people accessing treatments.*[152]

In retrospect, maybe it wasn't so smart to hand the keys of public health over to mad-scientist virologists, hypochondriacal epidemiologists, and megalomaniacal science bureaucrats.
— *Dr. Jay Bhattacharya*

Despite claiming that mass infection of unvaccinated people under age 60 would end the pandemic in three to six months, Dr. Bhattacharya scolded public health officials for their supposed errors. He posted on social media in 2023, "It's a virtue when scientists change their minds in light of new evidence. It's a vice when they lie about the evidence changing as an excuse for being wrong before."[153]

Dr. Bhattacharya excoriated public health officials, claiming they had tried too hard to limit COVID. He made YouTube videos designed to spread mistrust about them. Some examples include:

- Stanford's Dr. Jay Bhattacharya on The U.S. Public Health System's Crisis of Confidence[154]
- Public Health Must Seek to Rebuild Trust[155]
- Public Health Got It Wrong | Dr. Jay Bhattacharya | Dr. Martin Kulldorff | Leaders on the Frontier[156]
- Dr. Jay Bhattacharya on COVID, Myocarditis, and Vaccines[157]

- A Sober Evaluation of COVID-19 Vaccines[158]
- Dr. Jay Bhattacharya Sets the Record Straight on Vaccine Myths and Mandates[159]

In that last video he said:

The public health community at large has in many ways failed us. They have politicized the vaccine, they have politicized the virus, and undermined trust in them.

In an interview from 2023, Dr. Bhattacharya had the following exchange:

Question: Jay, let's begin with a clip from your last appearance on this program, which took place on October 13, 2021. My question to you was: what needs to happen?

Dr. Jay Bhattacharya: I think the first thing that has to happen is that public health should apologize. The public health establishment in the United States and the world has failed the public.

Question: "The first thing that has to happen is that public health should apologize." Dr. Anthony Fauci, now retired but, during the lockdown, the director of the National Institute of Allergy and Infectious Diseases, has he apologized?

Dr. Jay Bhattacharya: No.

Question: Dr. Francis Collins, again, now retired but, during the lockdown, director of National Institutes of Health, has Dr. Collins apologized?

Dr. Jay Bhattacharya: No, unfortunately.

Question: Federal public health officials, state public health officials, county public health officials, put them all together, and you get several thousand public health officials in this country who are responsible for locking counties down, states down, the country down. As far as you're aware, have any of them apologized?

Dr. Jay Bhattacharya: *Think very, very few have acknowledged any errors at all.*[160]

In one interview titled "Dr. Jay Bhattacharya: How to Avoid 'Absolutely Catastrophic' COVID Mistakes," he described Drs. Anthony Fauci and Francis Collins as being "like mob bosses,"[161] and in another interview with right-wing influencer Jordan Peterson, he again spoke about scientists who tried to limit COVID as organized criminals, saying:

> *Interesting because the science on COVID, on the lockdowns, on the mitigation measures, on a whole host of topics, if the public was listening, they would hear this idea that there was this sort of universal conclusion that you had to do lockdowns, you had to wear masks, you had to social distance, you had to put plastic barriers up...*
>
> *All of these ideas were sold as if there was a scientific consensus in favor of them. That was a lie. There was never a scientific consensus on almost any of the topics... In fact, the preexisting narrative, the preexisting idea among most scientists before the pandemic was quite the opposite direction.*
>
> *What happened was a relatively small group, a cartel almost, of very powerful scientific bureaucrats, took over the whole apparatus of science, at least as far as the public eye was concerned, dominated the media, dominated the message to politicians. And as a result, we had a catastrophic response to COVID. And we're going to be paying the cost of that for a very long time.*[162]

It's true that we had a catastrophic response to COVID, and we're going to be paying the cost of that for a very long time.

Dr. Bhattacharya also deluged his 525,000 social media followers with messages of doubt about science and public health. Here are just a few examples:

- *Everyone sane has lost trust in @CDCgov because of its covid failures and embrace of pseudo science. Their plan to regain trust? Panic monger new bugs to relive the halcyon days of 2020.*[163]

- *Once upon a time, I thought it reasonable for public health to expect not to be contradicted. You know, *smoking is bad for you" and the like. But that idea was based on public health telling the truth about science. Post covid era, my trust they will do that is gone.*[164]

- *Public health should not have a propaganda budget.*[165]

- *The people currently in charge of public health oversaw the disastrous response to covid. Now these same experts blame the public for their myriad failures and demand more authoritarian power to censor the people. Public trust has, very understandably, collapsed.*[166]

- *The American medical and public health establishments threw away public trust in them during the covid era. Their support for a government Ministry of Truth is a sign of weakness. And what makes them think they would control the ministry forever?*[167]

- *During the covid era, the government was the number one source of misinformation, with "noble" lie after "noble" lie told to manipulate the population into doing things public health, in its infinite wisdom, deemed good. Lockdowns could never be enacted without propaganda.*[168]

- *The scope of the gov't misinfo campaign in the covid era is mind boggling. No recovered immunity, the vax stops infection and transmission, no vax side effects, the @gbdeclaration advocated to let it rip… Lie after lie after lie.*[169]

- *Public health criminalized normal human interactions.*[170]

- *The next time public health officials tell you that you are not essential, tell them to go take a flying leap. Who do they think they are?*[171]

- *Public health put the interests of children dead last in the covid era.*[172]

- *Science journalists took dictation from science bureaucrats and their well-funded virologists because they feared losing access to sources. So they spread a lie: that The Science(tm) proved that the bureaucrats and virologists did not start the pandemic. @thackerpd has receipts.*[173]

- *Birx says the idea that the vax prevents infection was premised on 'hope'. Vax mandates were premised on this false 'hope'. The government had no evidence it was true, yet Fauci, Walensky, and even Biden repeatedly told the American public this lie.*[174]

- *It's amazing to watch public health professionals who pushed vaccine mandates and discrimination befuddled by the fact that people no longer trust them, and now question other vaccines. It is public health malpractice, by people not very good at their job.*[175]

- *Only ~2% of Americans have taken the new covid booster. The result is the fruit of US public health torching its credibility with its support for school closures, toddler masking, vax mandates, not asking pharma for an RCT, & other anti-science nonsense.*[176]

- *Fauci and Collins owe the country an apology... [Two] of the nation's top public health officials obstructed the proper deliberative process essential to fashioning proper policy responses to the emergency.*[177]

- *It's time for a new generation of leadership in public health. This time with a better appreciation of the scientific method and less prone to panic and authoritarian excess. This generation failed its key test and cannot be trusted with the public's health.*[178]

- *In retrospect, maybe it wasn't so smart to hand the keys of pub-*

lic health over to mad-scientist virologists, hypochondriacal epidemiologists, and megalomaniacal science bureaucrats.[179]

- *Tony Fauci's particular genius is the cultivation of a cult following among credulous, fawning, scientifically illiterate media poohbahs.*[180]
- *In 2022, @MartinKulldorff and I warned that public health's embrace of covid vax mandates, political partisanship, and the "noble" lie would increase public skepticism about other vaccines, including essential ones. Alas, this prophecy has come true.*[181]
- *Fauci and Collins poisoned the well of debate over lab leaks, social distancing, the vax, and lockdowns, causing untold damage to the public's health. The primary sin of the public health establishment was unwarranted hubris in the name of science.*[182]
- *During the covid era, the world had the misfortune of leadership by a deeply unethical scientific bureaucracy, led by people like Tony Fauci and Francis Collins. They abused their power to smear dissenting scientists. They wanted to create an illusion of consensus. It worked.*[183]
- *There is no such thing as a short lockdown. Once a government implements one, it sets in motion a cycle of panic leading to pointless damaging actions, leading to more fear that takes years to unwind, if ever. 'Two weeks to flatten the curve' will always be a lie.*[184]
- *Though the #1 source of misinformation in the covid era was public officials -- e.g. Dr. Fauci -- I firmly support their right to speech. I wish they would reciprocate the support so that the public could be warned about government misinformation.*[185]
- *I'm shocked by the dehumanizing language of some public health writers. Experts who think school closures were bad have a 'stink.' The unvaxxed deserve 'despair and death.' All who are not 'covid conscious' deserve shame. No wonder the public has no trust left in public health.*[186]

- *Great @TracyBethHoeg thread compiling the ways that the public health and medical establishments ignored science and ethics in the covid era. No wonder trust in medicine is so low these days.*[187]
- *Scientists embraced pseudo science in the covid era, including school closures and toddler masking. Scientists pushed censorship and authoritarian power. Scientists are likely the cause of the pandemic itself. The collapse in trust is well earned.*[188]
- *If the @CDCDirector is serious about building back trust, she should meet publicly in conversation with prominent lockdown critics like @MartinKulldorff and hire scientific advisors with a broader range of expertise, representative more of science than The Science(tm).*[189]
- *Very simple rule for frustrated public health officials and bureaucrats, retired and active: if you want the people to trust you, become worthy of trust. Actually embracing science would be a good first step.*[190]
- *Imagine a public health worthy of trust. That never told lies, noble or otherwise. That reasoned with the public based on solid science. That never sought to manipulate the public. That never took political sides. That did not look down on the people it is supposed to serve...*[191]
- *The problem has been more a small cabal of arrogant, petty, and powerful science bureaucrats who were the primary drivers of the destructive zero covid fantasy. They never deserved our trust, but they came in the name of The Science(tm) and panicked a lot of reasonable people.*[192]

This was nothing more than emotive bleating designed to trigger doubt and anger.

In one article, "A Covid Commission Americans Can Trust," Dr. Bhattacharya spoke about the lack of trust. He said:

The country has lost faith in experts, but a thorough review free from conflicts of interest could help. Trust in science has eroded, and the damage won't be limited to epidemiology, virology and public health. Scientists in other fields will unfortunately also have to deal with the fallout, including oncologists, physicists, computer scientists, environmental engineers and even economists.[193]

This article was published in June 2021, just before Delta arrived, causing mass death and disability, especially amongst unvaccinated people. In a stark example of the disconnect between the real and mirror worlds, the first line of this article, about the lack of trust in science, said, "The pandemic is on its way out."

In 2022, he recorded a podcast with *Reason*, which described the interview by saying:

The anti-lockdown Stanford public health professor on being attacked by Fauci, the loss of trust in medical experts, and how to save science going forward.

I sat down with Bhattacharya to talk about what it was like to be at the very center of an official effort to suppress heterodox thinking about the pandemic, why he believes he and his Great Barrington Declaration co-authors have been vindicated, and whether the public health establishment can ever recover from ongoing revelations of incompetence, malfeasance, and politically motivated decision-making. He also discusses how the centralization of science funding encourages dangerous groupthink, why he believes in mRNA vaccines but remains staunchly anti-mandate, and why he stopped wearing masks a long time ago.[161]

Read that again—*incompetence, malfeasance, politically motivated decision-making, and dangerous groupthink.*

Like Dr. Prasad, Dr. Bhattacharya was clear about his political goals regarding public health institutions, stating in a 2023 interview, "The fact that public health did not actually end up protecting people, ended up harming people, that demands a political response, which, I think, will inevitably come."[160]

In a *Newsweek* article, he stated:

> *Over the past three years, the public has seen first-hand the tremendous power the public health establishment wields. Using emergency power that most people never realized an American government possessed, public health violated Americans' most fundamental civil rights in the name of infection control. We endured three years of useless and divisive policies, including lockdowns, church and business closures, zoom schools, mask mandates, and vaccine mandates and discrimination. […] Legislation is crucial to combatting this grave abuse of the public, especially given how public health's tyrannical playbook is now the accepted norm among public health leaders at the national and international levels.*[194]

He concluded:

> *Public trust in public health has cratered due to over-zealous enforcement of its guidance far past diminishing returns. It can only recover once public health authorities face the same checks and balances as other parts of government. […] If public health opts for the latter, rejects authoritarian power, and restores its commitment to basic ethical principles, it may regain the public's trust so that it can creatively address the challenges to health that the American people now face.*

Despite spreading disinformation and mistrust for years, Dr. Bhat-tacharya performatively lamented the lack of trust in public health saying in an interview on Fox News:

> *And I think one of the things I think I'm most concerned about is how do we regain that trust? Public health has to be trusted. It serves a really important role. And during the pandemic, it's squandered much of that public trust.*[149]

In 2024 he recorded a podcast, "Dr. Jay Bhattacharya on COVID Lies, Vaccine Truth, and the Breakdown of Science," which said:

> *Dr. Bhattacharya also outlines how he believes we can reform the NIH, CDC, FDA, and the American healthcare system more broadly to improve outcomes and restore trust in our institutions.*[195]

In the mirror world, doctors who spoke about "COVID lies" claimed to be both upset by the lack of trust and to have valuable ideas on how to restore it.

When younger, healthier people get infected, that's a good thing because that's exactly the way that population immunity develops.
— *Dr. Scott Atlas*

Dr. Scott Atlas is a Stanford neuroradiologist who was a ubiquitous media presence early in the pandemic. He speculated that COVID would kill 10,000 Americans and that the worst was over in April 2020. His willingness to tell people what they wanted to hear led him to serve as Trump's COVID advisor in the fall of 2020, where he undermined nearly all efforts to contain the virus, believing that the best way to get rid of it was to spread it.

According to *The Atlas Dogma*,[196] a report from the U.S. House Select Subcommittee on the Coronavirus Crisis:

The herd immunity strategy pushed by Dr. Atlas was premised on the theory that the best response to the pandemic was to expose enough people to the virus—without any vaccines and few effective treatments—so that a large enough portion of the population would become immune and stop the virus from spreading widely. A central element of the strategy was so-called "focused protection," which assumed that "high risk" individuals—such as the elderly and individuals with underlying medical conditions like obesity, diabetes, or heart disease—could be easily identified and effectively isolated while the rest of society resumed pre-pandemic life and were even encouraged to become infected. Then, when enough of the "low risk" individuals had been infected and developed immunity (a threshold that was unknown and, as it turned out given waning immunity and the emergence of new variants capable of evading prior immunity, likely unattainable), the "focused protection" could end and everyone could resume their normal lives with the protection of herd immunity.

The report contained multiple sections that detailed how Dr. Atlas undermined attempts to limit the virus:

- *Outspoken Proponents of a Dangerous and Discredited Herd Immunity Strategy Attempted to Influence the Trump Administration's Pandemic Response from the Earliest Months of the Coronavirus Crisis*
- *The Trump Administration Secretively Hired Dr. Atlas in July 2020 and Initially Concealed His Role Before Giving Him Sweeping Access to Top White House Officials*
- *Dr. Atlas Advanced His Dangerous and Discredited Herd Immunity Strategy Within the Trump Administration*

- *Dr. Atlas Successfully Pressed the Trump Administration to Weaken CDC's Testing Guidance and Reduce Coronavirus Testing, Without Any Countervailing Mitigation Measures, Well Before Vaccines Became Available*
- *Dr. Atlas Sought to Undermine the Use of Masks to Curb the Spread of the Coronavirus*
- *Top Trump Administration Officials Ignored Multiple Warnings About the Potential for Harm and Embraced Dr. Atlas's Herd Immunity Strategy, Resulting in Preventable Illness and Death*

It further reported that:

Dr. Atlas also used his newfound position of power to recruit herd immunity proponents to come to Washington, D.C., to meet with multiple senior Administration officials and, according to (CDC) Director Redfield, "convince people that herd immunity was going to save us, and this thing was going to go bye-bye."

Dr. Deborah Birx, former White House Coronavirus Response Coordinator, also testified that:

Dr. Atlas' view was that anybody who was not going to have severe disease should be allowed to become infected. I do believe that he thought that there was long-term protection from reinfection, but we didn't know that. And so he really was trying to, and it was a team, it wasn't just Dr. Atlas, there was a team of physicians and PhDs who strongly believed that the virus was innocent to the majority of the American people and somehow you could magically separate the 50 or 60 million vulnerable Americans from that infection at a high level.[197]

While other doctors worked in hospitals, Dr. Atlas was eager to get on TV and share his belief that the mass infection of unvaccinated youth would lead to herd immunity. He wrote it down and recorded it in multiple interviews.

In an article from March 2020, Dr. Atlas lamented that "current strategies prevent the development of immunity among the population."[198] He said:

> There is massive uncertainty, but using Ioannidis' mid-range fatality rate, this virus could cause about 10,000 deaths in the United States overall, overall, a number that would not be extraordinary news in the total of flu-like deaths every season.

He added:

> We know that up to 99% of positive cases have nothing beyond mild symptoms. […] More importantly, whole-population isolation is not medically ideal and will lead to less effective elimination of the infection threat. Population immunity for every disease like this can only be achieved by letting people who are not at risk for anything serious, who are not immune-compromised and elderly (the vast majority of people), get exposed to it. This allows their bodies to put forth the immune response, so the virus is controlled and transmission to others is eliminated. That's biology — not politics, not economics, and not non-medical risk assessment. We are preventing the development of immunity that is essential to stop the illness, and prevent a second wave when people are free to mingle.

In an article from April 2020, "The Data Is In — Stop the Panic and End the Total Isolation," Dr. Atlas said, "the tragedy of the COVID-19 pandemic appears to be entering the containment phase."[199] He continued:

> **Fact 3:** *Vital population immunity is prevented by total isolation*

policies, prolonging the problem.

We know from decades of medical science that infection itself allows people to generate an immune response — antibodies — so that the infection is controlled throughout the population by "herd immunity." Indeed, that is the main purpose of widespread immunization in other viral diseases — to assist with population immunity. In this virus, we know that medical care is not even necessary for the vast majority of people who are infected. It is so mild that half of infected people are asymptomatic, shown in early data from the Diamond Princess ship, and then in Iceland and Italy. That has been falsely portrayed as a problem requiring mass isolation. In fact, infected people without severe illness are the immediately available vehicle for establishing widespread immunity. By transmitting the virus to others in the low-risk group who then generate antibodies, they block the network of pathways toward the most vulnerable people, ultimately ending the threat. Extending whole-population isolation would directly prevent that widespread immunity from developing.

In another article from April 2020, "Reentry After the Panic: Paying the Health Price of Extreme Isolation," Dr. Atlas stated:

With a world-wide sense of relief, progress continues in containing the COVID-19 pandemic. Projections have been revised downward for virtually every major negative consequence of the disease.[200]

He added, "We now need to reenter normal life" and lamented not having "a population protected by a naturally developed immunity." He wrote:

But a bigger price might now be paid from choosing extreme isolation. In the absence of immunization, society needs circulation of the virus, assuming high-risk people can be isolated. Infection itself allows people to generate an immune response — natural antibodies. Given the estimated contagiousness of COVID-19, about 60 percent of people in the community need to have antibodies to stop the spread by "herd immunity." Remember, medical care is not necessary for the vast majority of people who are infected. We also infer from testing in Iceland and Vo, Italy, that half of infected people are asymptomatic. That has been mis-leadingly portrayed as a problem requiring mass isolation; those infected people are an important vehicle for establishing immu-nity by transmitting the virus to the low-risk group. Preliminary testing in Germany shows that perhaps 15 percent of people are immune; no doubt this varies greatly by region. It is very possible that whole-population isolation prevented natural herd immunity from developing.

We now need to reenter normal life. Yet, instead of having a population protected by a naturally developed immunity, we are faced with a perilous decision — how to prevent a second wave when people are free to mingle. We should not wait for vaccines.

Though he later claimed to be merely a champion of learning, the words "school," "classroom," and "education" did not appear in these articles.

During an interview from April 2020 with Steve Deace, Dr. Atlas stated:

We can allow a lot of people to get infected. Those who are not at risk to die or have a serious hospital-requiring illness, we should be fine with letting them get infected, generating immunity on their own, and the more immunity in the community, the better we can eradicate the threat of the virus, including the threat to people who are vulnerable. That's what herd immunity is. That's a basic principle.[201]

In Senate testimony from May 2020 Dr. Atlas said mitigation measures prolonged the pandemic:

We also know that total isolation prevents broad population immunity and prolongs the problem. *We know from decades of medical science that infection causes individuals to generate an immune response – antibodies – and the population later develops immunity. Indeed, that is the main purpose of widespread immunization in other viral diseases – to assist with "herd immunity". In the Covid-19 epicenter New York City, higher immunity is likely, although undoubtedly muted by the extreme isolation policies, as more than 20 percent of those tested had antibodies. A similar finding was reported in Boston. That fact has been incorrectly portrayed as an urgent problem requiring mass isolation. On the contrary, infected people are the immediately available vehicle for establishing widespread immunity. By transmitting the virus to others in lower-risk groups who then generate antibodies, pathways toward the most vulnerable people are blocked, ultimately eradicating the threat.*[202]

As he didn't want to "prevent broad population immunity" or "prolong the problem," Dr. Atlas mentioned schools in this testimony. He viewed schools as an opportunity to infect children and said, "Open all K-12 schools. If under 18 and in good health, you have nearly no risk of serious illness from Covid-19."

During a June 2020 interview with Tucker Carlson, Dr. Atlas said:

We expected more cases with more social mingling. [...] But the fact is the overwhelming majority of these cases are in younger healthier people. These people do not have a significant problem. They do not have the serious complications. They do not die. And so it's fantastic news that we have a lot of cases, but we don't see deaths going up, and what that means is A: we're are doing a better job of protecting the vulnerable, B: We're in good shape here.

We like the fact that there's a lot of cases in low- risk populations, because that's exactly how we're going to get herd immunity, population immunity, when low-risk people, with no significant problem handling this virus, which is basically 99% of people get this, they become immunity and they block the pathway of con-nectivity of contagiousness for older sicker people. […] Children have virtually zero risk of getting a serious complication, virtual-ly a zero risk of dying. […] Children only rarely if ever transmit the disease.[203]

During a Fox News interview in July 2020, he said:

When younger, healthier people get the disease, they don't have a problem with the disease. I'm not sure why that's so difficult for everyone to acknowledge. These people getting the infection is not really a problem, and in fact, as we said months ago, when you isolate everyone, including all the healthy people, you're prolonging the problem because you're preventing population immunity. Low-risk groups getting the infection is not a prob-lem.[204]

In another interview from August 2020, Dr. Atlas stated:

It doesn't matter if younger, healthier people get infected. I don't know how often that has to be said. They have nearly zero risk of a problem from this. When younger, healthier people get infected, that's a good thing because that's exactly the way that population immunity develops.[205]

Unsurprisingly, Dr. Atlas specifically credited the GBD with influencing his pro-infection philosophy. In October 2020, shortly after it was signed, he stated:

The prolonged lockdowns must end, and I just want to point out that now this is really meshing quite precisely with a growing body of some of the world's top epidemiologists and scientists who this past week signed something called the Great Barrington Declaration. Scientists led by people from Harvard, Stanford, and Oxford University, would-renown infectious disease and epidemiology scientists, have completely aligned with the President's policy and with everything that I have been advising him on, and this really refutes this sort of strange narrative that this is purely politically based, that somehow the President doesn't listen to the science. This is the science, this is what he's been advised by me and others.[206]

However, in January 2022, during his testimony to the House Select Committee, he spoke *very differently* about the GBD. Once it became clear their vision of herd immunity via mass infection was just a fantasy, Dr. Atlas testified, "he wasn't familiar with it at all."[207] He had this exchange:

Question: Do you view the Great Barrington declaration to outline the same strategy as the targeted protection strategy that we have been discussing throughout today?

Dr. Atlas. Well, the Great Barrington, I don't speak for what Great Barrington Declaration represents. I didn't write it. I didn't

*sign it and it didn't exist when I arranged this meeting. So I
wasn't familiar with it at all. I didn't even, know there was going
to be any kind of declaration written, when I arranged this meeting. So I'm familiar with the broad parts of it that I just stated.*

Question. *Sitting here today, do you believe that it's outlining the
same general strategy that you referred to as targeted protection?*

Dr. Atlas. *I think it's outlining the general strategy of increasing
the protection of the high-risk people and ending the harms of the
lockdowns. So in that sense, yes.*

Question. *Are there any differences between the two?*

Dr. Atlas. *I'm not — I don't really — you know, like I say, I didn't
sign the Great Barrington Declaration. I haven't really — I don't
know what's the details of it. I never read the full Great Barrington Declaration website and everything.*

Question. *Did you review or provide any input on the Great Barrington Declaration prior to its release?*

Dr. Atlas. *No. Like I said, I wasn't even aware it was being written.*

Question. *Did you have any conversations about it at a broad
level prior to its release?*

Dr. Atlas. *No. In fact, I was never — I'm not even sure there was
a known intent to write something. I don't know what they were
doing. I wasn't involved, they being the group of people who were
writing the Great Barrington Declaration.*

Question. *Sitting here today, can you recall if there's anything
that you disagree with in the Great Barrington Declaration?*

Dr. Atlas. *Well, like I say, I haven't read the detail of it. I'm not* *intimately familiar with every single detail. I've never really read through everything in the Great Barrington Declaration, but the general thrust of Great Barrington Declaration that I said already of increasing the protection of the high-risk people and reducing and getting rid of the massive harms of the lockdowns, those two things, I absolutely agree with.*

The GBD is one page long.

America's COVID Response Was Based on Lies
— *Dr. Scott Atlas*

Despite claiming that it was a "good thing" when young people contracted COVID, Dr. Atlas also spoke about the importance of trust. For example, in 2024 he said:

A peaceful society is built on trust. That won't continue if it's filled by people who lack the moral compass to admit their errors and who refuse to allow views counter to their own.[208]

However, Dr. Atlas simultaneously spread doubt for the purpose of undermining trust in public health, saying that only liars opposed his plans for mass infection. Some examples from social media include:

- *We have a crisis of competence & integrity. They were wrong on lockdowns, schools, mask & vax mandates - so destructive - yet ppl in govt, unis inc @Stanford, unwilling to say they were wrong. We can't have closure, a cohesive society, an ethical society if they continue to **lie**.*[209]

- *It's a shock so many are willing to **lie** for him- falsehoods, denial of all data. Maybe I'm naive that truth matters? Fauci was completely wrong on lockdowns, masks, vaccines - so harmful, destructive, the legacy so horrendous- yet ppl still pushing it as true. It frightens me.*[210]

- *Immoral corrupt inept bureaucrats. **Lies**, stonewalling, denials, the **lie** "we didn't know". Lockdowns & mandates were pseudoscience; millions died & suffered. I knew, said it over & over again. Demand they beg for forgiveness -Fauci, Birx, Redfield, media, academia #TruthStands[211]*

- *Still amazed some ppl perpetuate the **lie** that advocating targeted protection (increasing protection of hi-risk, ending destructive lockdowns & school closures) meant unmitigated spread. Can't be that stupid; they simply won't admit they were wrong & destroyed millions #Integrity[212]*

- *Misinformation. Disinformation. **Lies**. Pseudoscience. False. Embarrassing incompetence. Proven wrong, over & over again. Or maybe... facts do not matter? Science is dead? Rational thought is finished? People are that fearful, that susceptible to propaganda?[213]*

- *#Fauci, why did you **lie** and push forward that the origin of COVID was 'definitely not from a lab' back in early 2020 when you could not have known that? Was it because Trump said it was from a lab? #QuestionsForFauci[214]*

- *School closure advocates are guilty - they got what they wanted, & inflicted massive destruction on our kids, esp poor kids. And we predicted it 6/2020↓ They cannot deflect blame or **lie**. They are a shameful disgrace, a black mark on America. #Shame[215]*

- *The risk to healthy children is extremely low—that was known in the earliest days of the pandemic, March 2020. It was a complete **lie** that teachers were high risk and schools had to be closed, or that any measures had to be done in schools to protect teachers.[216]*

- *The first step is to clearly state the harsh truth ... **Lies** were told. Those **lies** harmed the public. Those **lies** were directly contrary to the evidence, to decades of knowledge on viral pandemics, and to long-established fundamental biology.[217]*

- *Academics pushed two **lies** on the public—if you're against* *lockdowns, you're choosing the economy over lives—that was a **lie**—and you are also for allowing the infection to spread without any mitigation. That is not what targeted protection meant.*[218]

This was purely emotive messaging designed to trigger rage and mistrust, and Dr. Atlas frequently blamed doctors. For example, he posted:

Doctors violated public trust - and the public knows it. They spewed out guidelines but didn't question it; b/c they're given (blind) trust, they needed to have higher degree of skepticism & know the data.[219]

In 2023, Dr. Atlas formalized his thoughts in an article, "America's COVID Response Was Based on Lies." He said:

The tragic failure of reckless, unprecedented lockdowns that were contrary to established pandemic science, and the added massive harms of those policies on children, the elderly, and lower-income families, are indisputable and well-documented in numerous studies. This was the biggest, the most tragic, and the most unethical breakdown of public health leadership in modern history.

In a democracy, indeed in any ethical and free society, the truth is essential. The American people need to hear the truth—the facts, free from the political distortions, misrepresentations, and censorship. The first step is to clearly state the harsh truth in the starkest possible terms. Lies were told. Those lies harmed the public. Those lies were directly contrary to the evidence, to decades of knowledge on viral pandemics, and to long-established fundamental biology.[220]

The "lies" that Dr. Atlas accused public health officials of spreading included "immune protection only comes from a vaccine" and "no one has any immunological protection, because this virus is completely new."

Dr. Atlas concluded his article by calling for some nebulous form of punishment. He said:

> But to ensure that this never happens again, government leaders, power-driven officials, and influential academics and advisors often harboring conflicts of interest must be held accountable.

In another interview, he spoke of the need to "clean house," saying:

> It's very sad that these people have power still. Again, I've said it before, Paul, but we have to vote these people out. We have to have people come in in charge who can put in clean house. The bureaucrats at the CDC, the NIH, and the FDA have really harmed our country. They have massive conflicts of interest. They're not thinking people. This is not very complicated, yet they're still in charge.[221]

After the election, Dr. Atlas repeated his call for purges of scientists in an article titled "Today's Public Health Emergency: Restoring Trust with Seven Steps." He spoke of a "cartel of NIH funding" and suggested "cleaning house of all heads of CDC, NIH, and FDA."[222] Dr. Atlas said:

> America's leaders imposed sinful harms and long-lasting damage on our children, the totality of which may not be realized for decades.

We'll Have Herd Immunity by April
— Dr. Marty Makary

Dr. Makary also has impressive credentials. According to his Johns Hopkins University faculty biography:

> Dr. Marty Makary is a surgeon and public policy researcher at

Johns Hopkins University. He writes for The Washington Post *and* The Wall Street Journal *and is the author of two New York Times bestselling books,* Unaccountable *and* The Price We Pay. *Dr. Makary served in leadership at the World Health Organization Patient Safety Program and has been elected to the National Academy of Medicine.*

Clinically, Dr. Makary is the chief of Islet Transplant Surgery at Johns Hopkins. He is the recipient of the Nobility in Science Award from the National Pancreas Foundation and has been a visiting professor at over 25 medical schools. He has published over 250 peer-reviewed scientific articles and has served on several editorial boards.

Dr. Makary is the recipient of the 2020 Business Book of the Year Award by the Association of Business Journalists for his most recent book, The Price We Pay. *It has been described by Don Berwick as "a deep dive into the real issues driving up the price of health care" and by Steve Forbes as "A must-read for every American."*

Dr. Makary serves as a professor at the Johns Hopkins School of Medicine and a professor, by courtesy, at the Johns Hopkins Carey Business School. His current research focuses on the underlying causes of disease, public policy, health care costs, and relationship-based medicine.[223]

Dr. Makary was also a public and influential presence during the pandemic. He testified before Congress and advised Virginia Governor Glen Youngkin.[224] He appeared 142 times on Fox News in 2021, according to "The Dishonest Doctors Who Were Fox News' Most Frequent Medical Guests in 2021."[137] He has a large social media presence and has made multiple podcasts and YouTube videos.

In 2021 alone, Dr. Makary authored numerous articles that aged poorly and were full of disinformation. A few examples include:

- **"We'll Have Herd Immunity by April"**: *Experts should level with the public about the good news. Some medical experts privately agreed with my prediction that there may be very little Covid-19 by April but suggested that I not talk publicly about herd immunity because people might become complacent and fail to take precautions or might decline the vaccine.*[225]

- **"Herd Immunity is Near, Despite Fauci's Denial"**: *Anthony Fauci has been saying that the country needs to vaccinate 70% to 85% of the population to reach herd immunity from Covid-19. But he inexplicably ignores natural immunity. If you account for previous infections, herd immunity is likely close at hand.*[226]

- **"Don't Buy the Fearmongering: The COVID-19 Threat Is Waning"**: *On a clinical level, we simply have not seen significant re-infections at any concerning rate. […] The public-health threat is now defanged.*[227]

- **"The Power of Natural Immunity"**: *The news about the U.S. Covid pandemic is even better than you've heard. Some 80% to 85% of American adults are immune to the virus: More than 64% have received at least one vaccine dose and, of those who haven't, roughly half have natural immunity from prior infection. There's ample scientific evidence that natural immunity is effective and durable, and public-health leaders should pay it heed.*[228]

- **"Natural Immunity to Covid Is Powerful. Policymakers Seem Afraid to Say So"**: *It's okay to have an incorrect scientific hypothesis. But when new data proves it wrong, you have to adapt. Unfortunately, many elected leaders and public health officials have held on far too long to the hypothesis that natural immunity offers unreliable protection against covid-19*

— a contention that is being rapidly debunked by science.[229]

- **"The Flimsy Evidence Behind the CDC's Push to Vaccinate Children"**: *The agency overcounts Covid hospitalizations and deaths and won't consider if one shot is sufficient.*[230]

- **"Risk Of COVID Is Now Very Low — It's Time To Stop Living In Fear: Doctor"**: *COVID cases are collapsing in front of our eyes.* […] *Yet some people want the pandemic to stretch out longer.*[231]

Of course, no one *wanted* the pandemic to stretch out longer. Dr. Makary just said that to spread anger and mistrust.

In May 2021, Dr. Makary said in two separate interviews, "We basically are in herd immunity right now"[232] and "most of the country is at herd immunity."[233] In June 2021, he claimed it's time to "move on and live a normal life."[234] He compared COVID to the flu, saying:

> *Right now we're about at 150th the daily cases of a regular seasonal flu in the middle of that flu season. So people have a distorted perception of risk.*

Dr. Makary repeatedly glorified "natural immunity" and berated people for not sharing his enthusiasm. He talked about "decades of protection"[235] and said, "Immunity is probably lifelong." Here's what he said in July 2021.

> ***Dr. Makary****: One of the biggest failures of our medical leadership has been ignoring natural immunity. It's about half of the unvaccinated, and they have a reasonable reason not to get the vaccine right now. They already have immunity. Many of them have circulating antibodies, and some of us doctors recommend one shot in those folks if they want to get a vaccine. But they've already got immunity. Now, there's two parts to immunity. One is the antibodies, but the other is the memory B cells and T cells. And that's probably what gives you decades of protection against*

severe illness. So COVID is going to turn into a seasonal virus that'll cause common cold -like symptoms, and that's going to be our future. We can't try to eliminate this with more restrictions.

Question*: And there are some people's cards that actually say that their shot expires within six months. I mean, are some of these shots good for a year or longer? Do we know? Did they tell us?*

Dr. Makary: *Immunity is probably lifelong. That's what many of us think. Certainly, the test of natural immunity over 19 months is showing that it's going strong and it's durable. Vaccinated immunity, we have suggestions now from Israel that it may start to wane six months and nine months into it.*

There are many more examples of Dr. Makary fawning over "natural immunity" from that time.

Dr. Makary repeatedly minimized Long COVID, writing articles or giving interviews such as "Don't Believe the Feds' Fearmongering About Long Covid,"[236] "Long Covid Real But 'Overplayed': Dr. Marty Makary,"[237] and "The Exaggeration of Long Covid."[238] In that first article, he said:

Public-health officials have massively exaggerated long Covid to scare low-risk Americans as our government gives more than $1 billion to a long Covid testing-industrial complex.

[...]

NIH and CDC also haven't had any interest in funding research on natural immunity, boosters in children or even vitamin D, which was discovered earlier this year to lower COVID mortality — a study that tragically came two years too late. Probably because it doesn't fit the White House narrative.

[…]

The CDC and NIH's constant fearmongering around long

COVID has also been used to support COVID restrictions.[236]

Like most WWTI doctors, Dr. Makary also greatly overhyped vaccines in early 2021. In March, he wrote an article in which he stated:

> *The CDC claims to be 'following the science,' but its advice suggests it's still paralyzed by fear.: An unpublished study conducted by the Israeli Health Ministry and Pfizer showed that vaccination reduced transmission by 89% to 94% and almost totally prevented hospitalization and death, according to press reports. Immunity kicks in fully about four weeks after the first vaccine dose, and then you are essentially bulletproof.*[239]

He spread this message on social media, posting:

> *If anyone hears of a person hospitalized or dead from Covid-19 after full vaccination, please let me know. The data show that vaccines confer near perfect protection against death and hospitalization from Covid. Can't we be honest about that?*[240]

He also claimed vaccines stopped transmission at that time, writing, "There has never been a documented case of a fully vaccinated person who is asymptomatic transmitting the virus."[231]

Additionally, Dr. Makary claimed vaccines would be effective against all future variants:

> *As the COVID pandemic wanes, Americans are being fed a distorted perception of the risks by the media and some experts. They continue to fuel fear by repeating speculation that variants will evade vaccines. Don't buy it.*[227]

When Delta and Omicron wrecked his declarations of herd immunity, Dr. Makary didn't change his messaging at all. He gave an interview in

June 2021 titled "Dr. Marty Makary Pans 'Fear-Mongering' Over Delta Variant,"[241] and, in August, he said:

> If you're one of the 99%+ of kids that are unvaccinated...those kids don't need to worry. [...] For most people right now, Delta is downgraded to a mild seasonal virus that causes mild common cold-like symptoms. [...] The vaccines have been perfectly consistent against all of the variants.[242]

Of course, Dr. Makary was wrong about Delta, which led to headlines such as "Florida Delta Wave Cases Plunge, Leaving Record Deaths in Its Wake."[243]

Predictably, he minimized Omicron as well. In December 2021, he lauded the variant as "nature's vaccine,"[244] and in an interview on Fox News titled "Omicron Fear Fueling a 'Second Pandemic of Lunacy'," he said:

> We're seeing this massive new wave of fear that is fueling our second pandemic after COVID-19, which is a pandemic of lunacy, which is omicron. Now I call it omi-cold. [...] This new scientific data from the lab explains the epidemiological data and the bedside observation of doctors that this is far more mild... and that's why I call it omi-cold.[245]

Of course, Dr. Makary was also wrong about Omicron, as explained by articles titled "During the Omicron Wave, Death Rates Soared for Older People,"[32] and "Hospitalizations of Young Children with the Virus Surged During the U.S. Omicron Wave."[246] It was not "nature's vaccine" or "omi-cold."

In addition to these poor predictions, Dr. Makary routinely botched basic facts, minimizing the harms of the virus while fearmongering about the risks of the vaccine. In an article from June 2021, Dr. Makary wrote:

In reviewing the medical literature and news reports, and in talking to pediatricians across the country, I am not aware of a single healthy child in the U.S. who has died of COVID-19 to date.[247]

A simple internet search revealed many such tragedies, and several research papers also showed that the virus had killed healthy children,[248] though death is not the only bad outcome from COVID.

In contrast, although the rate of vaccine-myocarditis is less than 1 in 10,000 young men,[249] Dr. Makary claimed that "hundreds of thousands of young ppl got myocarditis for no good reason,"[250] an obviously fabricated number. However, in the mirror world, vaccine side effects were more consequential than death from COVID.

Public health officials actively propagated misinformation that ruined lives and forever damaged public trust in the medical profession.
— *Dr. Marty Makary*

Though Dr. Makary said we had herd immunity in May 2021, he repeatedly excoriated public health officials and called on them to admit to errors. During an interview on Fox News that month, he dismissed any concerns about variants, saying they were "all encompassed by the vaccine in preventing serious outcomes"[251] and said the main priority was to not "scare people." "People need something to look forward to," he said. Dr. Makary said that anyone who disagreed was trying to "manipulate the public," and had this exchange:

Question: You talked about this a couple of months ago. You said look, we are two months away from herd immunity. Are we there, are we closer, is it ever going to be fully realized in your estimation?

Dr. Makary: Well unfortunately, we have this perception now that's being created by some public health leaders that we reach to total eradication. And we're not going to get to total risk elimination. That is a false goal and quite honestly it's being used to manipulate the public. We heard today if [we] get to 70% vaccination, then we can see restrictions. That's dishonest. Most of the country is at herd immunity. Other parts will get there later this month. […] I call that herd immunity, and I think what's happening is that our public health leaders are dismissing natural immunity from prior infection.

No one was talking about "total risk elimination" in May 2021. Dr. Makary just made that up to make public health leaders look foolish to his followers.

He frequently lambasted public health officials for not joining him in spreading disinformation. For instance, he published an article in February 2021, which said:

Scientists shouldn't try to manipulate the public by hiding the truth. […] Herd immunity is the inevitable result of viral spread and vaccination. When the chain of virus transmission has been broken in multiple places, it's harder for it to spread—and that includes the new strains.[225]

In an article from March 2021, "Covid Prescription: Get the Vaccine, Wait a Month, Return to Normal," he blamed the CDC for not overhyping brand new vaccines. He said:

The Centers for Disease Control and Prevention has lost a lot of credibility during the Covid-19 pandemic by being late or wrong on testing, masks, vaccine allocation and school reopening. Staying consistent with that pattern, this week—three months

after the vaccine rollout began—the CDC finally started telling
vaccinated people that they can have normal interactions with
other vaccinated people—but only in highly limited circumstanc-
es. Given the impressive effectiveness of the vaccine, that should
have been immediately obvious by applying scientific inference
and common sense.[239]

According to Dr. Makary, anyone who disagreed with him about the inevitability of herd immunity in April 2021 was trying to *"manipulate the public by hiding the truth."*

In May 2021, he said in a podcast with Dr. Damania:

Yeah. It's crazy that we've been moving the ball post so much in
this long race; it's why people don't have trust in public health
officials anymore. So we basically are in herd immunity right
now, and we're basically, we have one tenth of the number of
daily cases in my health flu season. We have one full season, and
we have about 400,000 cases a day, or about 25,000 cases a day.
We're below one tenth of the number of daily cases of the flu and
the same case fatality rate.[232]

We weren't "basically at herd immunity" then.

In his May 2021 article, "Don't Buy the Fearmongering: The COVID-19 Threat Is Waning," Dr. Makary wrote:

With far fewer susceptible people and a younger cohort, we're
dealing with a different risk level than even just a few months
ago. Despite this good news, Americans are being told variants
and hesitancy will prevent "herd immunity." Yet noticeably
absent from their calculations is the contribution of natural
immunity from prior infection or exposure. Dr. Anthony Fauci
and Dr. Rochelle Walensky simply don't talk about the percent of

Americans they estimate have natural immunity. That omission
creates a perception that the race to 70 to 85 percent immunity is
more desperate, resulting in a prolonged timeline, talk of vaccine
mandates and an imperative that young kids get the shot.[227]

He was worried about a *"prolonged timeline, talk of vaccine mandates*
and an imperative that young kids get the shot." He believed the virus
was gone in the spring of 2021, but he was worried that measures to contain it might remain. The reverse happened.

In another article, "Why America Doesn't Trust the CDC," Dr. Makary wrote about the pediatric vaccine and said:

If the CDC is curious as to why people aren't listening to its rec-
ommendations, it should consider how it bypassed experts to put
the matter before a Kangaroo court of like-minded loyalists. The
Biden administration should insist that we return to the standard
process of putting all major vaccine decisions before a vote of the
FDA's leading vaccine experts.[252]

Dr. Makary didn't follow this "standard process" once he became
head of the FDA and had the power to limit COVID vaccines for children
and pregnant individuals.[253] Under the direction of Robert F. Kennedy Jr.,
he and Dr. Prasad simply decreed it instead of waiting for the advisory
board to make the decision.

Dr. Makary also spread this message—*damaging the trust with an*
absurd position[254]—on social media. Though there are countless examples, in one such post he shared his article "The CDC Keeps Pushing
Covid Boosters on Kids Despite Real Health Risks"[255] and said:

"A few wks ago public-health officials beclowned themselves by
blocking Djokovic from traveling to Florida to play tennis out-
doors." This Biden admin position embodies everything wrong

with public-health policy today:

- *Ignoring natural immunity*
- *Downplaying vax-induced myocarditis in young males*
- *Ignoring the extremely low risk of Covid in healthy young people*
- *Ignoring data that vaccines do NOT prevent transmission*
- *Creating vax hesitancy through mandates*
- *Damaging the trust with an absurd position*
- *Crying wolf by endlessly renewing the state of emergency[254]*

Dr. Makary often spoke about "public trust" and how to rebuild it. Predictably, he felt the blame lay with people who tried to stop COVID and didn't join him in spreading disinformation about it. A few examples are:

- *The cozy relationship between gov't health agencies and Pfizer & Moderna evidenced by closed door meetings and the lack of transparency around clinical trial outcomes data has damaged public trust. It's clear why the top 2 vaccine experts at the FDA quit last year in protest.[256]*
- *Great piece by Carl Schramm on what Walensky's apology really meant. Blaming the "CDC's slow response" when the pandemic hit was really just blaming the prior administration. More humility and less blame gaming would go a long way to rebuild public trust.[257]*
- *An ancient trait of the medical profession is to speak up when we believe something is not in the best interest of our patients. Less absolutism and more humility by health agencies would go a long way in rebuilding public trust. My piece w/ @TracyBethHoeg[258]*

- *The Ignore Natural Immunity Policy of public health officials has been convenient for pushing a simple vaccine message. Its also been highly profitable to Pharma. But its scientifically dishonest & resulted in a collapse in public trust in health agencies.*[259]
- *Public health officials changing their position on natural immunity, after so much hostility toward the idea, would go a long way in rebuilding the public trust, as I explain in today's @washingtonpost*[260]

Even after variants demolished his declarations of herd immunity and homages to "natural immunity," Dr. Makary continued making podcasts such as "The Credibility of Public Health Has Been Shot,"[261] which aired just before Omicron arrived. The next year he recorded a Fox News segment titled "Dr. Marty Makary on CDC Statement: The Public Is Hungry for Humility."[262] He recorded a podcast in 2024 called "Dr. Marty Makary: 'The Reason People Don't Trust the Medical Establishment Is Because It Lied to Them.'"[263] "The public's rising distrust is warranted," it said.

In 2024, he published a book, *Blind Spots: When Medicine Gets It Wrong, and What It Means for Our Health*. According to its description on Amazon:

> *From Johns Hopkins medical expert Dr. Marty Makary, the New York Times-bestselling author of The Price We Pay-an eye-opening look at the medical groupthink that has led to public harm, and what you need to know about your health.*
> *How could the experts have gotten it so wrong? Dr. Marty Makary asks, Could it be that many modern-day health crises have been caused by the hubris of the medical establishment?*[264]

In interviews promoting it, he said:

> *The biggest topic in our medical journals right now is mistrust*

in the medical establishment. They're scratching their heads. "People don't trust us, and it must be because of those spreading misinformation." ... No, the reason they don't trust the medical establishment is because it was lying to them for three years during the Covid pandemic.[265]

He recorded podcasts about his book titled:

- Restoring Trust in Medicine: A Call for Transparency and Reform[266]
- How Medical Establishment Keeps Americans Sick, and Evils of Censorship[267]
- Exposing Medical Blind Spots: Health, Truth, And Accountability[268]
- One Of the Biggest Screw-Ups in Modern Medicine[269]
- 'Blind Spots' Author Dr. Marty Makary on Chronic Disease and The Failures of Modern Medicine[270]
- Blind Spots: Exposing Groupthink in The Medical Establishment[271]
- Medical Establishment Wants to Keep Americans Sick Through Perverse Incentives[272]
- Exposing The Truth of Big Pharma[273]
- Modern Medicine and its Blind Spots[274]
- The Biggest Lies in The History of Medicine[275]
- What's Wrong with American Medicine?[276]
- Why Your Doctor Is Misleading You[277]
- Groupthink And Its Effect on Modern Medicine[278]
- What Modern Medicine Gets Wrong[279]

Dr. Makary promoted one of these on social media by saying:

Trust in the healthcare system has plummeted over the last four years—from 71.5% to 40.1%. In my new book Blind Spots, I explain how decades of medical groupthink have shaken the public's confidence. As physicians, we must acknowledge our mistakes and work to rebuild the trust our profession once held.[280]

One of the core examples in Dr. Makary's book was about peanut allergies. The Amazon description said:

> *More Americans have peanut allergies today than at any point in history. Why? In 2000, the American Academy of Pediatrics issued a strict recommendation that parents avoid giving their children peanut products until they're three years old. Getting the science perfectly backward, triggering intolerance with lack of early exposure, the US now leads the world in peanut allergies-and this misinformation is still rearing its head today.*[264]

Dr. Makary even wrote an article promoting his book, "How Pediatricians Created the Peanut Allergy Epidemic."[281] "By recommending that children avoid exposure to peanuts until age 3, doctors inadvertently turned a rare issue into a major health problem," he said. Yet, in his book about *"medical groupthink that has led to public harm,"*[264] Dr. Makary neglected to mention his essay "We'll Have Herd Immunity by April."

Actual Nuremberg Execution, Hanging
— *Dr. Paul Alexander*

At least one WWTI doctor took an incredibly dark turn. In 2020, Dr. Paul Alexander, the doctor in the first Trump administration who actually said, "We want them infected," produced content like:

- *Actual Nuremberg execution, hanging...I want proper legal inquiries, courts, juries, tribunals & under oath, of all involved in COVID fraud non-pandemic, from virus to lockdowns, to DEADLY medical treatment of our precious elderly in hospitals (the death COVID protocol).*[282]
- *Hang them high I say, hang them all! all medical doctors! If we take them to court room with judges & juries*

& the verdict is they caused deaths negligently & know-
ingly, then we hang all, millions of doctors if we have to,
we hang them all! We show them no mercy like they did
to our parents, grand-parents...we punish them...I am
not accepting para "but we were following CDC, NIH,
FDA etc."[283]

That's horrifying, and it should be unequivocally condemned.

Public health agencies have seen a staggering exodus of personnel, many exhausted and demoralized, in part because of abuse and threats.

— The New York Times

While WWTI doctors castigated public health officials for "under-mining natural immunity" or not letting Novak Djokovic play tennis, they *never* reflected on their own failed forecasts. Though Dr. Makary was eager to call out pediatricians for supposedly botching peanut allergies, I've never seen him apply that level of scrutiny to his article, "Herd Immunity Is Near, Despite Fauci's Denial."[226] Dr. Prasad has never reflected on his message that "vaccines reduce transmission and will lead us back to normal life."[9] Dr. Bhattacharya has never revisited his pronouncement that "the central problem right now I think is the fear that people still feel about COVID."[143] Dr. Atlas never paused to look back on his statement that it was "fantastic news that we have a lot of cases."[203]

None of these doctors ever honestly grappled with the consequences of blasting out their false message in major media outlets for months on end. Millions of Americans trusted these highly credentialed doctors who spoke with great confidence when they said COVID was all going away, and it only threatened the elderly and infirm. Many people stopped taking COVID seriously because they were told public health officials were lying to them. *How are they doing today? Did they all turn out OK?*

Having prominent doctors repeatedly call them lying tyrants wasn't helpful for public health officials either. Hundreds of them resigned or retired rather than face abuse and threats. According to news reports, "some have become the target of far-right activists, conservative groups and anti-vaccination extremists who have coalesced around common goals: fighting mask orders, quarantines and contact tracing with protests, threats and personal attacks."[284] According to a survey from *The New York Times*, "public health agencies have seen a staggering exodus of personnel, many exhausted and demoralized, in part because of abuse and threats."[285] They reported "more than 500 top health officials who left their jobs in the past 19 months." Additionally, those working in public health weren't the only ones targeted:

- A *Nature* survey of 321 scientists found that "more than two-thirds of researchers reported negative experiences as a result of their media appearances or their social media comments, and 22% had received threats of physical or sexual violence. Some scientists said that their employer had received complaints about them or that their home address had been revealed online. Six scientists said they were physically attacked."[286]
- Dr. Anthony Fauci needed "personal security from law enforcement at all times, including at his home."[287] According to news reports, "he and his family have required continued security in the face of harassment and death threats from people angry over his guidance on the coronavirus pandemic."[288]
- Vaccine-advocate Dr. Peter Hotez has been doxed and subject to coordinated campaigns of harassment for his vaccine advocacy.[289] According to Dr. Hotez, the hate mail he received

"was filled with all sorts of Nazi imagery, Nuremberg hangings and terrible, terrible stuff. It was pretty upsetting."[290] Dr. Hotez was stalked at home by an anti-vaxxer.[291] Prior to the pandemic, Dr. Richard Pan was assaulted in the street for advocating for vaccines,[292] and Dr. David Gorski has been the victim of harassment campaigns.[293]

- Anti-vaxxers have protested outside hospitals in Canada and elsewhere. According to news reports, "A crowd rallying against vaccination for COVID-19 clogged the streets outside a Vancouver hospital this week, haranguing and, in one case, assaulting health care workers, slowing ambulances, delaying patients entering for treatment, and disturbing those recovering inside."[294]

- Pro-fascist groups opposed to vaccines have staged violent rallies in Italy. This included storming an emergency room and attacking nurses and police officers.[295]

- In France, "demonstrators carried signs evoking the Auschwitz death camp or South Africa's apartheid regime." In Russia, an actor wore a yellow star at an awards ceremony and spoke of "waking up in a world where [COVID-19 vaccination] became an identification mark." Across the world, Jewish stars are used as a symbol of anti-vaxxer "persecution."[296]

- In Australia, "Anti-vaccine and extreme right-wing groups have led violent rallies" while "prominent fascists were among the crowd."[297] In Germany, an "anti- lockdown, anti-vaccine movement with links to the far right has recruited hundreds of children into a private online group."[298] Anti-vaccine protesters in Berlin yelled "Hands off our children."[299]

- Anti-vaccine rallies turned violent in Los Angeles[300] and anti-vaxxers disrupted vaccination sites there.[301] They did the same thing in Georgia.[302] In New York City, they attacked a COVID-19 testing station.[303]

- A man in Maryland killed his brother, who was a pharmacist, as well as his sister-in-law because they were "killing people with the COVID shot."[304]

- A principal in Arizona was confronted by men carrying zip ties and was threatened with a "citizen's arrest" after the child of one of the men was told to quarantine because of a possible exposure to the virus.[305] The principal also received threats such as, "Next time it will be a barrel pointed at your Nazi face."[306]

- According to news reports, "a parent in Northern California barged into his daughter's elementary school and punched a teacher in the face over mask rules. At a school in Texas, a parent ripped a mask off a teacher's face during a 'Meet the Teacher' event."[307]

- In Georgia, "a customer who argued about wearing a face mask at a Georgia supermarket shot and killed a cashier on Monday and wounded a sheriff's deputy who was providing security at the store."[308] This is an extreme example of a sadly common occurrence.

- A pharmacist in Wisconsin destroyed COVID-19 vaccines as he believed that the "COVID-19 vaccine was not safe for people and could harm them and change their DNA."[309]

- Doctors in Idaho "have been accused of killing patients by grieving family members who don't believe COVID-19 is real."[310] A hospital spokesperson said, "Our health care workers are almost feeling like Vietnam veterans, scared to go into the community after a shift." Hospitals are installing extra "panic buttons" to protect their workers from assaults.[311]

- According to news reports, "the Hawaii lieutenant governor watched in horror as protesters showed up outside his condo, yelled at him through bullhorns and beamed strobe lights into the building to harass him over vaccine requirements."[307]

- In Canada, a man "punched a nurse in the face multiple times, knocking her to the ground after she administered a COVID-19 vaccine to his wife without his permission."[312] Nurses have also been attacked in Guatemala by anti-vaccine residents of a village.[313]

- Anti-vaxxers have harassed children and their parents. In the UK, one yelled at a mother, "She'll have immunity, you shouldn't be getting the vaccine since you have natural immunity. You shouldn't be using her as a lab rat."[314] In California, an anti-vaxxer yelled at children walking to school, "They're trying to rape our children with this poison. They're going to rape their lives away,"[315] while another compared masking to "child abuse."

- Rep. Marjorie Taylor Greene (Georgia) suggested that citizens use their "Second Amendment rights" to greet community members knocking on doors to encourage vaccination.[316] Rep. Madison Cawthorn (North Carolina) suggested that such vaccination campaigns could be a pretense to "take" people's guns and Bibles.[317]

- Tucker Carlson said the Pentagon's vaccine mandate was an attempt to weed out "men with high testosterone," that it was "anti-Christian," and that the military is "doing PR for Satanists."[318] He also said that "Buying a fake vaccination card is an act of desperation by decent, law- abiding Americans who have been forced into a corner by tyrants."[319]

- Some people apparently believe that "COVID-19 vaccines are called Luciferase, have the patent number 060606, and come from a digital program called Inferno."[320] Republican officials in Florida[321] and New Hampshire[322] have likened the vaccine to Satanism as have several religious leaders in the US[323] and Bolivia.[324] The imagined connection between vaccines and Satan is also not new.

- According to news reports, "anti-vaccine demonstrations across Ohio in recent weeks are drawing extremists that include conspiracy theorists, white supremacists and people who misappropriate the Holocaust."[325]

- In Washington "anti-mask protesters that included the Proud Boys attempted to gain entry" to three schools, forcing them to lockdown.[326]

- After anti-vaxxers showed up at health officials' homes in Los Angeles, "city leaders approved an ordinance Tuesday that would bar protests within 300 feet of the residence belonging to the person being targeted, a move that came following months of demonstrations outside the homes of public and elected officials."[327]

- In Texas, "a man has been charged after allegedly threatening to gun down a Maryland doctor who urged the public to take the coronavirus vaccine."[328]

- Countless school board meetings have been disrupted by anti-vaxxers, often linked with the Proud Boys and other right-wing extremist groups. According to news reports, "drawing false equivalence between COVID regulations and Nazi fascism is popular among anti-vax, anti-mask groups, including some local teachers and school board members."[329]

- In California, "a breast cancer patient says she was sprayed with bear mace, physically assaulted, and verbally abused outside a cancer treatment center in West Hollywood, Los Angeles by far-right activists who were angry over the clinic's mandatory mask policy."[330]

WWTI doctors alone were not responsible for this, but they never spoke out against it, and instead of trying to lower the temperature, they poured fuel on the fire. They never defended Dr. Fauci, even when the headlines read, "Anthony Fauci Says He Still Needs a Security Detail After Ron DeSantis Threatened to 'Grab That Little Elf and Chuck Him Across the Potomac'."[331] Instead, they compared him to a fascist dictator. Dr. Martin Kulldorff said on social media:

> *Faucism and Fascism are not the same, but there are some similarities*
>
> *- Blind belief in an all-knowing leader*
>
> *- Government-corporate partnership*

- Censoring and blacklisting opponents

- Disregarding scientific principles and knowledge

- Harming workers and the poor

- Scapegoating[332]

In the mirror world, it was Dr. Fauci who was guilty of scapegoating.

Similarly, WWTI doctors never stood up for vaccine-hero Dr. Peter Hotez, and they often insulted him in intentionally provocative ways. For example, after Dr. Hotez won an award, Dr. Prasad shared this news on social media with the message, "If you can't get everything wrong and win awards, is it even public health?"[333] Here were some of the responses this single post generated:

- *How long will Official US Public Health defy gravity? How long will media cover for them?*

- *Following the party line is the only thing that matters.*

- *Why does the system reward itself? Because it can.*

- *Most doctors just want to stay part of the club. It's more comfortable, lucrative and strokes the ego more than doing critical science and being kicked out of the system.*

- *The criminals reward each other*

- *Oh, boy... if I didn't have reason to ignore experts coming out of Yale before, I sure do now.*

- *Generals in the failed war on covid giving each other medals as public trust in the biomedical establishment is plummeting. Not helpful.*

- *It's really unbelievable at this point. Hard to trust institutions that bestow awards - for public health no less - to people like Hotez.*

- *This is the upside down world we are living in. Truly*

1984 stuff.

- *It's remarkable how many schools and other medical institutions are still in on this BS. There is NO trust in them anymore. And they wonder why it will continue*
- *Trust in physicians and hospitals decreased substantially over the course of the pandemic, from 71.5% in April 2020 to 40.1% in January 2024*

This sort of mistrust permeated the social media feeds of WWTI doctors. Anyone who might have stood up for Dr. Hotez was blocked from commenting long ago. The echo chamber echoed.

Dr. Prasad also shared a headline, "Lockdown Child Sexual Abuse 'Hidden by Under-Reporting'," with the message, "Hope Peter covers this when he explains his support for lockdowns."[334] One person commented:

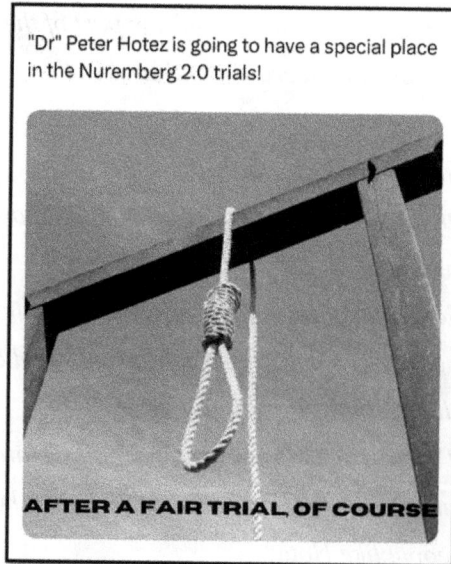

"Dr" Peter Hotez is going to have a special place in the Nuremberg 2.0 trials!

AFTER A FAIR TRIAL, OF COURSE

A routine death threat on social media towards Dr. Peter Hotez

*The thing is, he couldn't care less about any of the collateral dam-
age, the harm to children & teens, the decimation of small businesses and jobs lost, and the massive inflation. He has no heart
and is a soulless being.*[335]

That sort of bile was normal in the social media feeds of many
WWTI doctors. It's no surprise that Dr. Hotez received hateful death
threats when influencers like Dr. Prasad accused him of indifference to
pedophilia for the sin of trying to stop people from dying of COVID.

**I've been yearning for an end to the pandemic. Now that it's here,
I'm a little afraid.**
— *Dr. Lucy McBride*

We can now return to Dr. McBride. With her warning of "harmful
medical advice" from "media personalities and internet influencers" in
mind, let's review some of her pandemic record.

Though many scientists doubted herd immunity to COVID was
possible in the spring of 2021,[336] Dr. McBride's message at that time was
that we were "post-pandemic," that brand new vaccines rendered people
essentially bulletproof against a brand-new virus, and variants were of no
concern. She shared her optimism on social media, podcasts, television
interviews, and editorials in widely read publications such as *The Washington Post* and *The Atlantic*. Here's a small sample.

- *March 2, 2021: COVID-19 cases are dropping, but anxiety is
  everywhere.*[337]
- *March 9, 2021: I've been yearning for an end to the pandemic. Now that it's here, I'm a little afraid. […] The pandemic will end. With dropping case rates and three incredible
  vaccines robustly protecting us from COVID-19, soon we'll be
  able to relax the restrictions of pandemic life.*[338]

- ***March 10, 2021:*** *I see it every day: ambivalence & #anxiety about reentry. After a year of #trauma, it's normal. Let's name, normalize, & navigate it. I was honored to speak about #FONO & my @washingtonpost opinion piece on @Morning_Joe today![339]*

- ***March 16, 2021:*** *Enjoyed talking with @ryanegorman of @iHeartRadio podcast about my @washingtonpost Op-Ed & how to safely and sanely navigate our post-pandemic transition to normalcy. I hope you take a listen![340]*

- ***March 26, 2021:*** *Further evidence that the variants are infinitely less scary than the lack of nuanced messaging about them. So many of my vaccinated patients – particularly the elderly – are PARALYZED by fear of the variants.[341]*

- ***April 3, 2021:*** *Wired and tired after months of COVID-19 distress, it's time to recover our mental health. To fully bounce back from COVID, we need a dose of reassurance and a plan for recovery. We need science under our feet and doctors at our back. The first steps toward post-pandemic health are seemingly simple yet vexingly hard for most of us. […]We have every reason to be hopeful. COVID-related deaths and hospitalizations are falling fast, and real world data confirms the stunning efficacy of our vaccines. The medical community has its hands on the science we need for reentry. To fully recoup from COVID, we now need our arms around our patients. The doctor is in; are you.[342]*

- ***April 3, 2021:*** *But as you know, once you've been vaccinated, your risk of death & severe disease essentially goes away. The risk is of getting milder illness. And even that risk goes down as herd immunity takes hold.[343]*

- ***April 3, 2021:*** *Post-pandemic health: To fully bounce back from #COVID, we need a dose of reassurance and a plan for recovery. We need science under our feet and doctors at our back.[344]*

- ***April 6, 2021:*** *The risks of getting #COVID19 and transmit-*

ting #SARSCoV2 both drop significantly after #vaccination. Neither risk is zero (zero isn't even on the menu). As we approach herd immunity, these risks will get even smaller than they already are.[345]

- *April 19, 2021: I've been using the "off-ramp" analogy with patients — both for how restrictions should END & how we can expect our brains to adjust post-pandemic. There's no on/ off switch for either. #FactsNotFear #Nuance #Context*[346]

- *April 21, 2021: I made these points on @MSNBC @Morning_ Joe today: #vaccines 1) essentially take death/severe dz off table; 2) drop risk of #COVID19 to 0.0005% (@CDC data), 3) reduce transmission (94% per Israeli data), 4) are powerful against all current variants. #FactsNotFear#ThisIsOurShot*[347]

- *April 21, 2021: Vaccines aren't 100% effective (though these are close!), but we don't need them to be 100% to gradually resume regular life as we head toward herd immunity.*[348]

- *April 22, 2021: My (humble) impression is this: nothing in life is risk-free. Certainly the risk of COVID transmission is higher w/ the circulating variants, but as we edge toward herd immunity, outdoor masking is less important (if at all) unless in a crowded space like a rally w/ shouting etc.*[349]

- *May 1, 2021: The real-world data on the Covid-19 vaccines is clear: they are stunningly effective. The vaccines essentially take death and severe disease off the table. They dramatically reduce the risks of getting Covid and transmitting the virus to other people. They are powerful weapons against all of the circulating variants. In short, they are the clear ticket to normality. […] People need to know, for example, that the risk of two vaccinated people sickening one another with Covid-19 is vanishingly small. […] Vaccinated grandparents should be reassured, for example, that seeing their unvaccinated grandchildren poses very little risk to themselves and that, in general, the risks of Covid-19 in kids are small.*[350]

- *May 1, 2021: The #vaccines are so effective at preventing*

#COVID & reducing transmission it can be hard to believe. Remember when we thought we might never get a #vaccine? Well, here we are with a near-perfect vaccine. Reminder: perfect isn't on the menu.[351]

- *May 4, 2021: The reason you would need booster shots is if the virus mutates in a way that escapes the immune protection conferred by the vaccines. That has not happened yet. Nor do we expect that to happen, given how quickly we are crushing the curve and how robust we know the immune response to be from these vaccines. It's just not anything that anybody should be worried about. [...] Why all the negative news about variants when it's just not important? [...] If you're in that tiny category of people that does get COVID after vaccination, you're going to get a cold or a mild illness, most likely. Are there exceptions? Yes. But the vaccines are stunningly effective against the virus. They take death and severe disease off the table. They prevent transmission and they cover all the variants.*[352]

- *May 26, 2021: Parents need to role model confidence and optimism about the end of the pandemic.*[353]

- *May 26, 2021: As covid-19 cases continue to fall and vaccines demonstrate vigor against even the most concerning variants, it's time to evaluate which pandemic restrictions are worth keeping in place. [...] This low risk for children nearly vanishes as cases plummet. As we saw in Israel and Britain, vaccinating adults indirectly protects children. The same trend is evident here in the United States: Adult vaccination has lowered COVID-19 incidence among children by 50 percent in the past four weeks.*[354]

- *June 2, 2021: What I'm telling you is I'm following the science and seeing the very low risk that COVID-19 poses to kids, and it's lower and lower every day. And then we also see that kids are really protected by the vaccination status of the staff, and faculty, and teachers at the schools. And so by the time fall rolls around, of course, depending on the local situation of COVID in the particular region we're talking about, it just isn't going to make sense for most schools to restrict kids. Now, there's lots of nuance here, right?*

Because I don't have a crystal ball and because could things change? Could case rates go up? They could. It's just very, very unlikely. Again, if you look at the UK and Israel as the seniors and we're the sophomores, we're going to be in so much better shape even next week than we are today, and in the fall, it should be a lot different. […] the vaccines that we currently have are so stunningly effective against all of the circulating variants. […] worst case scenario, we need boosters and Pfizer and Moderna will crank them out.[355]

All this from a doctor who said in April 2021:

As physicians, dispensing false hope is dangerous & unethical; but when hope is rooted in scientific data, it's our obligation to dispense it.[356]

I'm A Doctor Seeing Patients with Coronaphobia. Here's What You Need to Know.
— Dr. Lucy McBride

While Dr. McBride announced we were "post-pandemic" as early as March 2021 and that variants were nothing to worry about, she was *very concerned* that strangers were trying too hard to avoid the virus. She had dozens of tweets using the hashtag *#FactsNotFear* and encouraged her audience to "abandon irrational fear."[357]

She even coined several new medical terms to pathologize cautious people. For example, in her article, "I'm A Doctor Seeing Patients with Coronaphobia. Here's What You Need to Know," from March 2021, Dr. McBride wrote:

"Coronaphobia" can be defined as an exaggerated fear of COVID-19 that is rooted in rational anxiety about the very real threat of COVID. […] Not dying is important (and is essentially guaranteed with COVID-19 vaccination); but what about living? […] COVID-19 cases are dropping, but anxiety is everywhere.[337]

She wrote the article, "I've Been Yearning for an End to the Pandemic. Now That It's Here, I'm a Little Afraid," a week later in which she created yet another term—Fear of Normal (FONO)—to further stigmatize those who didn't agree that the pandemic was over.[338] She elaborated on these articles in an interview from May 2021:

I wrote an article for The Huffington Post about what I call "coronaphobia," and I also wrote a piece for The Washington Post about what I call "fear of normal," or FONO. What I'm seeing is an epidemic of unbridled fear that is basically the reverberations of the anxiety that we all experienced when the pandemic was happening in full force. As the pandemic comes under much better control, we need to shift our thinking and then our behaviors to reflect reality.[352]

COVID has since injured millions of Americans and killed over 600,000 of them. Coronaphobia has never appeared on a death certificate. In his article, "'Coronaphobia: How Antivaxxers and Pandemic Minimizers Pathologize Fear of Disease," Dr. David Gorski, an expert in the anti-vaccine movement, discussed how Dr. McBride's rhetoric mirrored pre-pandemic anti-vaccine propaganda. He wrote:

During the pandemic, everything old is new again and antivaccine talking points keep popping up again and again from pandemic minimizers and COVID-19 contrarians like Dr. McBride. In this case, it's the pathologizing of the fear of infectious dis-

*ease, representing it as an anxiety disorder, specifically a phobia,
that might even need treatment. In other words, if you are afraid
of COVID, you might be mentally ill. It is not my intention to
deny that there are people out there suffering from anxiety and
depression due to the consequences of the COVID-19 pandemic,
some of whom might even require treatment. There are.*

*What I am going to point out is how the messaging that Dr.
McBride is doubling down on a year after she first promoted
it is very similar to messaging that I've been encountering for
many years coming from the antivaccine movement. Although Dr.
McBride probably doesn't realize it, she is echoing an old antivax
trope that does exactly the same thing: Seeks to shame those who
fear vaccine-preventable diseases.*[358]

Once Delta arrived, invalidating Dr. McBride's optimistic declarations that we were edging "toward herd immunity," she continued to
be afraid of fear. In August 2021, as Delta caused a spike in pediatric
hospitalizations, she authored an article titled "Fear of COVID-19 in
Kids is Getting Ahead of the Data," as if this was necessarily a bad thing.
"Shielding children from danger is a fundamental instinct. Tolerating risk
for them is hard—but necessary—emotional work,"[359] she said.

Pediatricians with actual responsibility for treating sick children
weren't so blasé. "This is different,"[360] one said. "What we're seeing now
is previously healthy kids coming in with symptomatic infection." Another said that "we're not only seeing more children now with acute SARS-
CoV2 in the hospital, we're starting also to see an uptick of MISC – or
Multisystem Inflammatory Syndrome in Children." Less than a month
after Dr. McBride published her essay, the CDC reported that Delta had
caused a 5-fold increase in pediatric hospitalizations.[361] Dr. McBride got

her data, though it was too late for many children. They *were* the data.[362]

Having used "coronaphobia" and "Fear of Normal" in 2021, Dr. McBride needed a new term to pathologize cautious people in 2022. In March, she wrote an article titled "Dealing With 'Post-Pandemic Stress': A Doctor's Guide," in which she stated:

> *It's what some medical professionals, including myself, are calling "post-pandemic stress" which is not an official diagnosis (nor does it mean that COVID is gone!) but is characterized by anxiety, mood instability, and mental exhaustion that is interfering with quality of life.*[363]

Fortunately, Dr. McBride knew the cure for "post-pandemic stress." In May 2022, she said, "I'm finding that the 'cure' for some of my patients' outsize fear of COVID is … COVID."[364]

The risk of COVID-19 is really, really small in kids. It's a smaller risk than the seasonal flu. [...] If you're under 11, the risk of getting COVID is teeny.
— *Dr. Lucy McBride*

Dr. McBride frequently minimized pediatric COVID, recording podcasts such as "Worry Less about Your Kids & COVID-19!"[365] She partnered with anti-vaccine doctors in January 2022 to found the group Urgency of Normal, which copied the GBD by advocating "focused protection for the vulnerable." It also spread disinformation to minimize COVID's risk to children. For example, the Urgency of Normal sought to pacify parents by saying that "COVID is a flu-like risk to unvaccinated children."[366] They used several statistical gimmicks to make this false claim.

- They compared COVID deaths when mitigation measures

were in place to pre-pandemic flu deaths.[367]

- They compared the raw tally of COVID deaths to *estimated* flu deaths, which inflated the flu death toll relative to COVID.[368]
- They compared the infection fatality rate of COVID to the flu, ignoring the *essential fact* that COVID is much more contagious than the flu.[369]
- They made factual errors, claiming that COVID had killed around 400 children, when in fact it had killed around 1,200.[370]

The Urgency of Normal did all they could to obscure the basic fact that from April 2020 to January 2022—when the Urgency of Normal was formed—COVID killed around 1,200 children, while the flu killed 15.[371] A single child died during the 2020-2021 flu season,[372] when mitigation measures were most stringent, while COVID killed several hundred children during that time. Currently, the CDC reports 1,955 COVID deaths[373] and 439 flu deaths[371] among children since the start of the pandemic, though obviously children should be vaccinated against both viruses, and death is not the only bad outcome from either. Despite the Urgency of Normal not mentioning it, COVID can hurt children without killing them, and COVID hospitalized many more children than the flu. Flu hospitalized just 9 children ages 5-11 years old in 2020-2021, while COVID hospitalized over 8,300 children that age during that time. [374]

However, that didn't stop Dr. McBride from saying in May 2021:

The risk of COVID-19 is really, really small in kids. It's a smaller risk than the seasonal flu. We don't close schools and mask kids in flu season. We have somehow as a society, quote-unquote, "tolerated" the fact that hundreds of kids die from the flu every year. This virus has generally spared children, particularly young children. […] If you're under 11, the risk of getting COVID is teeny.[352]

Not only was Dr. McBride wrong about the relative risks of COVID and the flu, schools would occasionally close for the flu before the pandemic,[375] pediatricians vaccinated kids against the flu instead of "tolerating" their death,[376] and babies have by far the highest COVID risk of all children.[377]

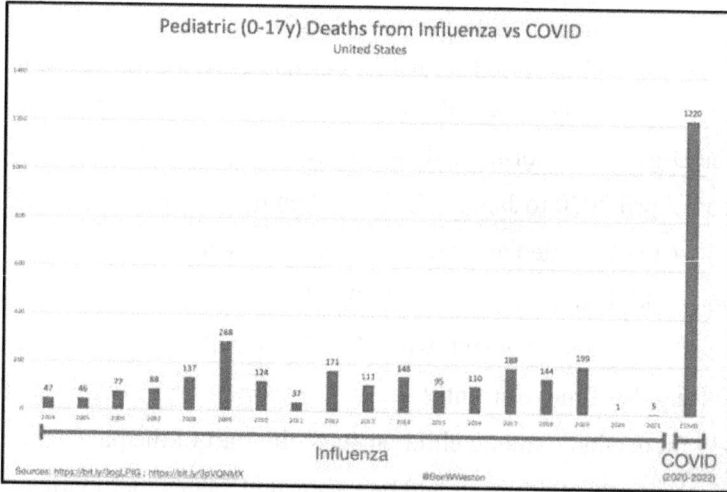

Chart by Dr. Ben Weston[378] Used with permission.

Though Dr. McBride refused to share these basic numbers, to her credit, she vaccinated her teen daughter and shared this publicly.[379] However, she also said, "I'm pro-vax but the risk/benefit ratio for healthy teen boys isn't yet clear,"[380] presumably because of rare cases of vaccine-induced myocarditis, which was already known to be mild in 95% of cases.[381] This aged almost as poorly as her declaration that we were "post-pandemic," though again, it was too late for some healthy teen boys. According to a news report from August 2021:

> *A Granville County 17-year-old who died after contracting COVID-19 is being remembered as a happy-go-lucky teen who loved to play baseball and was deeply involved in his church. Matthew Kirby died late Thursday after spending nine days in*

intensive care. His father, Stephen Kirby, posted on Facebook
that the coronavirus infection led to myocarditis, an inflammation
of the heart.[382]

The Urgency of Normal also exaggerated the supposed harms of mitigation measures. One article about the Urgency of Normal noted:

The physicians and scientists of the Urgency of Normal are cherry-picking data in their push to end pandemic precautions, but are getting favorable mainstream media attention and support from wealthy, white communities that never felt the full brunt of Covid-19.[383]

It continued:

Tyler Black, a child and adolescent psychiatrist and suicidologist at BC Children's Hospital in Vancouver, hadn't heard anything about the Urgency of Normal group or its "tool kit" until it came out. But when he saw it go up on Twitter, he was appalled. "Their document was so poor, with so many mistakes, that it required immediate public correction," he said. He messaged some of the signers directly on Twitter, he said, and when no one responded, he went public, in a detailed Twitter thread that focused on his area of expertise: child mental health. Several other subject-area experts did the same, debunking comparisons to the flu and diving into the dismissal that many kids are fine. The central problem he saw was that the group claimed that masks harm children's mental health and social development—something he's seen no evidence for in his own work.

"It was really, really gross to see what they did with the mental health science. It's a true perversion of what science communication is supposed to be," Black said. "They had mis-cited the

*CDC—I'm not talking about they made a mistake, I'm talking
about mis-citing. Academic misconduct." The Centers for
Disease Control and Prevention study found that there was no
significant increase in child suicide, yet the group used that study
to claim the opposite—an increase in suicide. After pushback, the
authors edited the tool kit to remove that mention of suicide, he
said, without noting what had been revised.*

Dr. Black also added, "I consider it ghoulish to wield child suicide
statistics inaccurately to make advocacy points."[384] Indeed, the next year,
an article titled "Teen Suicide Plummeted During Covid-19 School Closures, New Study Finds" was published. It said:

*Rates of suicide and suicide attempts among teenagers were at
their lowest when schools were closed for the Covid-19 pandemic, a new study published Wednesday shows, pointing to an overall pattern that shows mental health in children and teenagers is
at its worst while school is in session.[385]*

The Urgency of Normal team attributed all childhood mental health
issues to remote schooling, without considering that some children were
profoundly affected by their bout with COVID or from losing a loved one
or teacher to it.[386] Despite early pandemic musings that children could not
spread the virus, there's no question that kids can and did bring the virus
home and spread it to more vulnerable relatives.[387] By the spring of 2022,
over 200,000 American children had lost a parent or caregiver to the virus.[388] In New York City alone, 8,600 children—1 in 200 children—have
lost a parent or caregiver.[389] Around the world, an estimated 10.5 million
children have lost parents or caregivers to COVID, and 7.5 million were
orphaned.[390]

This can be a disaster for children. As Tim Requarth said in his article
"America's Pandemic Orphans Are Slipping Through the Cracks":

Losing a parent may be one of the most destabilizing events of the human experience. Orphans are at increased risk of substance abuse, dropping out of school, and poverty. They are almost twice as likely as non-orphans to die by suicide, and they remain more susceptible to almost every major cause of death for the rest of their life.[391]

He's right. After the death of her father, 15-year-old Elizabeth George said, "I didn't want to go to school. I just wanted to stay at home."[386] Charles Nelson, a professor of pediatrics and psychology at Harvard University who has studied separation from caregivers, said, "Honestly, it makes me sick to my stomach to think of the hurt so many kids are experiencing. We could have done better to protect these kids." The Urgency of Normal doctors never mentioned COVID orphans. They pretended these children didn't exist.

"I worry most about peoples' confusion and resulting anxiety about not knowing who to trust in a global health crisis."
— Dr. Lucy McBride

In January 2024, three years after many WWTI doctors declared the pandemic over, a headline asked, "Why Are 1,500 Americans Still Dying from COVID Every Week?"[392] The article answered by saying, "Americans aren't accessing available vaccines and treatments." That's absolutely true and very important. But I think Dr. McBride gave a deeper answer in her Congressional testimony. She said:

But at its core, I worry most about peoples' confusion and resulting anxiety about not knowing who to trust in a global health crisis. Specifically, I worry about the risk that the erosion of trust in medicine and in public health poses to our individual and collective health.

This pandemic is about a virus; it's also about information, messaging, and the contagion of mistrust. To build back better we must start with trust. In patient care, trust is hard-won and easily lost. [...] Trust is born when doctors first acknowledge uncertainty—and then lean into things that are certain. [...]

That vacuum of trust has been and continues to be filled with a cacophony of voices calling out from across a variety of platforms, from celebrities, media personalities, and internet influencers. Without a source of truth, people look to the showy salesmen and get easily tangled in webs of harmful medical advice.[2]

It's hard to argue with any of that.

Chapter 5: There's No Vaccine That Is, You Know, Safe and Effective

One thing RFK Jr. did is he would post true stories of children who died immediately after the vaccine.
— *Dr. Marty Makary*

In 2024, Robert F. Kennedy Jr. promoted and distributed the anti-vax propaganda movie *Vaxxed 3: Authorized to Kill: The Groundbreaking Film They Don't Want You to See.*[1] Graphics advertising the movie warned of "Deadly protocols. Tragic outcomes. Powerful testimonies." It was promoted on social media, with claims the film "exposes what really happened during COVID, behind hospital closed doors and beyond."[2]

This is par for the course for Kennedy, who is perhaps America's most famous and influential anti-vaccine advocate. As Dr. Paul Offit said, "What, exactly, has Robert F. Kennedy, Jr. accomplished? Using the platform of a famous name, he has chosen to lie about vaccines and vaccine safety, no doubt putting children in harm's way."[3]

For many years, Kennedy has spread disinformation and doubt. His website, Children's Health Defense (CHD), publishes a deluge of anti-vax articles, such as the following: "Are Public Health Authorities the Authors of Fake Measles News?"[4]; "The Vaccine Program: Betrayal of Public Trust & Institutional Corruption"[5]; "Why Won't the CDC Do Proper Safety Trials on Childhood Vaccines? Follow the Money"[6]; and "CDC Lies About, and Media Repeats, Risk of Dying from Measles."[7] Kennedy wants his audience angry, scared, and full of mistrust. Other of his site's incendiary anti-vaccine content includes:

- Mercury and Autism Relationship Confirmed in Longitudinal Study[8]
- Evidence of Harm: Mercury in Vaccines and the Autism Epi-

demic: A Medical Controversy[9]

- Vaccines Can Spread Diseases Through Shedding[10]
- New Study: Gardasil HPV Vaccine Contains Chemical Used in Biological Warfare[11]
- New Data Shows DNA From Aborted Fetal Cell Lines in Vaccines[12]
- 'Dissolving Illusions': 225 Years of Lies and Cover-Ups Behind Vaccines[13]
- Vaccines Contain Dangerous Ingredients. Small Doses Can be Unhealthy. Disease is a Product of Genetics and Environment[14]
- Vaccine Rhetoric v. Reality — Keeping Vaccination's Unflattering Track Record Secret[15]
- Read the Fine Print: Vaccine Package Inserts Reveal Hundreds of Medical Conditions Linked to Vaccines[16]
- Natural Measles Immunity — Better Protection and More Long-Term Benefits Than Vaccines[17]
- Vaccines and Autism—Is the Science Really Settled?[18]
- Vaccine Injury Touches Families Throughout the U.S.[19]
- Vaccines Do Not Deserve the Credit for Reducing Contagious Diseases[20]
- Vaccine Boom, Population Bust: Study Queries Link Between HPV Vaccine and Soaring Infertility[21]
- Mercury Toxicity: Highly Toxic, Cumulative and Still in Vaccines[22]
- Unvaccinated Children Have Much Lower Rates of Chronic Illness[23]
- Vaccine Mandates for Everyone, Everywhere—A Globally Coordinated Agenda[24]
- CDC's Latest Tuskegee Experiment African American Autism and Vaccines[25]
- CDC Scientist Still Maintains Agency Forced Researchers to Lie About Safety of Mercury Based Vaccines[26]
- Don't Fall for the CDC's Outlandish Lies About Thimerosal[27]
- Worse than Nothing—How Ineffective Vaccines Enhance Disease[28]

- MMR Vaccine's Poison Pill: Mumps After Puberty, Reduced Testosterone and Sperm Counts[29]
- Mercury, Vaccines and the CDC's Worst Nightmare[30]
- Japan Leads the Way: No Vaccine Mandates and No MMR Vaccine = Healthier Children[31]
- It's Been 10 Years Since a Whistleblower Exposed the CDC's Cover-Up of the Link Between Vaccines and Autism. The Agency Has Done Nothing[32]
- Kids, Vaccines and Autism: Will a New Legal Strategy End the Decades-long Battle for Truth and Justice?[33]
- Measles Vaccine Narrative Is Collapsing[34]

In his book, *The Real Anthony Fauci*, Kennedy cast doubt on germ theory and embraced "miasma theory," which he said, "Emphasizes preventing disease by fortifying the immune system through nutrition and by reducing exposures to environmental toxins and stresses."[35] After reading this, Dr. Paul Offit responded with:

> *I thought "It all makes sense"… I mean, it all adds up. […] It's so unbelievable, because you can't imagine that someone who's the head of Health and Human Services doesn't believe that specific viruses or bacteria cause specific diseases, and that the prevention or treatment of them is lifesaving.*

At least when he is in front of mainstream audiences, Kennedy brazenly lies about his anti-vaccine advocacy, and he doesn't flinch when his lies are revealed. He had the following exchange on CNN:

> **Question:** *You have gained notoriety for your skepticism about vaccines, and over the summer in an interview you said quote, "There's no vaccine that is, you know, safe and effective." Do you still believe that?*
>
> **Kennedy:** *I never said […]*
>
> [The host played a clip of Kennedy saying, *"There's no vaccine*

that is, you know, safe and effective. "][36]

Kennedy has plans and a more influential platform to spread this attitude and disinformation within the federal government. Shortly after Trump won the election, Kennedy made the following statement:

> *So there's no vaccine on that schedule, that 72 vaccines, that has ever gone through a pre-licensing safety study placebo-controlled trial against a real placebo. And that's wrong because that means that nobody knows what the risk profiles are. […] And nobody can tell you whether that product is averting more problems than it's causing.*
>
> *And what I will do, you know, if I'm given this job in the White House, is I'll make sure that those studies get done, that there are people on the panels that approve these products that are not loaded with conflicts of interest. So it's real science. disinterested people and that doctors and patients and Americans know exactly what the costs and benefits of every vaccine are and can make a rational decision.*[37]

In reality, nearly all vaccines were tested against placebos.[38]

Most tragically, Kennedy's 2019 visit to Samoa helped worsen a measles outbreak that sickened 5,700 people and killed 83 of them, mostly young children.[39] While there, he met with local anti-vaccine activists and the Samoan prime minister. He later wrote a letter to the prime minister suggesting the measles vaccine was responsible for the whole thing and used Facebook to spread gross disinformation about the outbreak. He has never expressed the slightest bit of remorse for this tragedy and tried to cover up his role in it.[40] These deaths should be mentioned *every time* Kennedy's name comes up.

However, calling Kennedy an anti-vaccine activist hardly captures the depths of his disinformation. From legitimizing chemtrails[41]—the belief that airplanes are spraying chemicals on the populace—to germ-theory denial,[42] Kennedy has been a firehose of dangerous, deluded nonsense for decades. He tries to spread fear and doubt about institutions and the entire concept of public health. Here are some of his "greatest hits" as compiled by the American media monitoring organization GLAAD:[43]

- *Made false claims that COVID-19 was "ethnically targeted" to attack certain ethnic groups while sparing Ashkenazi Jews and Chinese people, a conspiracy theory that drew accusations of antisemitism and racism.*[44]

- *Told Joe Rogan that Wi-Fi causes cancer and "leaky brain."*[45]

- *Falsely linked vaccines to various medical conditions, including the scientifically discredited belief that vaccines for children cause autism. Kennedy advertised misleading information about vaccine ingredients and circulated retracted studies linking vaccines to various medical conditions.*[46]

- *At an anti-vaccine rally in Washington, D.C., compared vaccination records to the persecution of Jews by the Nazis. He said, "Even in Hitler Germany [sic], you could, you could cross the Alps into Switzerland. You could hide in an attic, like Anne Frank did. [...] I visited, in 1962, East Germany with my father and met people who had climbed the wall and escaped, so it was possible. Many died, true, but it was possible." In fact, Frank and some 6 million other Jews were murdered by Nazis. Frank and her family hid in an attic in the Netherlands, not Germany, before she was caught and was sent to a concentration camp, where she died.*[47]

- *Falsely told Louisiana lawmakers in 2021 that the coronavirus vaccine was the "deadliest vaccine ever made."*[46]

- *His nonprofit organization Children's Health Defense was removed from Facebook and Instagram for repeatedly violating guidelines by spreading medical misinformation.*[48]

- *Claimed that chemicals in our water are causing kids to be transgender. He told anti-trans conspiracy theorist Jordan Peterson that kids are "swimming through a soup of toxic chemicals,"*[49] *including atrazine, a common herbicide, and that, "A lot of the problems we see in kids, and particularly boys, it's probably underappreciated that how much of that is coming from chemical exposures, including a lot of the sexual dysphoria that we're seeing." There is no evidence to indicate that the herbicide causes gender dysphoria in humans. The Centers for Disease Control and Prevention says, "Most people are not exposed to atrazine on a regular basis."*[50]
- *Suggested that poppers, not HIV, causes AIDS and that, "But for [Director of the National Institute of Allergy and Infectious Diseases Anthony] Fauci, it was really important to call it a virus because that made it an infectious disease, and it allowed him to take control of it."*[51]
- *Falsely and repeatedly endorsed the idea that mass shootings have increased because of heightened use of antidepressants.*[46]

No one is more elite or part of the establishment than Kennedy. Yet he rails against the "Democratic elites"[52] as if he were an outsider, and his presidential campaign was designed to help Trump.[53] Everyone knew this, as explained by the article "RFK's Voters Know They're Not Electing the Next President. They're with Him Anyway."[54] After a judge kicked him off the ballot in NY for lying about his residence,[55] he responded by saying, "The Democrats are showing contempt for democracy."[56] Kennedy did everything he could to get Trump elected, and no reasonable person ever thought he had any other goal.

He takes testosterone,[57] hung out with Jeffrey Epstein,[58] and claims to have brain worms—likely a disease called neurocysticercosis.[59] He promotes quack COVID cures.[60] He is American Loon #204[61] and one of the Disinformation Dozen, the twelve anti-vaxxers who are "responsible for almost two-thirds of anti-vaccine content circulating on social media platforms."[62]

He is paranoid and aggrieved, as described in the article "RFK, Jr. is Even Crazier Than You Might Think."[63] An article about one of his speeches titled "'Our Country Is Under Attack': RFK Jr. Speaks on CIA and Totalitarianism" began by saying:

> *In his speech — described by the Ron Paul Institute as "a compelling indictment of the mad push to total control" — Kennedy said the techniques used by government officials during the COVID pandemic to "edge people into subservience" come straight out of the Central Intelligence Agency (CIA) manuals he researched for his book, "American Values."*[64]

Kennedy is grandiose and enamored with himself. He's cast himself in the role of the brave hero and is eager to slay his enemies. Ten days before the 2024 election, he posted:

> *FDA's war on public health is about to end. This includes its aggressive suppression of psychedelics, peptides, stem cells, raw milk, hyperbaric therapies, chelating compounds, ivermectin, hydroxychloroquine, vitamins, clean foods, sunshine, exercise, nutraceuticals and anything else that advances human health and can't be patented by Pharma. If you work for the FDA and are part of this corrupt system, I have two messages for you: 1. Preserve your records, and 2. Pack your bags.*[65]

Kennedy also has a sordid personal life,[66] and while normally this would not be worth mentioning, it reveals fundamental defects in his character. Kennedy has hurt[67] and taken advantage[68] of people close to him. His own family disavowed him.[69]

He's not compassionate or humble. He is a deeply unwell crank who did well for himself during the pandemic, as explained by the article "Robert F. Kennedy Jr. Is Making Millions Off His Anti-Vax Crusade."[70] The ridiculousness of his exploits with dead bears and whales obscures the grave threat he poses. His buffoonery is a *distraction* from his danger. As the pundit Charlie Sykes said, "a clown with a flamethrower still has a flamethrower."[71] Children are already dead because of his disinformation. If it weren't for his famous last name, you'd likely move far away from him if you heard him ranting in the park.

Even if Kennedy occasionally makes some reasonable points about our regulatory agencies and pharma malfeasance, I would only consider him on "my team" if space aliens invaded, which, based on his statement, "RFK Jr.: We Need Disclosure on UFOs,"[72] wouldn't surprise Kennedy. Everyone has a right to make informed decisions about their health, and fundamentally, Kennedy robs people of this basic right. Above all else, he is *dangerous*. No ethical or serious person, especially a doctor, should praise or legitimize him.

Yet, several WWTI doctors did exactly that. They shared Kennedy's disdain for mitigation measures and his enthusiasm for infecting unvaccinated children with SARS-CoV-2. Mostly, they—rightly—recognized him as an ally for spreading doubt about public health and a vehicle by which they could achieve political power. In service of these larger, common goals, they were willing to overlook many things about Kennedy, including dead children.

I really think the way to engage with RFK is the way you're doing, actually, and the way I'm trying to do, which is not to insult him and to give credence to what his root concerns are.

— *Dr. Vinay Prasad*

In 2022, Dr. Vinay Prasad claimed to be *very worried* about the fate of routine vaccination when he sensed an opportunity to spread doubt about the COVID vaccine, and I'll return to that at the end of the chapter. However, soon after expressing concern about measles and polio, Dr. Prasad was happy to praise Kennedy and dunk on vaccine advocates. On social media, Dr. Prasad often defended Kennedy, writing:

> *In many ways (regulatory capture) he really embodies where Dems should be. He is spot on. Yet I share this sentiment. I think mainstream media is covering him poorly. He is a major political force going forward. Unfair coverage will backfire.*[73]

He used aggressive terms to fantasize that Kennedy would beat public health officials and vaccine experts in an imaginary debate. He said:

- *RFK Jr will flatten most public health experts in debate bc public health has become tribal, unable to use brain to read science.*[74]
- *Most in public health will lose a debate to RFK Jr Making 2 year olds wear a cloth mask is just as nutty as thinking wifi opens blood brain barrier leading to influx of toxins*[75]
- *RFK Jr would destroy Hotez. I would be happy to have a conversation with RFK Jr. I think it is important to acknowledge what RFK is saying about regulatory capture that is very right and then I would probe the parts I disagree with*[76]
- *An establishment figure who got most COVID19 policy wrong is going to get obliterated by RFK Jr.*[77]
- *So RFK Jr was going to be 'defeated' by pro toddler masking, pro school closure, scared of #barbieheimer- Peter Hotez in a debate... Riiight*[8]

In an interview with Brianna Joy, titled "What RFK Jr. Gets Right/Wrong About Vaccines." Dr. Prasad described himself as a member of the "progressive left"[79] and had the following exchange:

> *Joy: And the claims have, you know, the claims for the quote*

unquote medical establishment have been so kind of more than they can prove or expressing more confidence than really exist in science, expressing more confidence than really exist in science that he has a legitimate concern about just, frankly, losing to RFK. Jr. and like losing face at this point?

Dr. Prasad: *That's a good question, and I think yes, a legitimate scientist who's in the establishment who holds a lot of these opposing viewpoints, should have a dialogue with RFK. I don't think it should be Peter Hotez. I think Paul Offit would be better, I actually think it would be better if you have a bunch of doctors who have slightly different shades of gray point of view and we get a roundtable, I think that would be better. The reason Peter Hotez I think wouldn't be that terrific is that I think RFK is going to mop the floor with him for some of his past views, particularly on school closure, on mandating the COVID vaccine to children. You know, so as to your point an establishment figure who got a lot of covered policy wrong is not going to go well in the eye of, you know, the Joe Rogan audience supporter and I really think the way to engage with RFK is the way you're doing actually, and the way I'm trying to do, which is not to insult him and to give credence to what his root concerns are, which is really the concern of the corrupting influence of money. That's his root concern; how can I trust the system?*

It's so corrupt with money that how can I trust that these vaccines are really best for my children, and if there was a safety signal, you wouldn't tell me anyway would you? And that root concern is a real concern that we on the progressive left have never, you know, we need to address that root concern, stop revolving door

politics, improve FDA, have some impartiality of the agencies.
And then I think we can come back to him with better studies and
say, look, these particular concerns were not valid, but we found
out this other drug out here on the market was doing a lot of
harm and thank you.

Kennedy's "root concern" is that vaccines kill and devastate children, not the "corrupting influence of money."

In another YouTube video, Dr. Prasad worried about rare, mild vaccine side effects while praising Kennedy. He said:

> *Let's turn to regulatory capture. RFK Jr. is worried that our regu-*
> *latory agencies do the work of the industry that they're supposed*
> *to regulate. […] And on this issue, I think he actually has a pretty*
> *good point, When you're in government and you rubber stamp*
> *a perpetual booster campaign and men who are 20 years old*
> *who've had COVID, that's a dubious decision. It's very likely*
> *they're going to have myocarditis.*[80]

Dr. Prasad also praised Kennedy's COVID stances, saying:

> *We combined the police state with the visible, the public com-*
> *mons, and we combined that in a very inappropriate way. So I*
> *think RFK Jr. is correct there. That's a misuse of public power*
> *and that is concerning and fits with this argument about lock-*
> *downs.*

In an article titled "What RFK Jr. Gets Right—and What He Gets Wrong," Dr. Prasad acknowledged that Kennedy was wrong about quack COVID cures, but felt that Kennedy was right on some points, "including deep truths about the public's current—and very understandable—epidemic of distrust, the corruption of our institutions, and more."[81]

Dr. Prasad felt that Kennedy was right about "regulatory capture." He said:

> *Kennedy is willing to say that Democrats have become captives of big industry—especially Big Tech—and that they have acted as shills for the pharmaceutical companies, especially Pfizer, the manufacturer of the most widely distributed Covid-19 vaccine in the U.S.*

Dr. Prasad was even eager to absolve Kennedy of responsibility for Samoa. In an article titled "The True Story of the Samoa Measles Outbreak," Dr. Prasad told a false story about the tragedy. He blamed "the government's poor response," and said:

> *What did RFK say in Samoa? I don't know but the time course makes no sense. He visited in 2019, but vax rates were already low. The die had been cast.*[82]

Anyone with internet access could have easily discovered what Kennedy said in Samoa. His trip was well-documented at the time—the article "Deadly Measles Outbreak Hits Children in Samoa After Anti-Vaccine Fears" was published in the *Washington Post* in 2019.[83] It mentioned Kennedy ten times and included his letter to the Prime Minister blaming a "defective vaccine" for the outbreak. However, Dr. Prasad had to feign ignorance about this to make Kennedy more palatable to his audience.

Dr. Prasad also felt that Kennedy was right about "The Death of Trust." Dr. Prasad didn't identify Kennedy's disinformation as a cause of mistrust, but rather that public health leaders were to blame because they tried to control COVID. Dr. Prasad favorably quoted Kennedy for saying the response to COVID was "militarized and monetized." Dr. Prasad spoke about "elites" and said doctors who aimed for herd immunity via mass infection were "silenced and demonized." He described himself as a Democrat whose only concern was the "future prospects of poor children." Dr. Prasad wrote:

I am largely sympathetic to Kennedy's views on the mishandling of the Covid-19 pandemic. In general, Kennedy thinks lockdowns were antithetical to public health, is critical of prolonged school closure, and is against Covid-19 vaccination mandates.

When Covid-19 emerged, Kennedy said that "instead of a public health response to a public health crisis, we had a militarized and monetized response, which is the inverse response you want." The Democratic Party—my party—used to pride itself on holding power to account. Instead, during the past few years, the party has reveled in its power to shut down society.

I think Kennedy is correct that lockdowns were a colossal failure, one that will especially harm the future prospects of poor children who lost years of school or left the education system for good. He also had early insight into the excesses of the lockdown, and how foolishly many officials responded. He said on one podcast, "Police were pulling surfers out of the ocean and ticketing them." He's right to point out the absurdity. There is no doubt that closing playgrounds and ticketing surfers were an abuse of power that provided zero public health benefit. Amazingly, those who put these policies in place have yet to apologize. He's also correct to fault the social media environment that has repeatedly, over the past few years, suppressed videos or speech raising questions about public health policies—and even the origin of Covid-19—that some elites found objectionable. Unfortunately for public debate and public health, people with great scientific expertise who objected to how Covid-19 was handled were silenced and demonized. This has been a black mark on science, public health, tech companies, and too many journalists.

Kennedy is not a scientist or a doctor—he's a lawyer and an activist. But one reason I think he is resonating is that he makes Americans feel that they are being spoken to honestly, answering a deep longing from a public who feels battered by officials and skeptical of "approved" experts.

Dr. Prasad worried about surfers who got tickets and said the Democratic Party "reveled in its power to shut down society," as if public health leaders tried to control COVID for pleasure and power alone.

During a podcast that aired the week before the 2024 election, Dr. Prasad again blamed "the establishment" for the loss of trust and wished Kennedy well in his mission to gut the "corrupt" FDA.[84] Dr. Prasad said:

I've had a number of people tweet at me and say that, you know, every once in a while, I say, Robert F. Kennedy Jr. has a point, because he often does have a point. The FDA is captured and doing a poor job. […]

And whether you like someone or not, we should all be honest enough to say, when you agree with someone, even if there's somebody who's, even if there's someone who on some other issue disagree about, and then they say, but he's doing a lot of damage to public health and trust in science.

I say, no one has done more damage to public trust in science. Then Rochelle Walensky, Anthony Fauci, Ashish Jha, Bob Califf, Peter Marks, the establishment, the IDSA, the CDC, the American Academy of Pediatrics, these organizations are supposed to not get things wrong, like should a two-year-old wear a cloth mask except for when they nap side by side in daycare.

They have to be held to the highest standard. They got things obviously and blatantly wrong. They've done more to damage public health than all the Joe Rogans, Weinsteins and RFKs in the world. It's not even a question. […]

But the establishment, the people who set the policies, they have to strive to get things right. They need to do studies. They need to course correct. They have to admit their errors. They need to be held to the highest standard.

So, to me, it's no contest. Fauci did much worse damage than RFK could ever have done, even acknowledging that some of his things he says, I think are incorrect. And I disagree with him on some things, particularly routine childhood immunization and the like.

But on regulatory capture, on the COVID -19 vaccine, on the FDA being a corrupt entity that needs to be, you know, entirely sort of renovated from a gut rehab job, I completely agree with him, and I wish him well in that pursuit.

Once Kennedy's nomination to lead the Department of Health and Human Services (HHS) was announced, Dr. Prasad said:

God gave people two arms… One to vote for Donald Trump, and the other one to give thumbs up to RFK Jr.[85]

Dr. Prasad's monetized Substack blog, *Sensible Medicine*, published an article by Dr. Joseph Marine titled "Why Doctors Should Learn to Stop Worrying and Love MAHA [Make America Healthy Again],"[86] which omitted Kennedy's anti-vaccine history. In addition, Dr. Prasad wrote an article titled "Sabotaging RFK Jr's Confirmation Will Increase Vaccine Hesitancy" that was rife with absurd claims:

The best way to curb vaccine hesitancy is to approve RFK Jr, and redirect his energies to generating more data. More data will answer the key questions that remain unanswered: which childhood immunization program is optimal. The worse thing we can do is tank his nomination. Then vaccine hesitancy will explode.[87]

In reality, no medical products have more data than vaccines; anti-vaxxers won't change their minds with more data; and Kennedy is literally the worst person in the world to generate more data. However, Dr. Prasad also wrote an article titled "Doctors Criticizing RFK Jr. Paved the Way for His Ascendency" and promoted it on social media:

> *It has been bizarre watching @ashishkjha & Marks & Califf and others criticize @RobertKennedyJr for being 'anti-science' These docs abandoned science to help Biden ram through unethical vaccine mandates, to cloth mask 2 year olds and boost young men.*[88]

According to Dr. Prasad, the best way to maintain confidence in vaccines was to put America's #1 anti-vaxxer in charge. At the same time, doctors like him—who praised, normalized, and sanitized Kennedy— bore no responsibility for his rise.

The term for this is *sanewashing*, defined as:

> *Attempting to downplay a person or idea's radicality to make it more palatable to the general public. This is often done by claiming that the radicals are taken out of context, don't truly represent the movement, or that opponents' arguments about its severity are wrong.*[89]

Dr. Prasad never discussed the fact Kennedy promoted the movie *Vaxxed III, Authorized to Kill.*[90] He doesn't want to associate himself with that, though that's exactly what he's doing. Doctors who praised Kennedy told the world that the man behind this movie is quirky perhaps, but basically normal and okay.

Dr. Prasad was not the only WWTI doctor to sanewash America's most powerful and influential anti-vaxxer.

In public health, we are supposed to be beyond politics, and what we say should be equally suitable and just for Democrats, Republicans, and independents alike.
— *Dr. Jay Bhattacharya*

Dr. Jay Bhattacharya also had kind things to say about Kennedy and even spoke at the announcement of his VP candidate, Nicole Shanahan:

> *Thank you, Mr. Kennedy, for the opportunity to speak on this important day in American history when you announce your vice-presidential candidate. I wanted to take the opportunity to explain why it is so vital for this country to maintain its firm commitment to free speech, which has come under such direct attack during the pandemic. I know this issue is near and dear to you since you have been the direct target of censorship by government regulators during the pandemic. I have, too.*
>
> *I am Professor Jay Bhattacharya, and I am a scientific dissident. I have been a professor at Stanford University's medical school for over twenty years. In October 2020, I wrote a document called the Great Barrington Declaration with fellow epidemiologists from Harvard and Oxford, telling the world that we did not need to close schools, churches, and businesses to deal with the pandemic. We proposed protecting vulnerable older people better and not disrupting the lives of the less vulnerable, especially children. [...]*
>
> *So, what is the punchline? Free speech is essential for our health. Free scientific dissent protects us against powerful government scientific bureaucracies that have gone down the wrong path. And especially in emergencies, free speech is essential, for that is when powerful government scientific bureaucrats most need a*

reminder that there is no high Pope of science. Support for free speech does not mean we agree on everything, but it does mean that I support everyone's ability to speak their mind without the government censoring them.

Since I work in public health, I am not here to endorse anyone for president. In public health, we are supposed to be beyond politics, and what we say should be equally suitable and just for Democrats, Republicans, and independents alike. However, I am glad to work with anybody who stands for free speech rights at a time like now when they are in peril. And I am delighted that Mr. Kennedy has lent his considerable voice to the cause.[91]

Although Dr. Bhattacharya said the GBD was concerned about "disrupting the lives of the less vulnerable, especially children," he neglected to mention it advocated for the purposeful mass infection of unvaccinated youth to have them serve as human shields to theoretically protect more vulnerable adults.

However, it's unlikely anyone in the audience would have minded had he been honest about this. Dr. Bhattacharya was introduced at the rally by Del Bigtree, a TV producer and anti-vax royalty:

They wrote a document called the Great Barrington Declaration. A document that will stand the test of time and be heralded as the path the world should have taken. It's my honor and pleasure to introduce you to one of the authors of the Great Barrington Declaration, Jay Bhattacharya.[92]

Del Bigtree had previously threatened doctors and politicians with trials during a rally in 2022. Bigtree said:

And mark my words, we will hold Tony Fauci accountable, we will hold Deborah Birx accountable, we will hold Joe Biden accountable. But unlike the Nuremberg trials that only tried those

doctors that destroyed the lives of human beings, we are going
to come after the press that lied to the world, that worked as a
propaganda machine to push this.[93]

As a reminder, ten Nazis were executed after the Nuremberg trials.[94]

Meanwhile, Ms. Shanahan, Kennedy's vice president pick, promoted a podcast called "COUNCIL of the CANCELED" with the founder of the modern anti-vaccine movement, Andrew Wakefield.[95] These are the people whom Dr. Bhattacharya celebrates and promotes.

After Kennedy's nomination to HHS Secretary was announced, Dr. Bhattacharya authored an article titled "RFK Jr. Will Disrupt the US Medical Establishment," which said:

> *Left-leaning medical establishment — were quick to lambast the*
> *choice, using selective quotations and a narrow focus to smear*
> *Kennedy. But establishment mandarins who focus on his some-*
> *times eccentric scientific claims, from vaccines to AIDS, overlook*
> *the single most important factor in his success: the anti-science,*
> *authoritarian policies of the Covid years. As a result, they miss*
> *what matters most in the Kennedy phenomenon: his broadly*
> *appealing, and thoroughly centrist, reform agenda.*[96]

According to Dr. Bhattacharya, Kennedy's belief that the FDA and USDA are "mass poisoning the American public" is "eccentric."[97]

One thing RFK Jr. did is he would post true stories of children who
died immediately after the vaccine.
— *Dr. Marty Makary*

Dr. Marty Makary also heaped praise on Kennedy. In an interview from 2023 titled "Dr. Makary on RFK Jr's Criticism of the 'Medical In-dustrial Complex': Saying Things 'People Know Are True'," Dr. Makary said:

> *[Kennedy Jr.] talked about guilt by association, that sort of mod-*
> *ern-day McCarthyism. He's talked about how asking questions*
> *is not allowed. He asked a lot of questions himself. But what's*
> *interesting is people really don't criticize the details of what he*
> *actually said when it came to the COVID pandemic. He's been*
> *a skeptic, and he may have a different opinion, but he wrote a*
> *500-page book on Dr. Fauci and the medical industrial complex.*
> *100% of it was true. He said that [Biden's] NIH nominee to*
> *direct the NIH ... received $200 million from Pfizer for research.*
> *100% true. So he's saying things that people know are true, but*
> *they just don't want to hear it.*
>
> *One thing RFK Jr. did is he would post true stories of children*
> *who died immediately after the vaccine. These were otherwise*
> *healthy children. Social media didn't like that. Facebook, Ins-*
> *tagram, LinkedIn, anyone who even associated with him was*
> *censored. And in his hearing yesterday, what I really appreciated*
> *is when he talked about the so-called toxic polarization of society*
> *and how we need to be kind to one another and restore civility.*
> *That is a message people are hungry for in the medical communi-*
> *ty and I think at large.*[98]

In reality, Kennedy used tragedies of dead children to spread an-
ti-vaccine disinformation.[99] According to the article, "RFK Jr. Spent
Years Stoking Fear and Mistrust of Vaccines. These People Were Hurt by
His Work":

> *When 12-year-old Braden Fahey collapsed during football prac-*
> *tice and died, it was just the beginning of his parents' nightmare.*
> *Deep in their grief a few months later, Gina and Padrig Fahey*
> *received news that shocked them to their core: A favorite photo*

of their beloved son was plastered on the cover of a book that falsely argues COVID-19 vaccines caused a spike of sudden deaths among healthy young people.

The book, called "Cause Unknown," was co-published by an anti-vaccine group led by Robert F. Kennedy Jr., President John F. Kennedy's nephew, who is now running for president. Kennedy wrote the foreword and promoted the book, tweeting that it details data showing "COVID shots are a crime against humanity." The Faheys couldn't understand how Braden's face appeared on the book's cover, or why his name appeared inside it.

Braden never received the vaccine. His death in August 2022 was due to a malformed blood vessel in his brain. No one ever contacted them to ask about their son's death, or for permission to use the photo. No one asked to confirm the date of his death — which the book misdated by a year. When the Faheys and residents of their town in California tried to contact the publisher and author to get Braden and his picture taken out of the book, no one responded.

"We reached out in every way possible," Gina Fahey told The Associated Press in an emotional interview. "We waited months and months to hear back, and nothing."

However, Dr. Makary's willingness to praise anti-vaccine disinformation agents and berate public health officials who didn't share his love of "natural immunity" opened many doors for him. He, along with Kennedy and several others, participated in a roundtable discussion[100]—promoted by Kennedy as a "Senate Hearing"—in September 2024 hosted by Wisconsin Senator Ron Johnson.[101]

Senator Johnson himself has spread copious COVID disinformation.

As early as March 2020, he opposed mitigation measures, comparing COVID to the "common flu" and traffic accidents. He later embraced quack COVID treatments and all manner of anti-vaccine conspiracies.[102]

Also present at the roundtable were Dr. Chris Palmer, who claims mental disorders are metabolic disorders of the brain; Casey Means, MD, who would become Trump's nominee for Surgeon General; her brother Calley Means, a co-founder of the online supplement store Truemed; Vani Hari, a.k.a. the Food Babe; right-wing influencer Jordan Peterson; and several other alternative medicine gurus and salesmen.

Poster published by Kennedy promoting the
September 2024 roundtable meeting as a
Senate Hearing

Predictably, Dr. Makary's core message was to not trust the "health care system." "Don't be fooled," he said. After stating his impressive credentials, lending legitimacy to the entire affair, Dr. Makary spoke as if he were an outsider to the medical establishment, including his own field. During his speech, Dr. Makary botched statistics about his specialty—pancreatic cancer—and wondered why other doctors weren't doing more research into it.[103] He spread classic alt-med tropes, saying, "We've gotta talk about food as medicine and research these areas," and that "we are not talking about the root causes of our chronic disease epidemic." He said:

> We have poisoned our food supply, engineered highly addictive chemicals that we put into our food. We spray it with pesticides that kill pests. What do you think they do to our gut lining and our microbiome? [...] The GI tract is reacting. It's not an acute inflammatory storm. It's a low-grade chronic inflammation. [...] and that inflammation permeates and drives so many of our chronic diseases that we didn't see half a century ago.
>
> Who's working on it? Who's looking into this? Who's talking about it? Our health care system is playing whack-a-mole on the back end, and we are not talking about the root causes of our chronic disease epidemic. We can't see the forest from the trees sometimes. [...] We cannot keep going down this path. We have the most overmedicated, sickest population in the world. And no one is talking about the root causes.

Notably, COVID is a "root cause" of illness in the U.S., though Dr. Makary repeatedly mocked people who tried to avoid it.

In a review of the roundtable, Dr. Andrea Love said:

> They demonized vaccines, medical interventions that improve our

health and save millions of lives every year. Because of vaccines, we have increased life expectancy and no longer die primarily of acute illnesses. Instead, they demonized "ultra processed foods" and blamed them for chronic illnesses, a claim that is not supported by causal evidence.

They conflate correlation with causation, and suggest that these foods are inherently harmful, instead of the confounding factor as it relates to overall lifestyle (diet patterns, exercise, access to healthcare,). They made no mention of the fact that illnesses that occur as we age like cancers and neurodegenerative disorders are a result of us living longer - and we live longer now BECAUSE of things like vaccines. They vilified processed foods while selling processed supplements and their own processed foods: protein bars, snacks, frozen foods. But processed is only bad when it serves your personal interests. They claim they want people to eat whole foods, but you gotta make sure to combine them with their supplement stacks! They vilified "processed foods" while omitting ANY nuance on what food processing mean. Processing is not linearly related to food quality. Processing methods can improve food access for many, especially those of lower socioeconomic status. This is a position that reeks of affluence and privilege.

This grotesque display is an insult to legitimate scientists, healthcare professionals, and members of the public who actually care about factual information. *It is an insult to everyone who paid taxes that funded this clown show. Platforming pseudoscience, chemophobia, and disinformation will continue to erode science literacy, public health, and our ability to actually live*

safe and healthy lives. Ron Johnson, Congress, and everyone that
enabled this should be ashamed.

Science disinformation is a global health threat. It must be
combatted. *With outbreaks of preventable diseases, refusal of*
evidence-based medical interventions, propagation of pseudosci-
ence by prominent public "personalities", it's needed now more
than ever.[102]

Donald Trump Has a Plan to Make America's Children Healthy Again. It's a Good One.
— Dr. Robert Redfield

Even Dr. Robert Redfield, the former head of the CDC, was willing
to sanewash Kennedy. In his article, "Donald Trump Has a Plan to Make
America's Children Healthy Again. It's a Good One," he wrote:

> *To heal our children, a president must see the possible and lead*
> *our nation to act. After more than 40 years in the public health*
> *arena, it might surprise some of my colleagues to know I think*
> *President Trump chose the right man for the job: Robert Kenne-*
> *dy, Jr.*[105]

Dr. Redfield added in an interview:

> *I think Kennedy is really passionate about this, about making*
> *America healthy again and I think Kennedy finally deciding to*
> *partner with President Trump is an opportunity to really devel-*
> *op, you know, you use the term and I agree with it. I think it's a*
> *moonshot opportunity to change our focus in healthcare from*
> *disease, disease and disease to health and health and health.*[106]

In another interview, he said:

> *I've started to work with Bobby Kennedy because Bobby Kenne-*

dy is not anti-vaccine. Bobby Kennedy wants to have an honest, open, transparent discussion about vaccines... I happen to have changed my view again. I practice two days a week and much of my practice now is Long COVID. And within that Long COVID, there's a subgroup that are there because they had bad reactions to the mRNA vaccines and I mean really bad reactions.[107]

In the mirror world, America's biggest spreader of anti-vaccine disinformation just w*ants to have an honest, open, transparent discussion about vaccines.*

It's time to fire President Biden's COVID-19 advisors and replace them with "pragmatists, realists and centrists — not extremists."
— Dr. Vinay Prasad

This relationship was not a one-way street. Kennedy appreciated the fact that highly credentialed doctors parroted his messages of doubt about vaccines and public health, so he was happy to amplify their voices. Kennedy's website posted several articles promoting Dr. Prasad and his calls to purge public health leaders and destroy the CDC. One article titled "'Joe, Let Them Go': Dr. Vinay Prasad Weighs in on Biden's COVID Advisors" said:

It's time to fire President Biden's COVID-19 advisors and replace them with "pragmatists, realists and centrists — not extremists," according to Vinay Prasad, M.D., M.P.H.

Referring to Drs. Anthony Fauci, Rochelle Walensky, Peter Marks, Vivek Murthy and Ashish Jha, Prasad said, "They all have to go. They have failed too many times in this pandemic."

In this week's no-holds-barred 30-minute rant, Prasad — a practicing hematologist-oncologist and professor in the Department

*of Epidemiology and Biostatistics at the University of California
San Francisco — ran through his short list of everything U.S.
public health officials got wrong.*

*Dr. Prasad provided his Substack readers with an even longer list
of reasons to dump Biden's COVID-19 team, writing:*

*"So as someone who has long believed in the value of the reg-
ulatory state, and long been a champion for increased funding
of public health, if the politician asks me 'should we destroy the
CDC,' I would have to say 'yes, please and let me help you.'"*

But in his video, he narrowed down the list to these:

- **Masking toddlers and school kids:** *"Did anyone think this was
  a good idea?"*
- **Zero cluster randomized control trials:** *"They kept saying
  follow the science, but they proved themselves to be ignorant
  scientists because they didn't take advantage of the greatest
  tool modern science has, which is randomization."*
- **The kids under 5 "vax disaster":** *"They ended up giving
  [Emergency Use] authorization for the kids under 5 for a
  vaccine they never had really credible data of a reduction in
  symptomatic disease."*
- **Adding COVID-19 vaccines to the Centers for Disease Control and Prevention immunization schedule:** *"A bone-headed
  policy."*
- **DoorDash Paxlovid:** *"They announced yesterday that they're
  going to use DoorDash to deliver Paxlovid ... Did you know
  the only available randomized control trial data for Paxlovid
  is in unvaccinated people who are at high risk of bad outcomes
  from COVID-19 who mostly didn't already have COVID-19?"*
- **Bivalent boosters without human data:** *"In the eyes of anyone
  who's actually paying attention to this they will look like fools
  to approve a bivalent booster based on mouse data."*
- **Boosting college kids who already had COVID-19:** *"This is*

258 Everyone Else is Lying to You

all a runaway train based on delusional thinking and very very bad medicine."

- **Mandates:** *"Mandates are always unethical for the young who have more to lose than gain."*

- **Myocarditis:** *"I wouldn't call that mild to take a 12-year-old and put them in the hospital for three days."*

Prasad said there's no point in being in charge of these agencies if you can't use science to minimize uncertainty. "They never provided evidence, they just kept saying louder and louder that they were right and that to me is not the hallmark of a scientist."

Prasad's parting words? "Joe, let go of these people. They are on the wrong side of every one of these issues."[108]

Even though nearly 800,000 Americans died of COVID under Biden's presidency, Dr. Prasad felt Biden's COVID advisors should be fired because they tried too hard to contain it.

Other examples about Kennedy promoting WWTI doctors and their message of doubt include:

- **"Media, Health Officials Should 'Just Tell the Truth' About COVID Shots for Kids, Physician Says":** Vinay Prasad, M.D., MPH, in a video released this week called out what he said were the *"lies and exaggerations"* about COVID-19 vaccines and kids being spread by media and public health officials.[109]

- **"'Crisis of Trust': Journalist Unravels Government's Secret Campaign to Censor Critics on Social Media":** In an interview with Jay Bhattacharya, M.D., Ph.D., investigative journalist Lee Fang exposed the *secret coordination* between government agencies, biotech firms, PR companies and social media giants to spread disinformation while censoring factual counternarratives.[110]

- **"Government Spending Millions on 'Cognitive Vaccines' to 'Protect' Public From 'Fringe' Viewpoints":** Dr. Jay Bhattacharya, Eric Weinstein, Ph.D., Nicole Shanahan, and

Mike Benz, on Wednesday discussed how government-funded "cognitive vaccines" and corporate interests are *stifling dissent and undermining public trust in science*, media, and democracy.[111]

- **"Dr. Marty Makary: Medical 'Groupthink' Harms Patients, Especially Kids":** Dr. Marty Makary, a public researcher with Johns Hopkins University and author of "Blind Spots: When Medicine Gets it Wrong, and What It Means for Our Health," said more doctors are "refusing to kiss the ring of the *medical oligarchs*, and instead are teaming up with creative people to redesign medical care."[112]

- **"Medical Mistakes Are a Leading Cause of Death in U.S. — Here's How to Protect Yourself":** The World Health Organization's surgical safety checklist, developed by Dr. Marty Makary — whose 2016 report estimated 250,000 Americans die annually from medical mistakes — has been proven to reduce adverse event rates and save lives.[113]

- **"'Many Lives Being Destroyed' by Government's Failure to Recognize Natural Immunity, Physician Says":** Dr. Marty Makary, a public health researcher at Johns Hopkins Bloomberg School of Public Health, on Tuesday accused government officials of practicing *"modern-day McCarthyism"* against anyone who suggests young healthy people, especially those who recovered from COVID, don't need booster shots.[114]

- **"Physician Speaks Out Against 'Vaccine Mandates for All' — Especially Children and Those With Natural Immunity":** In an interview with U.S. News & World Report, Dr. Marty Makary said the CDC's relentless focus on vaccine-induced immunity and its *"demonizing"* of those who choose not to get the vaccine make the agency "the most slow, reactionary, political CDC in American history."[115]

Read that again: *"lies and exaggerations," "secret coordination," "stifling dissent and undermining public trust in science," "medical oli-*

garchs," *"modern-day McCarthyism,"* *"demonizing."* This language was used to inflame and provoke Kennedy's audience.

COVID19 vaccines linked to myocarditis, pericarditis, ITP, Guillain Barre Syndrome, Bell's Palsy, ADEM, PE, Febrile seizures & more.
— The National Vaccine Information Center

Kennedy was not the only anti-vaxxer who recognized that WWTI doctors were kindred spirits in their mission to spread doubt. The National Vaccine Information Center (NVIC), America's oldest anti-vaccine organization, also shared their approval of Dr. Prasad on several occasions and used his credentials to bolster their anti-vax. They posted an article about him on social media and said:

> *COVID19 vaccines linked to myocarditis, pericarditis, ITP, Guillain Barre Syndrome, Bell's Palsy, ADEM, PE, Febrile seizures & more UCSF Professor of Epidemiology and Biostatistics and Medicine Vinay Prasad MD MPH, not some "misinformation spreader."*[116]

Other anti-vaccine social media accounts frequently shared videos of WWTI doctors, often with an introductory sentence of their own and an excerpt from the video. Below are just two accounts—@TheChiefNerd[117] and @newstart_2024[118]—who have over a million followers between them. This shows how anti-vaxxers spread the WWTI doctors' message of distrust to millions of people for years on end.

- **Dr. Jay Bhattacharya & Dr. Joseph Fraiman on Why the Vaccine Injured Were 'Public Enemy Number One' for the Biden Administration:** *"Essentially those people were public enemy number one in 2021 because the existence of those people... were a threat to the government's goal of making 80-90% of the population get the vaccine."*[119]

- **Gov. Ron DeSantis Hosts a Roundtable Discussion on the First COVID Grand Jury Report w/ Dr. Joseph Ladapo, Dr. Jay Bhattacharya, Dr. Bret Weinstein, & Dr. Joseph Fraiman:** *"With COVID it seems like there is not any commission on the horizon, there is not anyone really wanting to have an accounting so this doesn't happen again. So this Grand Jury is really serving that function for the country... and then if there is any accountability that needs to be done, they will have the ability to potentially pursue that as well."*[120]
- **Dr. Jay Bhattacharya Explains How Fauci & Birx Sabotaged Trump's Pandemic Response:** *"So he [Scott Atlas] gets called by President Trump to be an advisor. Tony Fauci and Debbie Birx basically view him as the enemy."*[121]
- **Dr. Jay Bhattacharya Debates Law Prof. Kate Klonick on Social Media Censorship During COVID Klonick:** *"This is an Orwellian telling of the actual factual record... What the factual record shows is that governments worked to suppress the speech of regular people using the leverage they had over the financial wellbeing of these platforms in order to suppress the speech of regular people."*[122]
- **Dr. Vinay Prasad Praises RFK Jr:** *"On regulatory capture, on the COVID-19 vaccine, on the FDA being a corrupt entity that needs to be entirely renovated... I completely agree with him, and I wish him well in that pursuit."*[123]
- **Dr. Vinay Prasad COOKS the Biden Administration for Pressuring Facebook to Censoring COVID Posts:** *"The ability for government to quiet people who disagree with their policies is horrific. In this case, they happened to be repeatedly wrong. I encourage Mark Zuckerberg to come further out and criticize that... And the more he tells us, I think we will find that it's going to be very bad for these people."*[124]

- **Dr. Vinay Prasad Says It's Time to Make Vaccine Makers Liable Again:** *"One of the things Robert F. Kennedy wants to do is remove a 1986 law that prevents parents from suing the company that makes the product only for vaccines. And I actually support that policy. I think vaccine makers should be able to be litigated for harms like myocarditis, which were suppressed."*[125]

- **Dr. Marty Makary & Dr. Vinay Prasad on How Dysfunctional the FDA Has Become "The FDA can be vindictive.":** *"They've done this to companies. If they don't like something you do with one study, they take it out on another submission. And that's why everyone's afraid to criticize the FDA... We talked so much previously about boosters for everybody. You had the two primary FDA reviewers, Marion Gruber and Phil Krause, resign at FDA. It actually came out they were fired. Peter Marks demoted them internally and the Biden administration put political pressure on FDA to directly approve boosters for young people, even though European nations didn't do it and even though these two reviewers felt that it was not justified, they were demoted for that. If Trump had done anything at all comparable, it would have been media armageddon."*[126]

- **Dr. Vinay Prasad Wrecks the 'Experts' Touting a New Paper Which Claims COVID Vaccinations LOWER the Risk of Heart Attacks, Clots & Strokes:** *"Here's the reality. Young men were harmed by mandates for COVID-19 vaccinations. We've proved that in a peer-reviewed paper, that the booster doses for young men had a higher risk of myocarditis than that vaccine could ever have prevented hospitalization from COVID-19. That's a clear harm... I think everyone's entitled to an opinion. But if you claim you're debunking someone and you are an idiot, which is what a lot of these people are, then I* *think it's a problem.*"[127]

- **Dr. Vinay Prasad on Regulatory Capture at the FDA & How Vaccine Mandates Led to 'Net Harm':** *"Is the [FDA's] real motivation to regulate these drug products in a way that's best for the American people, or is their real motivation an audition to some way work across the table and take that bureaucratic technical expertise and sell it to the companies — to create the hurdles they themselves know how to jump over and sell that expertise to the companies later."*[128]

- **Dr. Vinay Prasad on Harvard Firing Martin Kulldorff Over Vaccine Mandates:** *"The people who are playing games with him being fired and saying it's not about his views, they are being dishonest... The President meanwhile of Harvard, of course she stays on faculty with her $900,000 salary even though at least half of her CV is full of rampant plagiarism."*[129]

- **Dr. Vinay Prasad Fires Back at Francis Collins' Takedown of the Great Barrington Declaration:** *"You were the NIH Director. You could have had a series of Town Halls where you invited people like Jay Bhattacharya and Martin Kulldorff and had an open discussion of the pros and cons. You could have put them on YouTube. You have the powers of the federal government. You held zero debates. You just went on TV and you said proclamation after proclamation... You never tried to minimize uncertainty. You never brought anyone to the table who might disagree with you. If you were a general in war, you would be the dumbest general on the planet. Because even a general in war wants someone at the table who says, 'Hey, you think maybe we shouldn't invade someone?..Let's hear that argument.'"*[130]

- **Dr. Vinay Prasad on Being Canceled by the ACCP for 'Spreading Dangerous Misinformation':** *"Their basic claim was that they disagree with my COVID-19 policy views.*

That I spread 'dangerous misinformation'... and as a result, I shouldn't be able to give a speech on this other topic... Her letter really doesn't have a point-by-point list of the 'misinformation' I spread. She doesn't name anything, it's all a game of rumor... They're just happy to see me lose a speaking opportunity. That's what they want. That's the only goal."[131]

- **Dr. Vinay Prasad Torches Ashish Jha's Promotion of the New COVID Boosters:** *"Everything he's saying in that clip is just, as a matter-of-fact, bulls--t... These anchors are not journalists. They're just empty shills just promoting the White House propaganda."*[132]

- **Dr. Vinay Prasad Exposes the Flawed Data Used by the FDA to Support Booster Mandate:** *"The FDA is like Pfizer's lap dog. It's a little puppy dog that does whatever Pfizer says. It's enriching Pfizer and screwing the American people... There is no credible data that ever supported the booster that I was compelled by my employer to get at the risk of being fired... We caught them red handed. They slipped up. They gave us a piece of data that they didn't want to give us."*[133]

- **Dr. Vinay Prasad on the FDA Potentially Approving a 7th COVID Vaccine Dose:** *"Is this Evidence-Based Medicine, or is this Peter Marks and the FDA just making sh*t up?"*[134]

- **Dr. Vinay Prasad Calls Out The FDA For Not Making Pfizer & Moderna Do Randomized Trials for Boosters:** *"We need to force the manufacturers to generate the data and not doing that is criminal!"*[135]

- **Vinay Prasad absolutely nails it here!** *"The real lesson of medicine is that in the face of Mother Nature, you are quite impotent. And often when you think you can control it, you make it a lot worse."*[136]

- **Dr. Vinay Prasad reviews the latest UK pre-print study which compares rates of Myocarditis in younger males for vax vs virus.**[137]

- **Rep. James Comer Highlights the 'Misinformation' Spread by Public Health Officials During the Pandemic Makary:** *"There was a lot of misinformation spread during the pandemic – a lot spread by the CDC."*[138]

- **Dr. Marty Makary Roasts CDC Dir. Rochelle Walensky for Ignoring Natural Immunity:** *"Even worse she dug into her position as the data were overwhelming even to this day! ... They're still ignoring natural immunity. Even at my university you can't go to school without the primary vaccine. Even if you've had COVID 3x and were in the ICU w/ myocarditis, you still need to get the COVID vaccine. That is intellectually dishonest."*[139]

- **Dr. Marty Makary Reveals Why the CDC & NIH Dismissed Natural Immunity:** *"Let's not be honest with the public, was that the idea? ...Public health officials, people at the CDC & NIH privately told me that's what their concern was."*[140]

- **Dr. Marty Makary on How the COVID Vaccine Was Recommended for Pregnant Women With Zero Data:** *"They mysteriously stopped the trial after 349 women enrolled in the study... the results of those 349 women have never been made public"*[141]

- **Johns Hopkins Professor Dr. Marty Makary on new data showing the superiority of natural immunity:** *"The NIH controls the currency of academic medicine"*[142]

- **Shocking...** *Dr. Vinay Prasad: FDA's Marks demoted Krause, so Biden could ram COVID vax approval & mandate it | Krause's testimony.*[143]

- **Dr. Vinay Prasad: The vaccine mandates were medically unethical.** *Source: ReasonTV*[144]

- **Vinay Prasad, MD MPH; Physician & Associate Professor:** *CDC admits natural immunity is looking good!*[145]

- **Marty Makary and Tucker Carlson** - *CDC investigating whether Pfizer Covid vaccine increases stroke risk*[146]
- **Marty Makary MD, MPH:** *America has herd immunity; Covid has now the same CFR as the flu*[147]
- **Marty Makary MD, MPH:** *There is more evidence on natural immunity than there is on vaccinated immunity; one of the great failures of our medical leadership is ignoring natural immunity which changes everything.*[148]
- **Dr. Marty Makary:** *Kids more likely to die from suicide than corona.*[149]
- **Jay Bhattacharya on America's Covid "Ministry of Truth": It was a massive censorship campaign.** *"The US Federal Government systematically went to social media companies and forced them, coerced them to silence and censor COVID dissidents like me, like Sunetra. Basically, almost anybody who spoke up against the COVID government narrative faced this kind of censorship and smearing attacks. And the US federal government was actually a primary player. they would go to social media media companies, say, here are the themes we want censored, here are the ideas we want censored. Here are the people we want censored. And what the federal court found, the lower court, when they looked at this evidence, they essentially characterized it as a Ministry of Truth. It's a massive censorship campaign launched in order to protect the government policy from criticism by effective criticisms from outside scientists."*[150]
- **The Ingraham Angle - DOJ begs SCOTUS to let WH censor online speech - Dr. Jay Bhattacharya:** *It was the government that was the primary source of misinformation during the pandemic. The First Amendment would have protected us against the government misinformation had it been operative during the pandemic. The argument to Supreme Court today*

was so frustrating to hear because it was if Supreme Court justices lived through different pandemic where the government didn't say that mask stop the spread of the virus, the government didn't say that vaccines stop you from getting and spreading Covid, the government didn't say that there is no such thing as natural immunity...[151]

- **Dr. Jay Bhattacharya and Laura Ingraham** - *Exposing the dangerous gain-of-function acolytes*[152]
- **Dr. Jay Bhattacharya and Laura Ingraham** - *Public health control freaks unmasked*[153]
- **Professor Jay Bhattacharya MD:** *The lockdown harms are worse than Covid. Scientists are being silenced.*[154]

The CDC's latest guidelines could wind up lowering vaccination rates for truly dangerous diseases, like polio and measles.
— *Dr. Vinay Prasad*

We can now return to Dr. Prasad's "concern" about measles and polio. He was not a vaccine advocate before the pandemic, and often mocked doctors who were. Yet, for a few brief months in 2022, he purported to be *very concerned* about the fate of routine vaccines. However, Dr. Prasad was not worried about Kennedy and his ilk. Rather, he sensed yet another opportunity to spread disinformation about the pediatric COVID vaccine. In an article titled "Covid Vaccines Shouldn't Be 'Routine' for Kids," Dr. Prasad fretted that:

The CDC's latest guidelines could wind up lowering vaccination rates for truly dangerous diseases, like polio and measles.[155]

In reality, no American child has died from polio during my lifetime, and prior to 2025, measles last killed American children—nine of them—in 1991[156]. COVID, meanwhile, killed over 150 children in January 2021 alone.[157]

Nonetheless, for the express purpose of encouraging apathy about SARS-CoV-2—the virus that was killing children daily—Dr. Prasad faked *great concern* about polio and measles, which *infected* 339 Americans[158] combined, killing none of them. Dr. Prasad's article continued:

> *In an effort to encourage Covid-19 vaccination, the CDC may wind up lowering vaccination rates for polio and measles. Why? Because by adding Covid-19 shots to the schedule, the CDC is tacitly implying that this new vaccine is as important to kids as the combination MMR one. This is absolutely false. Measles can be a devastating childhood illness, but vaccination provides durable, sterilizing immunity. When vaccination rates are high, measles outbreaks can be averted.*[155]

Elsewhere, Dr. Prasad said:

> *A singular focus on COVID and pushing covid shots in kids, who mostly had covid (based on weak evidence/ w low yield <5% parents <5) has resulted in neglect for routine childhood immunization, which is disastrous. Many of us saw this coming.*[159]

In a "debate" on his Substack, Dr. Prasad argued that vaccinating children against COVID would lower measles vaccination rates. He said:

> *Third, and finally, doctors' time is limited. Routine childhood vaccine rates are slipping. Contrary to COVID-19 shots, the measles vaccine is sterilizing and high rates are needed to halt spread. Doctors must realize that pro-vax does not mean zealotry, but evidence first. [...] To the proposition: Should doctors encourage healthy kids (11 and under) to be vaccinated against COVID-19?*
>
> *I say, "No, Save your breath for routine vaccination."*[160]

Dr. Prasad presented no evidence that pediatricians didn't have enough time to vaccinate children against COVID and measles. However, he was right that childhood vaccine rates are slipping, and that measles can be a devastating childhood illness.

COVID can also be a devastating childhood illness, and the facts on the ground support the common-sense notion that mistrust of COVID vaccines will invariably seep into all vaccines, especially in the MAGA demographic that is listening to Kennedy. "Worst U.S. Whooping Cough Outbreak in a Decade Has Infected Thousands"[161] headlined an article from October 2024, while another article from April 2024 read, "This Year's Measles Case Total is Now the Highest in the U.S. Since 2019."[162] Meanwhile, a report published by KFF from September 2024 said:

This edition highlights vaccine hesitancy and misinformation around MMR (measles, mumps, and rubella) vaccines as children return to school and measles cases resurge in parts of the U.S. We also examine emerging narratives around COVID-19 vaccine misinformation following the FDA approval of COVID-19 boosters and false claims linking mpox to the vaccines. Additionally, a review of recent research explores strategies to combat MMR vaccine hesitancy. [...]

As students return to school, state health departments have urged families to make sure their children are up to date on recommended vaccinations. Without these immunizations, children risk contracting preventable diseases such as measles, which has seen a resurgence in several states. However, a KFF analysis highlights that routine immunization rates for kindergarteners have not returned to pre-pandemic levels, in part due to vaccine hesitancy fueled by misinformation and partisan politics. Persistent false claims include the debunked link between vaccines and autism, which has falsely led some to believe that vaccines are more harmful than the diseases they prevent. These claims downplay the severity of measles and dismiss it as rare or harmless. They also commonly suggest delaying or skipping vaccines for children to avoid unfounded risks, despite the CDC's evidence-based schedule. These misleading narratives erode public confidence in vaccines, fueling larger and faster outbreaks.[163]

Before joining the government, Drs. Prasad, Makary, and Bhattacharya were professors at the University of California, San Francisco; Johns Hopkins; and Stanford, respectively. They have impeccable credentials and claim to be "pro-vaccine" scientists who simply follow the evidence. Yet during a pandemic where 1.2 million Americans died, they developed a symbiotic relationship with America's most prominent anti-vaccine luminaries and cranks. In so doing, they showed their willingness to throw *all* vaccines under the bus to promote SARS-CoV-2 infections in unvaccinated children, spread doubt about anyone who objected, and gain power.

Sanewashing Kennedy sent a dangerous message, and it will have real-world consequences. It has already happened in Samoa[40] and in Europe,[165] and it's happening now in the U.S. According to an October 2024 NPR article titled "Worse US Whooping Cough Outbreak in a Decade Has Infected Thousands":

> *Whooping cough is spreading nationwide at the highest levels since 2014. There have been more than 16,000 cases this year — more than four times as many compared to the same time last year — and two confirmed deaths. And experts are concerned that the outbreak could worsen in the fall and winter months.*
>
> [...]

"There still is a lot of vaccine hesitancy and anti-vaxers out there that will not vaccinate their kids," said Dr. Tina Tan, a pediatric infectious disease physician at Northwestern University and the president-elect of the Infectious Diseases Society of America.[161]

The article quoted Dr. Eric Chow, the chief of epidemiology and immunization at the Seattle and King County public health department, as saying, "Sometimes you require a kind of sit-down conversation with the patient who may be a little bit more hesitant or may have encountered misinformation so it just requires a longer time to build trust and rapport."

Whooping cough is a horrible disease,[165] recently killing two infants in Louisiana,[166] and the CDC *currently* has valuable information about it.[167] In contrast, Kennedy spread anti-vaccine disinformation about it.[168] Measles is also a horrible disease. It is also surging;[169] the CDC *currently* has valuable information about it,[170] and Kennedy spread anti-vaccine disinformation about it.[171] This is a precarious moment.

Dr. Bhattacharya was right about one thing, though: If given the chance, Kennedy *will* disrupt the U.S. medical establishment. Specifically, he'll do everything he can to undermine vaccines, and when that happens, children *will* suffer. It's a law of nature. Do you think he'll let the CDC suggest the MMR in the middle of a measles outbreak? Do you think he'll suggest the HPV vaccine? Does the article from October 2024, "Kindergartener Vaccination Rates Slide Further as Exemptions Continue to Rise in the U.S."[172] concern him? Would he work to contain a bird flu outbreak? The answers are obvious, and all the doctors who gushed over and sanewashed Kennedy brought us to this moment. They own this already.

However, their journey has just begun. Although WWTI doctors advised presidents and governors during the pandemic, they absurdly felt they had the right to complain about the "medical and public health establishments,"[173] as if they were completely separate from it. Today, Drs. Prasad, Makary, and Bhattacharya have power, and they are the pinnacle of the medical establishment. Not only is COVID their responsibility, outbreaks of once-controlled diseases are happening on their watch, and it is their job to contain them.

Meanwhile, their boss, the man watching their every move, is the man behind *Vaxxed III: Authorized to Kill,* and his supporters are expecting them to deliver big results now that they have power. They were pleased that they banned the COVID vaccine for healthy people under age 65, including pregnant women. However, now that they have real-world responsibility, Drs. Makary and Prasad allowed it for older, vulnerable people. These doctors never *really* doubted the vaccine's value for this population, and they don't want their deaths on their hands.

Yet, the damage is done. Drs. Prasad, Makary, and Bhattacharya told people not to trust the medical establishment, and largely thanks to their efforts, many people no longer trust the medical establishment. Not only will many vulnerable people skip the booster and suffer as a result, but anti-vaxxers want the COVID vaccine banned for them too. Since Drs. Makary and Prasad don't want to do this, their anti-vax base, the people they cozied up to and legitimized for the past 4 years, has turned on them with a vengeance. As the saying goes, if you lie down with dogs, you get fleas.

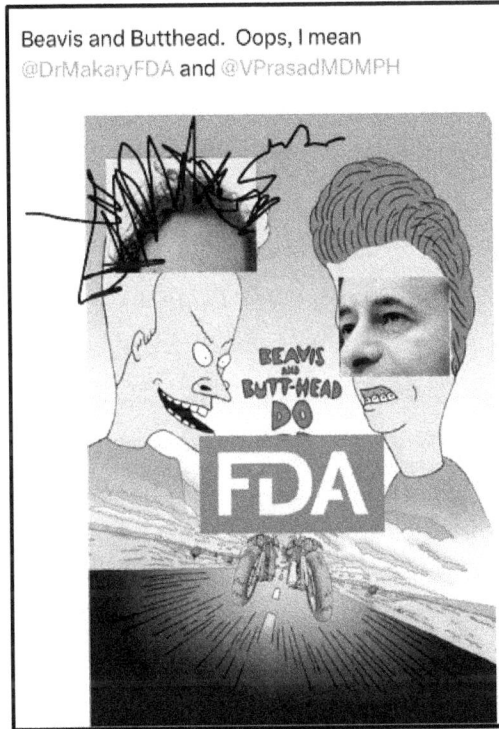

An anti-vax meme mocking Drs. Vinay Prasad
and Marty Makary after they approved the
Moderna vaccine for vulnerable populations

Chapter 6: The Historical Record is Critical. We Have Seen a Macabre Orwellian Attempt to Rewrite History

Straight out lies by @JamesSurowiecki
— Dr. Martin Kulldorff

According to Wikipedia:

> *Nikolai Ivanovich Yezhov was a Soviet secret police official under Joseph Stalin who was head of the People's Commissariat for Internal Affairs from 1936 to 1938, during the height of the Great Purge. Yezhov organized mass arrests, torture and executions during the Great Purge, but he fell from Stalin's favour and was arrested, subsequently admitting in a confession to a range of anti-Soviet activity including "unfounded arrests" during the Purge. He was executed in 1940 along with others who were blamed for the Purge.*[1]

After his death, Yezhov was removed from pictures where he was standing next to Stalin as part of Soviet propaganda. It was as if he never existed at all. A similar movement is under way to erase the history of the pandemic.

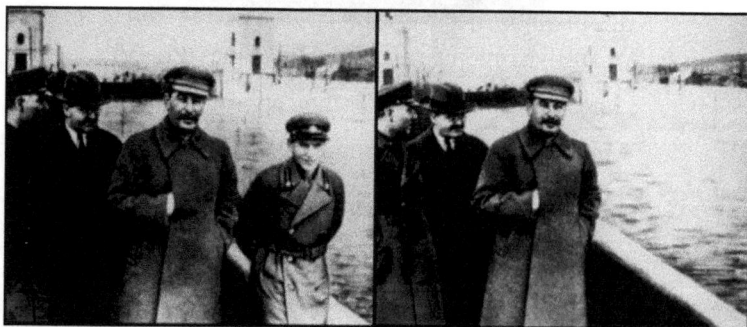

The erasure of Nikolai Ivanovich Yezhov. Source: *Wikipedia*

In December 2022, journalist James Surowiecki posted a quote from Dr. Jay Bhattacharya that blamed others for spreading disinformation. According to Dr. Bhattacharya:

> *Governments have been the most important and damaging source of misinformation during the pandemic.*[2]

Mr. Surowiecki was not impressed. He said:

> *Sunetra Gupta, co-author of the Great Barrington Declaration, claimed in May 2020 that the pandemic was "on its way out." In June 2021, Bhattacharya and Martin Kulldorff said exactly the same thing, right before Delta hit. They're in no position to talk about "misinformation."*[3]

Dr. Martin Kulldorff, one of the three authors of the GBD, responded with:

> *Straight out lies by @JamesSurowiecki. We wrote the @gbdeclaration correctly expecting a second wave in winter 2020/21, while many lockdowners thought lockdowns had worked. And, said anything of the kind in June 2021.*[4]

Mr. Surowiecki replied in turn:

> *Amazing Twitter moment. Martin Kulldorff calling me a "straight-out" liar, and denying that he and Jay Bhattacharya claimed in June 2021 that the pandemic was on its way out. June 27, 2021, WSJ article by Kulldorff and Bhattacharya begins: "The pandemic is on its way out."*[5]
>
> *I don't use the word gaslighting that often, but denying you said something that you literally published in* The Wall Street Journal, *and calling someone else a "straight-out" liar for citing it, definitely counts as "gaslighting."*[6]

So is Mr. Surowiecki a "straight-out liar?" No, he is not. In June

2021, just before Delta arrived, Drs. Kulldorff and Bhattacharya wrote an article titled "A Covid Commission Americans Can Trust" that began, *"The pandemic is on its way out."*[7] Delta arrived immediately after that.

This blatant denial of obvious reality became commonplace during the pandemic. As the virus obliterated doctors' predictions that "natural immunity" was "powerful" and that herd immunity was imminent, WWTI doctors denied their own words and committed verbicide, rejecting the idea that words have objective meanings. Language itself became a pandemic casualty.

As the pandemic progressed, WWTI doctors tried to erase the entire WWTI movement and ultimately the virus and its victims. Many aspects of the pandemic suffered the same fate as Nikolai Ivanovich Yezhov's photo. It's worthwhile to go over several examples to show that this was not an isolated incident, but part of a coherent pattern to rewrite the history of the pandemic and deny its horrors.

> **The piece was not about vaccinating young kids.**
> — *Dr. Stefan Baral*

My first article[8] for *Science-Based Medicine* was a rebuttal to a paper published in *The BMJ* by Drs. Wesley Pegden, Vinay Prasad, and Stefan Baral. The central thesis of their article was that "the likelihood of severe outcomes or death associated with COVID-19 infection is very low for children, undermining the appropriateness of an emergency use authorization for child COVID-19 vaccines."[9] Dr. Prasad further elaborated on this by posting:

> *Vast majority of kids recover quickly from SARS cov 2. And after all adults are vaccinated their risk of covid will decline precipitously. It's ok to acknowledge that covid19 is not an emergency for kids.*[10]

That aged poorly. Delta and Omicron arrived before the end of the year, each causing an unprecedented wave of illness in children. Fortunately, regulators issued the emergency use authorization and millions of children were able to be safely vaccinated. Meanwhile, the vaccine was found to save children from rare but grave outcomes. One study found:

> *During the period of time in which the Delta variant of the SARS-CoV-2 virus emerged and became dominant, the researchers found that adolescents (defined as patients who were 12- to 20-years old) who received the vaccine were approximately 98 percent less likely to be infected or have severe disease compared to those who did not receive it, with no evidence of increased cardiac complications or significant waning infection protection over the subsequent four months.*
>
> *Vaccination proved strongly protective against the Omicron wave, albeit at a lower magnitude than during Delta. Among adolescents, those who were vaccinated were roughly 86 percent less likely to be infected compared to unvaccinated peers, and their protection against severe illness and ICU admission was similarly high, being approximately 85 and 91 percent less likely, respectively, than the unvaccinated.*[11]

Yet the authors of the article, "Covid Vaccines for Children Should Not Get Emergency Use Authorization,"[9] later claimed the article had nothing to do with vaccines or children. In response to critics, Dr. Pedgen said, "The accusation doesn't even seem to be that we argued against vaccinating kids (which we didn't)."[12] Dr. Baral similarly responded by saying:

> *With all due respect, all we called for is the ACIP to meet and discuss. The piece was not about vaccinating young kids as*

compared to going through due diligence in deciding whether to
vaccinate young children.[13]

In an article for the Brownstone Institute, Dr. Prasad stated:

In May of 2021, Wes Pegden, Stef Baral and I argued in the BMJ
that kids vaccination should proceed via biological licensing
agreement pathway and not the emergency use authorization. Be-
cause these risks were so low, we must demand robust evidence
and large trials to show that the potential benefits of vaccination
outweigh potential harms. […] We wanted large randomized
trials.[14]

None of this was true. In reality, their article did not call on the Advisory Committee on Immunization Practices (ACIP) to "meet and discuss" as Dr. Baral claimed. It didn't mention the ACIP at all. Similarly, it did not propose "large randomized trials" as Dr. Prasad claimed. Rather than defend their idea that the emergency use authorization was a mistake, and the vaccine should have been unavailable to children when Delta and Omicron emerged, Drs. Pegden, Prasad, and Baral claimed their article didn't say what it said.

If it's true that the novel coronavirus would kill millions without
shelter-in-place orders and quarantines, then the extraordinary mea-
sures being carried out […] are surely justified.
— *Dr. Jay Bhattacharya*

In March 2020, Dr. Bhattacharya wrote an article in which he claimed, "Projections of the death toll could plausibly be orders of magnitude too high."[15] He speculated COVID would kill 20,000–40,000 Americans. This article began by saying:

If it's true that the novel coronavirus would kill millions without
shelter-in-place orders and quarantines, then the extraordinary

measures being carried out in cities and states around the country are surely justified.

That's a *much stronger* defense of shelter-in-place orders and quarantines than I ever wrote. Yet, when Dr. Bhattacharya was reminded of his eminently reasonable justification for shelter-in-place orders and quarantines, he denied his own words and claimed to be a victim because people accurately quoted him:

> *I wrote that sentence in the WSJ piece. But the extraordinary measures I advocated was not lockdown, but rather a rapid seroprevalence study and a focused protection approach. The people who keep that blog* [Science Based Medicine] *you show are lockdowners & have slandered me throughout the epidemic. [...] They excel in taking quotes out of context and spinning false conspiracy stories about funding.*[16]

So according to Dr. Bhattacharya, "shelter-in-place orders and quarantines" *really meant* a "rapid seroprevalence study and a focused protection approach." Dr. Bhattacharya became upset when I suggested to him that "shelter-in-place orders and quarantines" *really meant* "shelter-in-place orders and quarantines."

> *You are tiresome joho. How many times have people corrected your misreading of my article, and how many times have you ignored the correction? You argue in bad faith. Go troll someone else.*[17]

I still maintain that "shelter-in-place orders and quarantines" *really means* shelter-in-place orders and quarantines; however, this was just one example of Dr. Bhattacharya's attempts to redefine words while avoiding admitting error.

Herd immunity occurs when enough people have immunity so that most infected people cannot find new uninfected people to infect, leading to the end of the epidemic/pandemic.
— *Great Barrington Declaration*

The Great Barrington Declaration (GBD) said the following about herd immunity:

> **What is herd immunity?**
>
> *Herd immunity occurs when enough people have immunity so that most infected people cannot find new uninfected people to infect, leading to the end of the epidemic/pandemic.*[18]

That's a reasonable and widely accepted definition of herd immunity. Herd immunity refers to *cases* and the risk a virus poses to people without immunity to it. Dr. Bhattacharya and WWTI doctors treated herd immunity to COVID as inevitable in 2020. Dr. Bhattacharya further elaborated on the meaning of herd immunity in May 2021:

> *Herd immunity means the disease isn't spreading at high rates. It doesn't mean the disease is gone. In that sense, we're kind of already there but the disease has mostly stopped spreading in the US. Now it may come back, because this is very clearly a seasonal disease.*[19]

Dr. Bhattacharya was right: *herd immunity means the disease isn't spreading at high rates.* However, we weren't "kind of already there" in May 2021. Delta arrived immediately after this, proving that COVID was not seasonal and ruining his fantasies of herd immunity through mass infection.

To avoid admitting this error, however, Dr. Bhattacharya later invented his own definition of herd immunity. In an interview from 2022, he said:

What herd immunity looks like is you've had COVID before and recovered, or maybe you've had the vaccine, or whatever, but now if you get COVID it's much less likely to produce severe disease and death, because you have that immunity.[20]

Thankfully, it's true that COVID is killing much fewer people than before. An article from August 2024 confirms the declining death toll:

Provisional data from the National Center for Health Statistics (NCHS) on the top causes of deaths in the United States in 2023 shows COVID-19 dropped to the tenth leading cause of death. In 2022, it was the fourth leading cause of death, meaning deaths from COVID dropped by 68.9% in one year.[21]

However, unless SARS-CoV-2 mutated into significantly more virulent forms, it was always the case that fewer people would die from it as the pandemic progressed. The actual term for this is mortality displacement,[22] *not* herd immunity, and it reflects how the underlying population has changed since 2020. Not only is the virus not encountering an immunologically naive population, people can only die once. Tragically, 1.2 million Americans, who were by definition "vulnerable," are no longer available for the virus to kill a second time. As one person put it on social media:

If a rampaging bear keeps attacking the campgrounds, all the people who weren't able to outrun the bear the first time he attacked will already be dead the next time the bear rampages through the campsite. The lower death count doesn't mean the bear became tamer.[23]

Indeed, much like a rampaging bear who picked off the easy victims first, COVID's lower death count doesn't mean SARS-CoV-2 has weakened over time. Even with vaccines, COVID is still killing many more people than the flu,[24] often over 1,000 Americans per week.[25] Most importantly, the virus is still infecting enough people to generate headlines in August 2024 like "Summer COVID Surge Hits at Least 84 Countries and Continues to Climb."[26] Yet, according to Dr. Bhattacharya, he was not wrong about herd immunity in 2020. This is because WWTI doctors reject the idea that words have objective meanings.

> **To me the most concerning issue is a lot of what was considered misinformation was and is true: vaccines don't halt transmission.**
> — *Dr. Vinay Prasad*

At other times, WWTI doctors did more than deny their own words; they blamed other people for them. In early 2021, Dr. Prasad was convinced that vaccines would end the pandemic, and that adult vaccination would obviate the need to vaccinate children. An article from May 2021 quoted him as saying:

> *For somebody who's already been fully vaccinated, they can wear the mask out of solidarity or in a symbolic sense, but their wearing a mask indoors is not benefiting anyone else. There's an infinitesimally low probability of even having an infection that can be detected on a PCR test, let alone being able to spread it to someone.*[27]

Yet, Dr. Prasad later blamed the vaccine manufacturers as well as the "government & its actors" for making this claim. He said:

- **April 2022:** *Ironically, some of the worst misinformation came from government & its actors -masks, myocarditis, do vaccines halt transmission.*[28]
- **October 2022:** *I hadn't noticed this Pfizer tweet, but it's pretty clear that the company engaged in illegal marketing. Trans-*

*mission was not a primary or secondary endpoint of the study.
They had no basis to speak about it. Normally, this would be
investigated.*[29]

- **October 2022:** *It was abundantly clear that the vaccine
trials did not include transmission as a primary or secondary
endpoint. And thus could not comment. This tweet does appear
to be violating US law around misleading information. In a
normal world, Pfizer would be investigated for this.*[30]

- **October 2024:** *To me the most concerning issue is a lot of
what was considered misinformation was and is true: vaccines
don't halt transmission.*[31]

He was not alone. In a podcast from April 2021, Dr. Bhattacharya
had the following exchange with Dr. Zubin Damania:

> **Dr. Damania:** *Now, you and I are both vaccinated. We shook
> hands. We don't wear masks. We're about three feet apart from
> each other. And in the early days of the pandemic that would've
> gotten us both hung. But now I can say with confidence because
> I've looked at the data, like our chances of giving each other
> COVID are-*
> **Dr. Bhattacharya:** *Are zero.*
> **Dr. Damania:** *Pretty much zero.*[32]

Yet, during Congressional testimony from 2023, Dr. Bhattacharya
said the following.

> *What this case has revealed is that a dozen federal agencies,
> including the CDC, the Office of the Surgeon General, and the
> White House, pressured social media companies like Google,
> Facebook, and Twitter to censor and deboost even true speech
> that contradicted federal pandemic priorities, including especial-
> ly inconvenient facts about the covid vaccines, such as its ineffi-
> cacy against covid disease transmission.*[33]

Elsewhere, Dr. Bhattacharya said such claims, at least when made by public health officials, were not "honest mistakes." In his article titled "It's Time for Laws Limiting the Power of Public Health Institutions," he wrote the following:

> *Contrary to what you hear these days from those making poor decisions throughout the pandemic, many of the errors were not honest mistakes. Public health embraced positions at odds with the scientific evidence throughout the pandemic, for instance, by pretending that immunity after COVID recovery does not exist, and by overstating the ability of the vaccine to stop COVID infection and transmission.*[34]

Dr. Bhattacharya often repeated this message on social media:

> *Just wondering. Did the fact checkers ever correct Tony Fauci, Rochelle Walensky, or Rachel Maddow for saying that the covid vax prevents you from getting and spreading covid? If not, why not? It was one of the biggest lies of the covid era.*[35]

According to Dr. Bhattacharya, who said vaccinated people have a "zero" chance of spreading the virus, the CDC, Office of the Surgeon General, The White House, Anthony Fauci, Rochelle Walensky, and Rachel Maddow were to blame for his statement, and this was not an "honest mistake."

I've never said nor thought, "we want them infected"
— Dr. Jay Bhattacharya

However, WWTI doctors' commitment to denying their own words is much larger than denying a couple sentences here or there. They are part of a movement to deny the entire plan for herd immunity via mass infection even existed. In 2023, upon learning that I had linked him with the WWTI movement, Dr. Bhattacharya said:

> *I've never said nor thought, "we want them infected", and yet what would a casual reader take away from this misleading juxtaposition? The piece creates a false impression about @gbdeclaration for cheap political points.*[36]

Elsewhere he said:

> *Jonathan, each element of your tweet is a lie. I never told anyone to contract covid, certainly not en masse. You misread the GBD and mistake the privilege some people have to be hermits with virtue.*[37]

Dr. Bhattacharya also often said, "The GBD is the antithesis of a 'let it rip' strategy."[38]

Those are harsh words. Am I a liar? Fortunately, there's an easily accessible record of what WWTI doctors said in 2020. They had six core beliefs at the time, many of which have since received the same treatment as Nikolai Ivanovich Yezhov's photograph.

Core Belief #1: Covid Was Only Dangerous for Vulnerable People and Those Over Age 60 or Maybe 70

The GBD was premised on the false notion that people could be dichotomized into "vulnerable" and "not vulnerable" categories and the two groups could be hermetically sealed off from each other for months on end. "Vulnerable" people would live in a world of zero COVID, while "not vulnerable" would live in a world of pure COVID. To numb people to the risk this posed, the authors of the GBD routinely minimized COVID's risk to children and young adults, often using fake statistics. The FAQ section of the GBD said:

It is important to distinguish between the risk of infection and the
risk of death. Anyone can get infected, but there is more than a
thousand-fold difference in the risk of death between the oldest
and youngest. For old people, COVID-19 is more dangerous than
the annual influenza. For children, the COVID-19 mortality risk
is less than for the annual influenza. [18]

In reality, at least 115 children had died of COVID by this point in
the pandemic[39], while nine children died of flu.[40]

The GBD also said that COVID posed a risk only to people over 60.
It said:

People in their 60s are at somewhat high risk, and many are still
in the workforce. [18]

In interviews from 2020, the GBD's authors often raised that number.
For example, in November 2020, Dr. Bhattacharya similarly said:

For people under 70, it's 99.95% survival. It's much less deadly
for people who are under 70, 99.95%. [41]

COVID became a leading killer of young adults in 2021, even though
vaccines were available, and while death is the only outcome recognized
by the GBD, it is not COVID's only harm, even to children. WWTI doctors have never revisited their claims that the virus spared young people.

15-24	25-34	35-44	45-54
Unintentional Injury 15,792	Unintentional Injury 34,452	Unintentional Injury 36,444	Covid-19 36,881
Homicide 6,635	Suicide 8,862	Covid-19 16,006	Heart Disease 34,535
Suicide 6,528	Homicide 7,571	Heart Disease 12,754	Malignant Neoplasms 33,567
Covid-19 1,401	Covid-19 6,133	Malignant Neoplasms 11,194	Unintentional Injury 31,407

Leading causes of death, 2021. Source: CDC[42]

Core Belief #2: Children Don't Spread COVID

In April 2020, Dr. Bhattacharya said, "It's very unlikely that kids will pass the COVID-19 infection to their parents or to adults. It almost always runs in the other direction."[43]

The FAQ section of the GBD said:

We know that older people living with working-age adults have higher COVID-19 risk than older people living with other older people. There is no further excess risk if also living with children though.[18]

As the pandemic progressed, the authors of the GBD continued to claim that children did not spread the virus. In an interview from May 2023, Dr. Bhattacharya stated:

> Teachers were actually at lower risk of COVID than the population of other workers at large. Being around kids actually protected them, in some sense, because the kids are not super-spreaders.[44]

Even if children did not spread early SARS-CoV-2 variants, it turned out that they spread newer variants quite effectively. One systematic review and meta-analysis from 2022 reported:

> Unlike with the ancestral virus, children infected with variants of concern spread SARS-CoV-2 to an equivalent number of household contacts as infected adults and were equally as likely to acquire SARS-CoV-2 VOC from an infected family member.[45]

WWTI doctors have never revisited their claims that children don't spread the virus.

Core Belief #3: Natural Immunity Was Powerful and Reinfections Were Rare

Although the virus was less than a year-old, WWTI doctors spoke about it with great confidence in 2020. The GBD said:

> **Antibodies fade after COVID-19 infection. Does that mean natural immunity fades?** That the antibody response fades over time after COVID infections was already known from a large body of literature.
>
> However, it is also true that antibody response is not the only response our immune systems have in response to infection, and these

other immune responses (e.g. the production of specific T-cells) ap-
pears to be quite long lasting. You can see this in the fact that that
despite an estimated 750 million worldwide to date after 10 months
living with the virus, we have seen only a handful of reinfections.
If the virus is like other corona viruses in its immune response,
recovery from infection will provide lasting protection against rein-
fection, either complete immunity or protection that makes a severe
reinfection less likely.[18]

During a recording at the time, its authors had this conversation:

Dr. Gupta: *But so, we might get these sorts of epidemics, but there*
are two issues here. One is that the people who will be exposed to
the virus in the, in the new epidemic will be the young, the newborns
who will be exposed to the first time. And for them, the risk is prob-
ably not terribly high from what we're seeing. And for those of us
who might be re -exposed, again, it's likely from looking at the other
coronaviruses, that reinfection will not carry the same risk of severe
disease and death. And that's also true for many other pathogens.
But the second exposure does not carry the same risks. I think in the
early days of the coronavirus, this novel coronavirus epidemic, there
was some worry about whether immunity actually was generated by
infection.

Dr. Bhattacharya: *It sounds like that's not so much of a word that*
we've seen immunity in the context of infections with SARS-CoV-2,
is that true? Yeah, I would certainly say so. How many reinfections
have there been today?

Dr. Gupta: *Well, I mean, even if we had seen one or two reinfec-*
tions, I mean, we know that people get reinfected with chicken pox.

It doesn't. We don't immediately abandon the idea that you get lifelong immunity to chicken pox or measles or anything from the few incidents.

Dr. Bhattacharya*: We're talking about a very small number.*

Dr. Gupta*: A very small number of reinfections. Do not indicate anything about the actual distribution.*

Dr. Bhattacharya*: So, in that sense, when we're talking about SARS-CoV-2, it fits into the picture of the natural history of the typical virus, as you've described. It's not a virus from Mars; it's a virus that, in that sense, we can set expectations from the modeling and the kind of analysis we expected. Eventually, it will go down; even without a vaccine, it will go down.*

Dr. Gupta*: Yes, I think so. I think it's not probably immunity is not lifelong if we go by the other coronaviruses, but it's long enough that it will result in this endemic state where the number of people infected at any point in time might be a bit higher than measles, but the effects on people, the actual death toll […]*[46]

We know now that COVID reinfections are common and not always benign. An NIH-funded study from 2024 found:

> *Using health data from almost 213,000 Americans who experienced reinfections, researchers have found that severe infections from the virus that causes COVID-19 tend to foreshadow similar severity of infection the next time a person contracts the disease.*[47]

WWTI doctors have never revisited their claims that "natural immunity" was powerful and long lasting.

Core Belief #4: Herd Immunity Was Inevitable

Because they thought that COVID reinfections were rare, the GBD claimed herd immunity was inevitable, mocking anyone who doubted its imminent arrival. The GBD itself said:

Do you believe in herd immunity?

Yes. Herd immunity is a scientifically proven phenomenon. To ask an epidemiologist if they believe in herd immunity is like asking a physicist if they believe in gravity. Those who deny herd immunity may also wish to join the flat-earth society.

With COVID-19, can herd immunity be avoided?

No. Sooner or later, herd immunity will be reached either through natural infection or through a combination of vaccinations and natural infection.[18]

They repeated this message often on social media in the first part of the pandemic, saying in December 2020:

For COVID-19, all strategies lead to herd immunity, making it nonsensical to denote one specific approach as a herd immunity strategy just as it does not make sense for airplane pilots to talk about a "gravity strategy" for safely landing a plane.[48]

They authored articles such as "We May Already Have Herd Immunity – an Interview With Professor Sunetra Gupta"[49] and "It's Mad That 'Herd Immunity' Was Ever a Taboo Phrase."[50] That last article, by Drs. Kulldorff and Bhattacharya, was from May 2021. It said:

The denial of a basic scientific concept by so many prominent authorities is stunning - and alarming.

Herd immunity is fundamental in epidemiological science.

COVID spreads in populations when infectious individuals come in contact with individuals who are not already immune. Herd immunity reflects the obvious concept that an uninfected individ-

ual is less likely to catch the disease when a larger part of the
population is immune. While COVID cannot be eradicated, herd
immunity assures that in the long run, it will stay at low levels
with few hospitalisations and deaths.

Just like gravity, herd immunity is a scientific fact. To the shock of
many infectious disease epidemiologists, politicians, some media,
and scientists turned it into a dirty word. Some talked about a
'herd immunity strategy,' but every strategy leads to herd immu-
nity, so that is as nonsensical as pilots using a 'gravity strategy'
to land a plane. The plane will reach the ground no matter what;
the key is to land safely.

Both Delta and Omicron arrived before the end of the year, and we
still do not have herd immunity to COVID.

WWTI doctors have never revisited their claims that herd immunity
was inevitable.

**Core Belief #5: Mitigation Measures Were Bad Not Because They
Didn't Limit COVID, But Precisely Because They Limited COVID.**

From the moment they were implemented, WWTI doctors objected to mitigation measures. In an interview from March 2020, Dr.
Bhattacharya worried not about schools but about suppressing the
economy. He said:

It could be that many, many places around the country, including
California, it's safe to lift the caps. So the next step to me is run
the studies everywhere, redo the models, and take a hard look
and ask, is it really worth it to suppress the economy if I'm not
going to stress the hospital systems and have COVID-19 patients

die as a result of it.[51]

As early as March 2020, some WWTI doctors began speaking about lockdowns in apocalyptic terms. Dr. John Ioannidis made the following statement at that time:

> *Locking down the world with potentially tremendous social and financial consequences may be totally irrational. It's like an elephant being attacked by a house cat. Frustrated and trying to avoid the cat, the elephant accidentally jumps off a cliff and dies.*
>
> [...]
>
> *One of the bottom lines is that we don't know how long social distancing measures and lockdowns can be maintained without major consequences to the economy, society, and mental health. Unpredictable evolutions may ensue, including financial crisis, unrest, civil strife, war, and a meltdown of the social fabric.*[52]

Dr. Scott Atlas echoed these sentiments in an interview with a Russian propaganda outlet in 2020. He said:

> *The lockdowns will go down as an epic failure of public policy. The argument is undeniable. The lockdowns are killing people.*[53]

Even though lockdowns ended long ago, WWTI doctors constantly speak about them in this way today. It's easy to find quotes such as "lockdowns are the biggest assault on workers since segregation and the Vietnam War"[54] and "the biggest public health mistake we've ever made... The harm to people is catastrophic."[55] WWTI doctors blame lockdowns for nearly every societal ill, including "Plummeting childhood vaccination rates, worse cardiovascular disease outcomes, less cancer screening, and deteriorating mental health."[56]

However, in 2020 WWTI doctors objected to mitigation measures not because they felt they didn't limit infections, but precisely *because* they limited infections. They feared that if enough people lacked "natural immunity," this would just prolong the pandemic. Some examples include:

- **Great Barrington Declaration, October 2020**: *Lockdowns do not reduce the total number of cases in the long run and have never in history led to the eradication of a disease. At best, lockdowns delay the increase of cases for a finite period and at great cost.*[18]

- **Sunetra Gupta, November 2020**: *I was also deeply concerned that lockdowns only delay the inevitable spread of the virus.*[57]

- **Dr. Martin Kulldorff, December 2020**: *Lockdowns just prolonged the pandemic while failing to protect the old.*[58]

Although WWTI doctors now claim they were mostly concerned about the plight of poor children and the working class, they continue to protest that lockdowns delayed infections.

- **Sunetra Gupta, April 2022**: *Community-wide interventions did very little to alter the natural course of the pandemic and served only to delay the inevitable.*[59]

- **Dr. Jay Bhattacharya, September 2022**: *I think lockdowns protected for short times. It moved the incidences of cases forward from March 2020 forward to maybe six months, a year.*[60]

- **Drs. Martin Kulldorff and Jay Bhattacharya, February 2022**: *Lockdowns just postponed the inevitable.*[61]

There is some truth to this. Very few people have avoided COVID entirely. However, much of medicine is about postponing the inevitable. A person who gets COVID today, especially if they are up to date on their vaccines, is in much better shape than someone who got it in March 2020 when hospitals were overflowing and the disease was brand new.

Core Belief #6: The Mass Infection of Unvaccinated Youth Would Rapidly Lead to Herd Immunity and End the Pandemic.

This was the one ring to rule them all. The previous five beliefs were in service of the belief that the mass infection of unvaccinated youth and middle-aged adults would rapidly lead to herd immunity. WWTI doctors spread this message widely in 2020. They recorded it on video, tweeted it out, and wrote it in their Declaration. As the GBD put it:

> The most compassionate approach that balances the risks and benefits of reaching herd immunity is to allow those who are at minimal risk of death to live their lives normally to build up immunity to the virus through natural infection while better protecting those who are at highest risk. We call this Focused Protection.[62]

In his article from August 2020, "Herd Immunity Is Still Key in the Fight Against Covid-19," Dr. Kulldorff wrote:

> As a society we should appreciate young adults who help generate herd immunity by living normal lives and keeping society afloat. Thank you, thank you, thank you. When people throw misguided complaints at you, falsely claiming that you are endangering others, remember that the opposite is true.[63]

The next month, Dr. Sunetra Gupta stated in an interview:

> But the best way we can protect lives, both of those who are vulnerable to COVID and those who are vulnerable to the measures that we're taking to protect ourselves from COVID, is by allowing the infection to spread among those who are not vulnerable, such that immunity is built up in the population, which then brings the risk of infection down, let's say by Christmas, for ex-

ample, to those who are vulnerable to COVID.

And in the process, during that period when immunity is going to be built up, and we don't know how much immunity we need to build up, we've previously suggested that there is already substantial amounts of immunity in the population.

But, you know, we don't know that, but let's, if we take the measure, the view that, okay, we don't know how much immunity there is, but we do know that we can build up enough immunity to keep the risks low. So why not go ahead and do that? And meanwhile, aggressively shield the vulnerable population.[64]

The GBD spread the virtues of "natural immunity" frequently on social media in 2020 and 2021. Examples include:

- *Clear and compelling arguments for why using vaccines to deliver focused protection and allowing natural immunity to do the rest provides a robust and sustainable solution.*[65]
- *Focused Protection would allow those who are at minimal risk of death to live their lives normally to build up immunity to the virus through natural infection, while better protecting those who are at highest risk.*[66]
- *The Declaration advocates a strategy that minimizes mortality until herd immunity is reached. That is done by minimizing the number of older high-risk people in the group that get infected while maximizing them among those that are still uninfected when herd immunity arrives.*[67]

There is no difference between "maximizing them (infections) among those that are still uninfected" and "we want them infected."

The GBD was dedicated to "natural immunity" at this time because they thought it would end the pandemic within 3 to 6 months. They claimed the whole thing could all be over by April 2021 at the latest if only infections were maximized. This required approximately 230 million or so unvaccinated Americans to contract COVID during this interval. After this, the GBD claimed the virus would no longer be a threat to vulnerable people. POOF! The world would be safe, and life could resume normally. The FAQ of the GBD promised this optimistic message:

> **For how long must high-risk individuals be careful and/or self-isolate?**
>
> *When herd immunity is reached, they can live normally again with minimal risks. How long that takes depends on the strategy used. If age-wide lockdown measures are used to try and suppress the disease, it could take a year or two or three, making it very difficult for older people to protect themselves for that long. If focused protection is used, it will likely only take 3 to 6 months.*[18]

They also promoted this optimistic message on social media. One exchange from December 2020 said:

> **Question:** *I'm in my 60s. As per Plan B and @gbdeclaration I would have been in my 8th month of isolation and home delivery. I am absolutely sure this would not have reduced the economic impact of Covid or saved lives. This was never an option in New Zealand. Am I wrong?*[68]
>
> **GBD Answer:** *No we do not believe that would have been the case. Within the Focused Protection strategy - comprehensive shielding of the Elderly and vulnerable - with resources directed to those people -to you, would have had to be in place for 3 - 6 months.*[69]

Dr. Kulldorff said in December 2020:

> *If the young live normal lives, some will be infected, but their risk is less than from lockdown collateral damage. Pandemic will then be naturally over in 3-6 months.*[58]

In 2020, WWTI doctors wanted to rapidly maximize infections in young people, believing this would end the pandemic in less than half a year. However, today Dr. Bhattacharya claims he *"never said nor thought, 'we want them infected'"* and that *"the GBD is the antithesis of a 'let it rip' strategy."* Meanwhile, the GBD's social media feed is a ghost town full of forgotten celebrations of "natural immunity" like this:

> We promote a strategy called Focused Protection that would use
> resources to properly and comprehensively protect the elderly
> and vulnerable in society. Whilst allowing natural immunity to
> build up within the "working well." Please do read further.[70]

WWTI doctors have never revisited their claims that allowing "natural immunity" to build up within the "working well" would protect the elderly and vulnerable.

It's important to acknowledge that in 2020, the focus was mostly about using the kids as guinea pigs [...] to achieve herd immunity + faster reopening.
— *Dr. Jerome Adams*

These examples are all just small parts of the larger project to deny the WWTI movement ever existed. Today, WWTI doctors excoriate anyone who accurately remembers their pro-infection rhetoric from 2020.

Dr. Jerome Adams, who served as Surgeon General in the first Trump administration, is often mocked and criticized by WWTI doctors for two reasons. His first sin is that he still tells people to take COVID seriously, and he models the cautious behavior himself. His second sin is that he remembers.

In 2023, Dr. Adams caused a stir on social media by posting the following:

The pandemic school closure debate is now often framed as being solely about the kids. However, it's important to acknowledge that in 2020, the focus was mostly about using the kids as guinea pigs (ie subjecting them to a new virus) to achieve herd immunity + faster reopening.

My intent isn't to attack Atlas or anyone else. It's to remind us the context at the time for these policy debates, and the tradeoffs people don't acknowledge or forget about in hindsight. Many were fine with exposing kids (and school workers) to a deadly virus, with no vaccine or treatment, in the name of herd immunity. That's a fact. It's also a fact that Atlas's (and GBD's) herd immunity push was supposedly explicitly predicated on a commitment to FIRST protecting the vulnerable. Over a million are dead- so clearly we didn't do a good job of that.[71]

Dr. Adams also posted a page of his book on the pandemic, which said:

In hindsight, put another way, people act as if the concern was always and solely about the welfare of kids. In real time, however, most of the conversation led by Dr. Atlas and others who focused on this concept of forcing schools to open and facilitate herd immunity was about how deliberately infecting the kids would ultimately help the adults who wanted the economy to open. All of the doctors on the task force considered Dr. Scott's ideas for achieving herd immunity by essentially using our children as guinea pigs to be a non-starter.

Totally dishonest. I watched most of @ScottAtlas_IT press conferences and, agree or disagree, he repeatedly said kids were at such low risk, they might as well go to school, and derive the massive benefit of education.

— *Dr. Vinay Prasad*

Despite Dr. Atlas's multiple declarations in 2020 that "natural immunity" would lead to herd immunity, WWTI doctors now try to pretend none of that ever happened. In their telling, Dr. Atlas wasn't a leader of a failed movement to purposely infect unvaccinated youth. Instead, he was a tireless warrior for education, who merely wanted to nurture and care for our precious children.

Dr. Prasad blasted Dr. Adams, saying:

> *Totally dishonest. I watched most of @ScottAtlas_IT press conferences and, agree or disagree, he repeatedly said kids were at such low risk, they might as well go to school, and derive the massive benefit of education.*[72]

Dr. Bhattacharya similarly said:

> *This quote from the former SG is simply untrue. I spoke regularly with Scott Atlas in spring & summer 2020. His motivation derived from his understanding of the importance of schools for the well being of children and from the Swedish success in spring 2020 with open schools.*
>
> *I'll go one step further. It was evident to me at the time and now that the people who pushed lockdowns and school closures had no concern whatsoever about the well being of children, thinking of them primarily as vectors of disease to be suppressed rather than precious young people to be nurtured and cared for.*[73]

In reality, Dr. Adams was right. Here's what Dr. Atlas said in July 2020:

*The last point I want to make is that when younger, healthier peo-
ple get infected, that's a good thing. Why? Why does that sound
like a good thing? Because that's exactly the way that population
immunity develops. When you have low -risk groups get infected,
become immune, that is how you break up the sort of connectiv-
ity pathways to riskier, older, sicker people. That's what's called
herd immunity. There's nothing wrong with having low -risk people get the infection as long as you protect the high -risk people,
which apparently is being done because this explosion of cases
has not caused increased deaths.*[74]

According to Drs. Prasad and Bhattacharya, people who accurately
report what Dr. Atlas said are *"totally dishonest."*

**That explanation is very different from proposing that people be
deliberately exposed and infected. I have never done that.**
— *Dr. Scott Atlas*

In his article, "America's COVID Response Was Based on Lies,"
Dr. Atlas said:

*The historical record is critical. We have seen a macabre Orwel-
lian attempt to rewrite history and to blame the failure of widespread lockdowns on the lockdowns' critics, alongside absurd
denials of officials' own incessant demands for them.*[75]

Dr. Atlas was entirely right about the *macabre Orwellian attempt
to rewrite history*; however, he is a major participant in it. He too
says people who accurately quote him are dishonest. In a 2021
interview he discussed herd immunity by saying:

*It's a biological phenomenon where enough people have immuni-
ty of some form to an infection so that the spread of that infection*

is blocked. The propagation of that infection is blocked, and therefore vulnerable people are prevented from getting exposed or getting the infection.

This is a biological phenomenon. I mean, this is decades and decades old. I never advocated; what people said was somehow I was advocating a quote herd immunity strategy. First of all, that's frankly an asinine statement because the only way that every virus is stopped is when enough people have immunity to it. That's why you give the vaccines. Vaccination is a herd immunity strategy. But what they really meant, what they meant to imply, which was a lie, was that I was advising that we should just let the infection spread and run rampant and survival of the fittest, and that's what we should do.

And that's not, I never said that. I don't know anyone who even said that. The same claims were made about the people who wrote the Great Barrington Declaration. They never said that. What I said was increase the protection of the people at high risk and stop killing the people who are low risk with the lockdowns.[76]

In another interview from 2021, Dr. Atlas said:

It is true that I have explained the fact that younger people have little risk from this infection, as well as the biological concept of herd immunity, the most radioactive term in the pandemic discussion.

Yeah. That explanation is very different from proposing that people be deliberately exposed and infected. I have never done that. To the contrary, I have repeatedly called for mitigation measures, including extra sanitization, social distancing, masks when appropriate, group limits, testing, and other increased protections to limit the spread and the damage from the virus.

I explicitly call for augmenting protection of those at risk in dozens of on-the-record presentations, interviews, and written pieces. Yet, one must question why these accusers ignore these explicit, emphatic denials of me beyond those presentations that I ever supported spreading the infection unchecked to achieve herd immunity.[77]

On social media, Dr. Atlas continues to portray himself as a mere advocate for "children & the poor." Although he predicted that COVID would only kill about 10,000 Americans in 2020, Dr. Atlas stated the following in July 2024:

Everything I said was 100% correct. Proud of that, proud I tried to help my country. Tragically, I had zero authority. Lockdowners got their policies & own the results - killed/harmed millions, esp children & the poor. They're so immoral, they will never admit it. #Shameful[78]

Drs. Prasad and Bhattacharya have similarly attempted to sanitize the entire WWTI movement. Its 2020 homages to "natural immunity" and the inevitability of herd immunity via the mass infection of unvaccinated youth get the Nikolai Ivanovich Yezhov treatment.

Today, WWTI doctors portray themselves as only having opposed the pandemic's most unpopular mitigation measures. In his 2023 article, "Public Health Should Lose Your Trust," Dr. Prasad said the GBD merely opposed "Lockdowns, prolonged school closure, masking toddlers, visitor restrictions, and perpetual hospital masking."[79]

Similarly, during his Congressional testimony in 2023, Dr. Bhattacharya said:

The declaration called for an end to economic lockdowns, school

shutdowns, and similar restrictive policies on the ground that
they disproportionately harm the young and economically disad-
vantaged while conferring limited benefits.[33]

This is always how Dr. Bhattacharya talks about the GBD today. He *never* mentions the part about encouraging young people "to build up immunity to the virus through natural infection."
It's true that WWTI doctors talked about the importance of schools in 2020. The GBD said:

> *All children have a right to a high-quality education. Adults have*
> *a moral obligation to make this happen, and it is morally wrong*
> *to ask children to bear a disproportionate burden of the costs*
> *of the epidemic. Yet the lockdown policy, and especially school*
> *closures, guarantees that children are especially harmed.*[18]

Likewise, in his June 2020 article, "Science Says: 'Open the-Schools,'" Dr. Atlas argued that because mitigation measures had successfully protected children at the start of the pandemic, they were no longer needed. He stated:

> *To stop COVID-19 dead in its tracks, many governors, mayors*
> *and superintendents are threatening to keep schools closed this*
> *fall, failing to consider the greater harm that comes from refus-*
> *ing to open them. [...] The irony in such language is that children*
> *are safe at school already.*[80]

However, Dr. Atlas spread myths about pediatric COVID at the time, saying children had zero risk of dying and nearly zero risk of spreading the virus. In an interview from July 2020, he said:

> *We're supposed to be educating the children. The schools are for*
> *the children. The children have virtually zero risk by the facts all*
> *over the world from a significant infection. They have zero risk*
> *of death. They have nearly zero risk of spreading infection, even*

to their parents. This is validated all over the world by the facts.
And we're sitting here saying, Oh, we better close schools.[74]

It's entirely possible that WWTI doctors were genuinely concerned about education in 2020. However, in their vision, schools weren't just for learning; they were a place where children and teachers could gain "natural immunity" and end the pandemic. Dr. Adams said:

> *Most of the conversation led by Dr. Atlas and others who focused on this concept of forcing schools to open and facilitate herd immunity was about how deliberately infecting the kids would ultimately help the adults who wanted the economy to open.*[71]

If all WWTI doctors cared about was education—as they now claim—shouldn't they have wanted healthy students learning from healthy teachers? Shouldn't they have wanted cautious parents to feel their children were safe at school too? Why did they devote great effort to removing the most trivial mitigation measures, years *after* schools were open? The answer, of course, is that they didn't just want them educated; they wanted them infected. They believed "that total isolation prevents broad population immunity and prolongs the problem."[81] In their vision, every uninfected child was a policy failure. Today, they want all that forgotten.

What kind of society uses children as human shields for adults? I am a shield for my children, they are not to be used as shields for me.
— Dr. Scott Atlas

Beyond denying their own words, several WWTI doctors inverted their pandemic role, absurdly casting themselves as protectors of children against villains who would use them as human shields. In a video from 2024, which Robert F. Kennedy Jr. shared on social media, Dr. Atlas made the following statement:

> **Question:** *Doctor, were the leaders of the teacher's unions aware of all this data that masks don't work, that the lockdowns don't work, that kids are not at high risk, that forcing them to vaccinate is unnecessary? They put so much pressure on parents and families. They kept the schools locked out. Were they given the data, or can they lean on the excuse that they just didn't know and they were so confused?*
>
> **Dr. Atlas:** *No, it's a lie. Okay, this is one of the greatest sins, in my view. The big sin, what we as a society did to children. Okay, I mean, and I, you know, I don't want to get choked up about that. I mean, I could just burst into tears right now. It's so awful. We broke the social contract we have as people by harming our children as a society and injecting, for instance, experimental drugs into children that have side effects, many of which are uncertain for a disease that those children, healthy children, did not have a significant risk from to use them as shields. I mean, this is almost unspeakable.*[82]

Dr. Atlas shared his opposition to using children as shields with
the vaccine multiple times. Some examples are:

- *I am absolutely pro-vaccine, but to me it's unconscionable that a society uses its children as shields for adults. So we're going to inject our children with an experimental drug that they don't have a significant benefit from to shield ourselves.*[83]
- *Even if it were true that the vaccine prevents transmission—it does not, by all of the world's data—what kind of society uses children as human shields for adults? Its hard to say that without getting emotional, but I am a shield for my children, they are not to be used as shields for me.*[84]
- *This is morality at stake... People injected young children*

*w/an experimental drug w/known side-effects for a disease
healthy kids had no significant risk for serious illness. To use
them as shields? I'm a father. My children are not shields for
me. Where are we as a civilization?*[85]

- *We became a culture that injected young children with an
experimental drug, with known side effects, for a disease
they didn't have a significant risk from, mainly to use them as
shields for adults. That is the most immoral, unethical display
of anything I have seen in my life.*[86]

Dr. Atlas was not alone in this. Although she advocated for infecting children to have them serve as a "barrier for infection," Dr. Gupta also objected to vaccinating children for this reason. She said:

*I absolutely do not think that is logical at any level. I mean,
leave alone the ethics of using 12-year-olds as barriers for
infection. The bottom line is that these vaccines do not prevent
transmission. In the case of a 12-year-old, it benefits neither
the individual who is not at risk of severe disease and death nor
does it benefit the community. So all we're left with is a risk of
vaccination. To ask children to bear that risk to me is just simply
unacceptable.*[87]

Of course, Drs. Atlas and Gupta were fighting a strawman of their own creation. No one proposed vaccinating children primarily to have them serve as "barriers for infection." Everyone was clear that the main reason to vaccinate children was to protect them from COVID. In May 2021, when vaccines were first approved for adolescents, Dr. Sara Oliver of the CDC's National Center for Immunization and Respiratory Diseases said:

*Adolescents 12-17 years of age are at risk of severe illness from
Covid-19. There have been over 1.5 million reported cases and
over 13,000 hospitalizations to date among adolescents 12 to 17
years.*[88]

Similarly, the American Academy of Pediatrics stated that when vaccines became available to elementary school children:

> *Vaccinating children will protect children's health and allow
> them to fully engage in all of the activities that are so important
> to their health and development.*[89]

In the mirror world, doctors who wanted to infect children with
SARS-CoV-2 to have them serve as human shields anointed themselves
as their champions to spare them from being used as shields with the
vaccine.

There's a gross exaggeration of hospitalizations and deaths for COVID.
— *Dr. Scott Atlas*

Beyond erasing their own words, WWTI doctors are now eager to
erase COVID's victims, though this process began as soon as the virus
arrived. Even as morgues overflowed in the spring of 2020, Dr. Ioannidis
claimed the death toll was inflated. He claimed people were dying *with*
COVID, *not* of COVID, that death certificates couldn't be trusted, that
doctors were killing patients through premature intubations, and COVID
only killed those who were about to die anyway. A typical quote from
him at the time was:

> *There is some contentious issue about what exactly should count
> as a COVID-19 death. For example, in the last few days (in
> New York City) we have seen a very large number of probable
> COVID-19 deaths being added to the figures, and these are
> deaths where we have not documented with laboratory testing
> the presence of the virus, so they are pretty presumptive in terms
> of whether these are deaths that were caused by COVID-19,
> COVID-19 was present, but not really a key player in the demise*

of the patient.

So, I think we need to wait and see some mature data on what exactly the contribution of the virus has been in different deaths that we have documented. In Italy, where we have some more mature data, we see that close to 99% of people have underlying diseases, actually in most cases multiple underlying diseases and underlying causes that could also have led them to death. In the US, it seems to be less, but we would need to get some more in-depth analysis of what exactly is killing these people and how. [...]

So, the data in Italy suggest that it's very difficult to differentiate between deaths by SARS-CoV-2 and deaths with SARS-CoV-2. Since we had close to 99% of people dying have other causes that may have contributed to their demise, it's very difficult to dissociate and say that these people specifically died because they were infected. It's very likely that many of them would have died anyhow, if not immediately within a very short period of time, because of these other causes of death that they had. I think this is an ongoing debate. [...]

Countries use very different systems of recording deaths, and we know, not just from the COVID-19 era, but also from the past, that filling out death certificates can be very tricky. We know that death certificates often are pretty inaccurate, and if you create an environment where people believe that this is the cause of death, that is really the most prominent at the moment, they may subconsciously or unconsciously prefer to list COVID-19 as a major cause of death in the certificate, even though it may be less significant contributor if not an innocent bystander in some cases.

*This is very difficult to tell at the moment because, as you realize,
the battle is still ongoing. But at some point, we need to go back
and check very carefully and try to understand what exactly did
the virus do to all these people.*

*If we do that, we will also be able to estimate how many years of
life were really lost, because it's not just the number of deaths,
it's the number of person-years lost that matters the most. If
you have someone who is young and healthy and has no other
problems and suddenly dies in their twenties, this is a very large
number of person-years lost compared to someone who is very
old and has multiple reasons to die, and is already dying from
something else and you just happen to find a PCR positive test
for SARS-CoV-2 in a nasal swab. The number of person-years
lost is very small and you're not even sure that SARS-CoV-2 really did contribute to their death substantially.*[90]

I provided a detailed refutation to these claims in *We Want Them
Infected* and won't repeat it here, except to make three key points. First,
no one who worked on a COVID unit would have said anything like
this. It was *obvious* that COVID was killing our patients. Second, excess
mortality, a measure of the increase in the number of deaths during a time
period, perfectly paralleled COVID waves. According to CDC data:

*During January 26, 2020–February 27, 2021, an estimated
545,600–660,200 more persons than expected died in the United
States from all causes. The estimated number of excess deaths
peaked during the weeks ending April 11, 2020, August 1, 2020,
and January 2, 2021. Approximately 75%–88% of excess deaths
were directly associated with COVID-19.*[91]

And third, there's evidence that COVID deaths may be undercounted.[92]

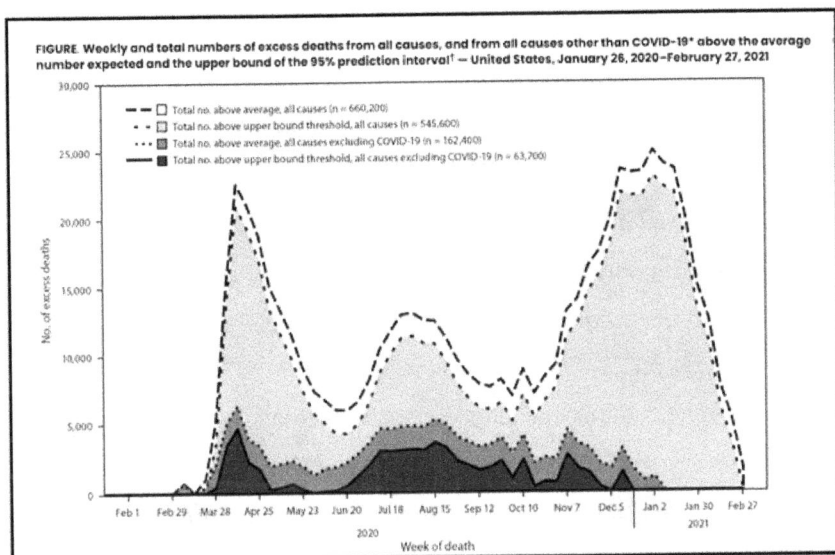

FIGURE. Weekly and total numbers of excess deaths from all causes, and from all causes other than COVID-19* above the average number expected and the upper bound of the 95% prediction interval† — United States, January 26, 2020–February 27, 2021

Excess mortality parallelled COVID waves in 2020 and 2021.

Source: CDC[92]

However, even in the pandemic's first days, Dr. Ioannidis was creating doubt. As forklifts were moving bodies into overflowing trucks, Dr. Ioannidis was preparing the public to disbelieve their own eyes. This has proved useful to WWTI doctors, as it allowed them to tell the public to disbelieve the pandemic's most basic numbers. They said not that many people would die of COVID, and now they claim they were right. In 2022, for example, Dr. Atlas gave a talk titled "The SARS2 Pandemic: Will Truth Prevail?" in which he said:

> So there's a gross exaggeration, predicting the pediatric side from the numbers you're reading of how many actually had COVID. What about deaths from COVID? It's the same sort of problem. This is CDC's data. [...] There's a gross exaggeration of hospitalizations and deaths from COVID in the United States. [...] It doesn't mean that people didn't die; I'm not minimizing COVID.[93]

In reality, Dr. Atlas was minimizing COVID.

In September 2021, after Delta ripped through much of the country, Dr. Prasad claimed greedy hospitals were inflating their numbers. He said:

> *Hospitals always run nearly full to maximize their "non-profits"*
> *If the severity of illness falls, they just admit less sick patients.*
> *This means however that using this as a fear monger tactic is*
> *inaccurate.*[94]

In 2024, he had this exchange on social media:

> **Question:** *How many of those "Covid deaths" were inflated for*
> *scaremongering tactics, or worse, fraudulent billing by hospital*
> *systems for the money?*[95]
>
> **Dr. Prasad:** *Maybe half.*[96]

Dr. Prasad never provided any evidence to back up this incredible claim.

Predictably, WWTI doctors will *never* remind their audience what happened at the start of the pandemic. They'll never share articles from 2020, such as "Hospitals Overflowing with Bodies in US Epicenter of Virus."[97] They want their audience to forget what the virus could do when it was allowed to spread unchecked. Not even the dead are spared the fate of Nikolai Ivanovich Yezhov and his photograph.

Chapter 7: Schools Would Have Opened. We Would Have Prioritized Protection of the Vulnerable

We are now defined more by what we say than what we actually do, and words, unlike deeds, are cheap and easy to counterfeit.
— Gurwinder Bhogal

The writer Gurwinder Bhogal contends that social media has elevated talkers over doers. He coined the term "Opinion Pageant" and defined it by saying:

> *The rise of social media as the primary mode of interaction has caused us to overvalue opinions as a gauge of character. We are now defined more by what we say than what we actually do, and words, unlike deeds, are cheap and easy to counterfeit.*[1]

That insightful observation accurately describes much of the discourse in the mirror world. WWTI doctors became famous for their *opinions*, not their *accomplishments*. With a couple of exceptions, they didn't actually *do* anything on the ground themselves. They weren't there in the trenches, figuring out how to staff a nursing home when employees called out sick. They didn't have to find a way to get kids to school when bus drivers got COVID. They didn't run any randomized controlled trials (RCTs), and most of them didn't treat any COVID patients.

However, this lack of real-world responsibility didn't stop them from incessantly saying what they *would have* done or *calling on* others to do things. WWTI doctors became pandemic celebrities by speaking about themselves entirely in the conditional tense and demanding that other people do things. Though they are currently failing to control measles and pertussis[2] now that they are the medical establishment and have real-world responsibility for the first time, many people genuinely admired WWTI doctors because they *called for* things to be done and listed all the wonderful things they *would have* done regarding COVID. Some examples include.

- **Dr. John Ioannidis:** *I would have used very draconian measures in nursing homes, so repeated testing, draconian hygiene.*[3]

- **Dr. Vinay Prasad:** *Many experts have called for more randomized trials during the pandemic. But they were ignored.*[4]

- **Dr. Martin Kulldorff:** *If we had done focused protection, as outlined in the Great Barrington Declaration, the pandemic would have been over now with fewer Covid deaths and less collateral public health damage.*[5]

- **Dr. Sunetra Gupta:** *The first is that we should have immediately shielded care home residents upon hearing that a new virus was abroad that was killing elderly people. This could have been achieved by redistributing the residents into smaller groups where they would be cared for by live-in staff. Permitted visitors would undergo routine testing and undertake periods of self-isolation to minimise the risk of introducing infection. The specific details would have to be worked out by the experts in the field. […] but it cannot have been harder than locking down the whole population and would certainly be achieved at a fraction of the cost.*[6]

- **Dr. Marty Makary:** *Just amazing to stop and think how hard the government was working to censor the private social media accounts of doctors who argued for public schools to be open as private schools were for wealthier children.*[7]

- **Great Barrington Declaration social media post:** *Focused Protection would have reduced the collateral harms that lockdowns. The harms of the lockdown are manifold and devastating, including plummeting childhood vaccination rates, worse cardiovascular disease outcomes, less cancer screening, and deteriorating mental health.*[8]

- **Dr. Jay Bhattacharya:** *A year ago, I called for the immediate opening of all schools in an interview with Paul Peterson. In*

Oct. 2020, in the @gbdeclaration_, we called for the opening of schools. Closing schools was a catastrophic public health failure.[9]

- **Dr. Jay Bhattacharya:** *We called for focused protection of vulnerable elderly and called for many policies, including paid sick leave.*[10]
- **Dr. Jay Bhattacharya:** *Add that to the fallacy that the @ gbdeclaration worked "against prevention." It literally called for focused protection of vulnerable people. […] The blindness to the devastating harms of lockdowns to children & the poor is also telling.*[11]
- **Dr. Jay Bhattacharya:** *If they've been adopted, the Great Barrington Declaration, but adopted schools would have stayed open, right?*[12]
- **Dr. Vinay Prasad:** *Just say you were lying. Just say you made shit up and then I also want them to admit they didn't run any studies. I want them to admit that they didn't run into this even though people told them to.*[13]

Dr. Vinay Prasad, like most WWTI doctors, was proud of himself for having *told* other people to do studies, not because he did any studies himself.

Why didn't they just protect the vulnerable and get on with life?
— *Dr. Jay Bhattacharya*

These "*I would have*" and "*called for*" statements have several features in common. First, they all state unambiguously good goals. No one could object to protecting vulnerable people, keeping kids in school, and RCTs.

Second, they all come from doctors who had no actual responsibility for making any of this happen. WWTI doctors won accolades for saying the words "protect the vulnerable," "open schools," and "do an RCT." However, they didn't do anything to *actually* advance these objectives.

They merely *called for* others to do the real work and treated this as a great accomplishment. Dr. Prasad boasted that he was "one of the few who called for RCTs."[14] He said, "You could have run many cluster RCTs of different masking strategies."[15]

However, WWTI doctors never expected anything of themselves. For example, Dr. Prasad said:

> *We should have studied whether social distancing works, and how much distance is ideal. We should know a lot more about who to test, why we're testing, and how often to test. Even school closure and reopening could have been studied. Randomized trials could have turned political fights into scientific questions. Not running them was a huge failure.*[4]

No one can argue with the statement "we should know a lot more," but why were the doctors who loudly *called for* things exempt from *actually doing* them? The sentence "not running them was a huge failure" was meant as an accusation, but it could be read as a confession. Why didn't Dr. Prasad run any RCTs? Is it truly impressive to *call for* others to do things?

Third, they were all much easier said than done. It's *really easy* to write the words "protect the vulnerable," "open schools," or "do an RCT." Anyone can do it. Of course, writing "I would have protected the vulnerable, opened schools, and run RCTs" is as impressive and believable as saying, "I would have kept SARS-CoV-2 out of the country entirely."

Yet, in the mirror world, a doctor who merely *called for* things expected to be credited as if they had *actually* done those things, and they made it all sound really easy. For example, Dr. Jay Bhattacharya said:

> *Not long from now, maybe 5 or 10 years, when covid is widely*

seen as a bad cold thanks to widespread population immunity,
people are going to look back and wonder at the panicked over-
reaction. They will say, why didn't they just protect the vulnera-
ble and get on with life?[16]

I think of what my clinical research team went through to enroll peo-
ple in that trial, and I thought my nurses were going to die.
— *Dr. Jeanne Marrazzo*

"Why didn't they just protect the vulnerable and get on with life?"
is an easy question to ask from a comfortable Stanford office. Here's the
answer.

In the real world, *actually* protecting the vulnerable was hard.
According to the article, "Nursing Home Staffing Shortages and Other
Problems Persist, U.S. Report Says":

> *Many Americans prefer to believe the Covid pandemic is a thing*
> *of the past. But for the nation's nursing homes, the effects have*
> *yet to fully fade, with staffing shortages and employee burnout*
> *still at crisis levels and many facilities struggling to stay afloat,*
> *according to a new report published Thursday by federal investi-*
> *gators. […]*
>
> *The inspector general's report described the staffing problems as*
> *"monumental," noting high levels of burnout, frequent employee*
> *turnover and the burdens of constantly training new employees,*
> *some of whom fail to show up for their first day of work. For*
> *nursing homes, the inability to attract and retain certified nurse*
> *aides, dietary services staff and housekeeping workers is tied to*
> *federal and state reimbursements that do not cover the full cost*
> *of care.*[17]

In the real world, *actually* keeping healthy kids learning from healthy teachers was hard. According to the article "COVID Hammers NYC School Attendance Among Students and Teachers" from January 2022:

> *The omicron surge is taking a toll on attendance in public schools all over New York City. Student attendance was 76% on Monday, the Department of Education told FOX 5 NY. Bronx Science 10th grader Roni Silverman said that when she returned from winter break she noticed many students and teachers at her school were out sick.*
>
> *"A lot of us are coasting right now, especially since we're supposed to have midterms, but they were canceled because too many people were not in attendance," Roni said. "So I think that everyone's trying their best to keep up but if our teachers aren't here, what are we supposed to do — learn ourselves?"*
>
> *Roni said that when a teacher doesn't show up, she and her classmates get sent to the auditorium. "One day since they had too many teachers absent, I actually just sat on the stage with my class because they didn't have enough space in the seats for us to sit," she said.*[18]

Even in 2024, headlines from Kentucky and Tennessee read, "Carroll County Schools Close After 25% of Teachers Contract Illnesses"[19] and "Mid-South Elementary School Shut Down Due to COVID Cases."[20]

In the real world, *actually* running RCTs was hard. According to the article, "Wartime Doctors Battling Covid-19 Rush to Treat the Ill — But Without Knowing What Really Works":

> *Jeanne Marrazzo, an infectious diseases specialist at the University of Alabama at Birmingham, oversaw testing of remdesivir, an antiviral drug tested in a randomized trial that has since been authorized and is one of the research success stories of the pandemic.*

She says hand-wringing about the lack of gold-standard evidence

simply does not take into account the situation on the ground.

"I think of what my clinical research team went through to enroll

people in that trial, and I thought my nurses were going to die.

One of them got covid and got sick," Marrazzo said. In those early

days, it took so long to get coronavirus test results that it could take

a full day to get a patient qualified and screened for the study.[21]

These tasks were made infinitely harder and often rendered totally

impossible when SARS-CoV-2 spread unchecked. That's just the sad

truth of what *the virus* did. This insistence on living in the hypothetical

world didn't just allow WWTI doctors to claim unearned greatness; it

allowed them to completely deny the reality of what happened in the real

world when the virus spread out of control.

Finally, because they incessantly uttered the words "protect the vul-

nerable," "open schools," or "do an RCT," WWTI doctors gave the im-

pression that only they were in favor of these measures. They portrayed

anyone who recognized the virus's impact on these laudable goals as ac-

tively opposed to them. Anyone who shared headlines like "At Least 45

Districts Shut Down In-Person Classes Due to Covid-19 Cases, Affecting

More Than 40,000 Students"[22] was accused of "advocating for school

closures," implying that these school district had other options and made

a bad choice. Here's what that article, from Texas in 2021, had to say:

Caseloads have left districts scrambling when many have said

they have fewer tools at their disposal to combat the spread of

the virus and have had to come up with their own strategies that

can differ from district to district. Administrators are tasked with

protecting students' and staff members' health, providing a quality

education and staying open enough days to avoid tacking on extra days at the end of the school year.

WWTI doctors claim *none of this would have happened* under their watch.

Similarly, Dr. Prasad penned an article titled "The Scientists Who Undermine Randomized Trials" that discussed an alliance between "pro-corporation entrenched interests, and left-wing public health,"[23] writing:

> In the last few weeks there have been several examples of scientists trying to undermine randomized trials— arguing they are not possible, not practical, or not useful.

Of course, scientists who recognized the limitations of RCTs weren't intentionally trying to "undermine" them. Dr. Prasad just portrayed them this way to spread doubt about their motives. As I discuss in another chapter, once he gained power, Dr. Prasad argued that RCTs were not always possible, practical, or useful.

Of course, WWTI doctors didn't make difficult or even wildly impossible things sound trivially easy just to cast themselves as heroes and win the Opinion Pageant. By claiming that they *would have* done great things, WWTI doctors sought to erase the virus and displace its consequences onto supposedly incompetent public health officials, who were *actually* supposed to do all the things they merely *called for*. For instance, when *the virus* forced schools to close in 2024, Dr. Prasad blamed *people*. He said, "Covid is just a cold; incompetent leaders forced schools to close."[24] Apparently, if Dr. Prasad had been in charge, he *would have* found ways to overcome sick teachers, bus drivers, and students that no one else figured out.

Likewise, the Great Barrington Declaration (GDB) *called for* public health officials to do dozens of impossible things, including delivering food to tens of millions of homebound seniors as the virus raged, as if this were a simple task. Later, Dr. Bhattacharya said the failure to actually do this "was a failure of imagination on the part of public health."[25] The GBD wasn't to blame, the virus wasn't to blame, only incompetent public health officials who couldn't do everything he *would have* done were to blame. In fact, Dr. Bhattacharya even said these forces were the *only* reason he didn't do these amazing things himself. He posted:

> *Imagine there hadn't been an @NIH -led "devastating takedown" of the @gbdeclaration in Oct 2020. Imagine no media/social media suppression. We would have won the policy argument. Schools would have opened. We would have prioritized protection of the vulnerable. Instead, lockdowns.*[26]

According to Dr. Bhattacharya, if it weren't for the all-powerful combination of the NIH and YouTube, he *would have* opened schools and protected vulnerable people. This fantasy version of Dr. Bhattacharya was extremely impressive.

Notably, WWTI doctors never criticized their own. Even though multiple WWTI doctors held positions of power and influence, they were never blamed for failing to "protect the vulnerable," "open schools," or "do an RCT." WWTI doctors only made these impossible demands from people they wanted to subvert and discredit, namely those who tried to limit COVID in any way.

They're not thinking people, they're told what to do, they just do it. Partly that's just really weak, dumb. [...] Partly they're just cowards.
— *Dr. Scott Atlas*

Winston Churchill is rumored to have said, "I no longer listen to what people say; I just watch what they do. Behaviour never lies." No one has to wonder what they *would have* done during the pandemic. There is no parallel universe where an alternate version of you was in charge of our pandemic response. What you *actually* did during the COVID pandemic is exactly what you *would have* done, and, as such, we can examine the real-world record of every doctor.

Along with countless others, I worked in a hospital. I've always described my COVID experience by saying that I didn't do a lot, but I saw a lot. Yet, this real-world experience meant nothing to WWTI doctors, nearly all of whom experienced the pandemic from their laptops.

Instead of trying to learn from doctors who operated in the real world, WWTI doctors undermined and berated them. They incited online mobs against Dr. Peter Hotez, who developed a low-cost, patent-free COVID vaccine. Other WWTI doctors launched vicious attacks on doctors who operated in the real world. For example, Dr. Scott Atlas said the following about doctors who suggested masks and vaccines:

> *I would say right to them they are a disgrace, a complete disgrace. I know that sounds very harsh, but I mean this is an example of a couple things. Number one, seems like most of our doctors are really sheep. They're not thinking people; they're told what to do, they just do it. Partly that's just really weak, dumb. I'm not being very articulate this morning, I'm sorry; but you know it's just I'm beside myself. Partly they're just cowards. We have a tremendous void in courage in our country. Doctors enjoy a position of huge prestige but, more importantly, trust.*[27]

Dr. Bhattacharya also attacked frontline doctors, saying they just wanted their jobs to be "easier." During an interview in 2022, he stated:

If you think about medicine as a vocation, you're supposed to devote your well-being to the life a patient that you are caring for [...] lockdowns actually reversed that and said look, 'You the population should suffer so that my job in medicine can be easier', so a reversal of the norms of medicine where medicine serves people, not people serve medicine. The fact that medicine, especially the leaders of medicine, were so strongly in favor of the lockdowns is a violation of the ethics of the medical profession. It essentially transforms the doctor-patient relationship to one where the patient serves the doctor rather than the other way around.[28]

In 2023, he posted a fake "review" of *We Want Them Infected*—which he later admitted he had not read—and said:

The unspoken root idea of his (Dr. Jonathan Howard) is that the general public owed it to doctors to not get covid because it would place doctors at risk of getting covid. Of course this is an inversion. Medical professionals serve the public, not the other way around.[29]

I never said anything like that. However, in the mirror world, doctors who treated zero COVID patients felt doctors who worked on COVID units were lazy, dumb, cowardly sheep. Although thousands of healthcare workers died of COVID, WWTI doctors feel we should have looked at the suffering and death that surrounded us and honored medical ethics by declaring *we need more people to get COVID.*

Dr. John Ioannidis even said frontline doctors were responsible for the death of their patients. During a podcast with Dr. Prasad, Dr. Ioannidis spoke as if he had been on the frontline himself. He said, "There is an effect of what we did, mostly wrong, in the first wave."[3] He then said that "a lot of lives" were lost at that time in part because of "not knowing how to use mechanical ventilation, just going crazy, and intubating people who did not have to be intubated." In another podcast, he said, "We have more treatments now; we know a little better what to do. You know, we just don't panic and start intubating everyone."[30]

In reality, Dr. Ioannidis did not treat any COVID patients, and the doctors who did knew that the virus killed our patients, not intubations. In fact, some evidence suggests that "delayed intubation is also associated with an increased mortality in a subset of COVID-19 patients."[31] However, rather than admit he underestimated COVID, Dr. Ioannidis opted to blame overwhelmed doctors dealing with a new virus for the demise of their patients.

> **If there's a scientist that is not willing to debate and discuss it with other scientists, you shouldn't trust them.**
> — *Dr. Martin Kulldorff*

We can also examine the real-world record of WWTI doctors. It turns out that what they *actually* did was write a lot of editorials and make a lot of YouTube videos listing all the incredible things they *would have* done. While other doctors worked in hospitals, they imagined a fictional world where all it took to protect the vulnerable and open schools was to utter the words "protect the vulnerable" and "open schools." In this fantasy world, they were in charge, and everything turned out just fine.

The authors of the GBD also presented their fantasy in many debates. Here are some examples:

- Seeking Common Ground in 'Herd Immunity' Debate[32]
- Be It Resolved, COVID-19 Is Everywhere, It's Time to Lift All Restrictions for Good. Guests Jay Bhattacharya and Jere-

my Faust Debate[33]
- Were COVID Lockdowns a Deadly Mistake? Jay Bhattacharya vs. Sten Vermund[34]
- COVID Debate: Martin Kulldorff and Eric Topol[35]
- End the COVID-19 Lockdowns? Two Epidemiologists Debate[36]
- Vaccine Mandates Debate[37]
- Surging COVID-19 Debate[38]
- Herd Immunity as a Coronavirus Pandemic Strategy[39]

In that last debate, from November 2020, Dr. Bhattacharya stated:

And so the Great Barrington Declaration is actually a call to return to [the] sort of principles that we had followed for many, many other infectious disease outbreaks. We protect the vulnerable with every single tool we have. We use our testing resources. We use our staff rotations on nursing homes. We use PPE. We do all kinds of things so that where people live, that are vulnerable, and older people are the main group, but also many other people with chronic conditions—again, we can talk about strategies to do that. We do that. That's why it's called focus protection.

Of course, Dr. Bhattacharya did not "do that." He just called for others to "do that" in podcasts, editorials, and debates.

However, this was not enough. WWTI doctors wanted more debates and more attention. Dr. Bhattacharya often called for more debates, saying, "Let's have a debate. Science works best when we have an open debate,"[40] while Dr. Martin Kulldorff said, "If there's a scientist that is not willing to debate and discuss it with other scientists, you shouldn't trust them."[41]

Dr. Sunetra Gupta gave interviews titled "Neil Ferguson Should Debate Lockdown with Me"[42] and "Social Media Attacks 'Stifling Coronavirus Debate.'"[43] In his article, "Public Health Should Lose Your Trust,"

Dr. Prasad berated public health officials for their "lack of debates," writing:

> *During the pandemic major universities held ~0 debates on lockdowns, prolonged school closure, masking toddlers, visitor restrictions, and perpetual hospital masking.*[44]

Dr. Prasad argued in another article that the government had an obligation to arrange such debates. He wrote:

> *Americans would have benefited from a broad debate among scientists about the available policy options for controlling the Covid-19 pandemic, and perhaps a bit of compromise. [...]*
>
> *In a world where scientists were trapped in their own homes for months, a series of dialogues — even virtual ones — made available for the broader scientific community, policy makers, and the public would have benefited us all.*[45]

Dr. Prasad concluded that had Dr. Francis Collins "chosen dialogue instead of contributing to animosity and combativeness, we might have been in a better place today."

Elsewhere, Dr. Prasad was even more emotional, calling Dr. Collins the "dumbest general on the planet."[46] He said:

> *You were the NIH Director. You could have had a series of Town Halls where you invited people like Jay Bhattacharya and Martin Kulldorff and had an open discussion of the pros and cons. You could have put them on YouTube. You have the powers of the federal government. You held zero debates. You just went on TV and you said proclamation after proclamation... You never tried to minimize uncertainty. You never brought anyone to the table who might disagree with you. If you were a general in war, you would be the dumbest general on the planet. Because even a general in*

*war wants someone at the table who says, 'Hey, you think maybe
we shouldn't invade someone? ..Let's hear that argument.'*

The right-wing media ecosystem predictably jumped in as well. *The
Wall Street Journal* published an article titled "How Fauci and Collins
Shut Down Covid Debate," which said, "They worked with the media to
trash the Great Barrington Declaration."[47]

In reality, debates are verbal jousts of wit and spectacles for public
entertainment, not for elucidating scientific truths. However, in the mirror
world, these onstage performances were vital to winning the Opinion
Pageant, and for this reason, WWTI doctors treated them with more
gravitas than anything that happened in hospitals, schools, and nursing
homes.

> **By far this is worse in terms of planning than last year. There's no
> question about it. Last year we had a lot of tools at our disposal [...]
> [Then], the delta variant really kind of appeared and just exploded
> on us.**
> — *Tim Savoy*

Although WWTI doctors didn't really *do anything* on the ground, this
does not mean they didn't do anything. They shared their opinions widely
and advised powerful politicians. Although they claimed they *would
have* protected the vulnerable, opened schools, and run RCTs, in the real
world, they undermined efforts to accomplish these vital tasks.

Though "protecting the vulnerable" was purportedly the entire point
of the GBD, Dr. Bhattacharya later cast doubt on the value of doing this
at all. His article "What Does Focused Protection Mean for Nursing
Homes?" was not about how to make nursing homes safe but rather to
question whether they should be kept safe at all. He wrote:

But, I have to admit that even the focused protection approach has its costs. What do the experiences of lockdown and focused protection mean for people living in nursing homes and care homes?[48]

Dr. Bhattacharya shared a sad story about a lonely man and concluded:

If abstractions like lockdown and focused protection are imposed without regard to the human costs, only inhumane outcomes can result. The control of COVID-19 spread, even to vulnerable people, is undoubtedly good – but it is not the only good.

WWTI doctors also opposed simple measures to protect the vulnerable. In addition to opposing boosters, Dr. Prasad also opposed masks in hospitals. He also made a long video about hospital masking and pitched it by saying:

A number of hospitals have winter mask mandates For staff, staff + visitors, on some floors but not others, inpatient but not outpatient, and all sorts of variations Is this evidence based? Or, as a wise professor recently told me, "just plain stupid."[49]

Dr. Prasad's Substack, *Sensible Medicine*, published an article which said:

I recently spent a week attending on the inpatient geriatric ward at our VA hospital. Most of our patients served in Vietnam. Many of them have lived hard lives and are in the hospital with a combination of severe illnesses and significant social problems. Many have little personal social support. I was happy to see that the VA no longer requires staff or patients to wear masks. Patients who are coughing are asked to wear masks, and staff who are sick are told to stay home.

I was unhappy to see that most doctors still wear masks.[50]

Sensible Medicine also published a "response" to this article that reached the same conclusion. It said:

> *There is a comfort to wearing a mask when I occasionally sniffle or sneeze and wonder if I might be harboring some virus – I can think I'm doing my best to protect my patients – but I also really like having my face uncovered for my patients, and that prefer-ence wins.*[51]

In the real world, hospital-acquired COVID is both common and not benign.[52] Preventing its spread in the hospital is protecting the vulnerable, and there is evidence that "stopping universal masking and SARS-CoV-2 testing was associated with a significant increase in hospital-onset respiratory viral infections relative to community infections."[53]

WWTI doctors also spread fear and doubt about measures to limit viral transmission in schools. Again, they did not object to these measures because they thought they failed to slow the virus, but precisely because they limited COVID infections in children. They saturated the media with articles such as "The Case Against Covid Tests for the Young and Healthy,"[57] "The Ill-Advised Push to Vaccinate the Young,"[58] "The Downsides of Masking Young Students Are Real,"[59] and "Kids Don't Need Covid-19 Vaccines to Return to School."[60] In 2023, Dr. Prasad even wrote an article titled "Do Not Report Covid Cases to Schools & Do Not Test Yourself If You Feel Ill" that said:

> *It's time to go dark with all COVID data. If enough people don't participate, the irrationality will stop. Eventually.*[58]

In the mirror world, ignorance is power.

The results were predictable. WWTI doctors' desire to infect unvaccinated children for the sake of herd immunity disrupted education in the real world. Sick children can't learn, and sick teachers can't teach. An excerpt from the article "At Least 45 Districts Shut Down In-Person Classes Due to Covid-19 Cases, Affecting More Than 40,000 Students" reads:

> *"By far this is worse in terms of planning than last year," said Tim Savoy, spokesperson for Hays Consolidated Independent School District, which closed some classrooms. "There's no question about it. Last year we had a lot of tools at our disposal: We could require masks, and we could provide a virtual option that was funded. [...] [Then], the delta variant really kind of appeared and just exploded on us."[22]*

There was nothing special about Texas. The virus also forced schools to close, not just in Democratic bastions but also in Kentucky,[59] Florida,[60] Georgia,[61] North Carolina,[62] Mississippi,[63] Alabama,[64] South Carolina,[65] Tennessee,[66] Missouri,[67] and West Virginia.[68] Doctors who said they *would have* kept schools open in the mirror world took away Mr. Savoy's tools and helped close them in the real world.

The pandemic affected educators as well. Although they weren't all infected in schools, we should not forget that COVID killed many of them. As early as May 2020, headlines from New York City read, "Coronavirus News: 30 Teachers Among 74 DOE Employees to Die of COVID-19."[69] A teacher at my child's school died. According to a December 2022 article:

> *Since the spring of 2020, Education Week documented 1,308 active and retired educators who succumbed to the virus. Among the total, 451 were active teachers. School staff members, including secretaries, food service workers, bus drivers, and others comprised the second biggest group of deaths at 332.[70]*

This was all bad for schools, but it never concerned WWTI doctors. In fact, WWTI doctors repeatedly blew off COVID's risk to teachers.

In October 2020, before anyone was vaccinated, Dr. Bhattacharya said teachers faced:

> *A very moderate risk should they become infected with dying, somewhere on the order of two in a thousand. You know, 998 of those 40-year-olds will survive should they become infected, out of a thousand.*[71]

When asked about long-term health, he replied:

> *I mean, every virus, the flu can have some long -term effects, but the fraction of the population you get, those are small.*

Meanwhile, Dr. Atlas said in March 2021:

> *There's zero reason to prioritize or insist the teachers get to the front of the line for vaccination.*[72]

Treating teachers as expendable didn't help children learn.

WWTI doctors also undermined RCTs in the real world. In a Fox News interview, Dr. Atlas said parents who had enrolled their child in a vaccine trial were "manipulated or brainwashed; they're psychologically damaged."[73] He said it was unethical to "inject experimental drugs into young children that have no significant benefit." This was not just a one-time comment. An article titled "At UChicago, Dr. Scott Atlas Condemns COVID Response's Victimization of Kids" stated:

> *Speaking at Friday's Academia's COVID Failures symposium, Dr. Scott Atlas highlighted the pernicious effects of the educational shutdown and COVID-19 vaccine trials on children and younger adults.*
>
> *In particular, Atlas claimed that Pfizer, a key actor in COVID vaccine development and distribution, used "infants and toddlers" in medical trials for a disease from which they faced little to no danger. He questioned what sort of society the United*

States was becoming, using children as "human shields" for adults.[74]

The Brownstone Institute also discouraged parents from enrolling their children in vaccine RCTs. An article titled "Kid Lab Rats" quoted Dr. Clayton Baker as saying:

> *Given the real and well-established risks of harm (including myocarditis and death), and given the functionally zero potential for benefit (since [Covid] is universally mild in children), the risk-to-benefit ratio for the [Covid] mRNA injections in children is infinitely bad. There is no ethical reason whatsoever to continue clinical trials of these products in children, and all such trials should be stopped.*[75]

Instead of loudly objecting to these attempts to undermine crucial vaccine research, many WWTI doctors teamed up with the Brownstone Institute. Dr. Prasad allowed them to publish his article "The Fragmented Trust in Public Health," which said:

> *Building trust in institutions is vital to their success, but as we enter the third year of the pandemic, public health still seems hellbent on destroying itself.*[76]

None of this helped enrollment in RCTs.

One place where we had some success was Florida.
— Dr. Martin Kulldorff

Defenders of the GBD will often argue that we never really tried it, implying that it *could have* worked if only we had the collective will to implement it. However, their plan for herd immunity via mass infection *actually* existed. The GBD was *actually* written and *actually* presented to the public. As such, we don't have to speak about it as a hypothetical entity. We don't have to wonder what *would have* happened in some parallel universe where we "tried the GBD" and everyone followed their policy recommendations and YouTube played their every video. We should not give credence to fantasies that everything *would have* been perfectly fine if only we had "protected the vulnerable" and let everyone get COVID in 2020. We can set aside the mirror world and discuss what *actually* happened in the real world.

In the real world, the plan to achieve herd immunity via mass infection failed. Many things went wrong with it. For "natural immunity" to lead to herd immunity in three to six months, 230 million or so unvaccinated and "not vulnerable" people had to be willing to catch COVID in that short time span. They wisely refused. Most "not vulnerable" people wisely choose to get vaccinated instead of being infected. Additionally, children turned out to spread the virus, many thousands of "not vulnerable" people turned out to be vulnerable, and "natural immunity" didn't turn out as "powerful" as they claimed it would be. Reinfections are trivially common and not always benign.

The obvious truth is that nowhere on Earth used focused protection to "protect the vulnerable" and achieved herd immunity in three to six months. As such, we don't have to ask if their plan *could* have worked; in the real world, it failed at every level.

Indeed, WWTI doctors had great influence in some areas, and in these places, we don't have to ask what *would have* happened there; we can examine what *actually* happened.

In October 2021, just after the Delta wave hit, Dr. Kulldorff, an author of the GBD, stated, "One place where we had some success was Florida."[77] Let's examine their record there:

- They **failed** to protect "vulnerable" people: "Florida Leads Nation in Number of COVID-19 Deaths of Nursing Home

Residents and Staff,"[78] August 2021.

- They **failed** to keep schools open: "School Closures Reported in Five Florida Counties; Districts 'Drowning' In COVID,"[79] August 2021.
- They **failed** to protect educators: "15 Miami-Dade Public School Staff Members Die of COVID In Just 10 Days,"[80] September 2021.
- They **failed** to protect "not vulnerable" people: "Child Covid Deaths More Than Doubled in Florida as Kids Returned to the Classroom,"[81] September 2021.
- They **failed** to end the pandemic: "Florida's COVID Deaths Reach Nearly 6,000 in 2024,"[82] January 2025.

In the mirror world, this was "some success." In the real world, when given the chance, WWTI doctors *failed* to do a single thing they said they *would* have done. This raises an obvious question: *Why didn't they just protect the vulnerable and get on with life?*

Chapter 8: mRNA Covid-19 Vaccines are Ruining Trust in Scientists and Public Health

What helps the elderly is if the young take this very minimal risk and live normal life until there's herd immunity, and […] then the older people can also live more normal lives.
— Dr. Martin Kulldorff

An article from September 2020 reported on a discussion Florida Governor Ron DeSantis had with several WWTI doctors. It quoted Gov. DeSantis as saying:

> *"Herd immunity I think implies the disease is done, but I think that the role that population immunity has played thus far in epidemics waning, it doesn't mean that the disease is gone, but it's driven the reproduction — it's been a big factor in driving the reproduction rate below 1 in a lot of these areas," the Governor said.*
>
> *Meanwhile, DeSantis acknowledged that the term has become politically charged.*
>
> *"I think it's being used to say that you should just do nothing and just let the disease do what it wants. I don't think that's what you're advocating," DeSantis said.*[1]

Florida still does not have herd immunity to COVID.

However, Florida's COVID experience serves as a cautionary tale about what happens when WWTI doctors run the show. In September 2020, before anyone was vaccinated, WWTI doctors told Gov. DeSantis what he wanted to hear: the virus was only harmful to older people and that measures to limit infections in young people only prolonged the pandemic. A few quotes from that meeting follow:

> **Dr. Michael Levitt:** *Everything we've heard here, for example, in treating age groups differently, makes complete sense. [...] The need to let young people interact with each other, both for social reasons and for herd immunity, makes perfectly good common sense. I think there should have been more of that.*
>
> **Dr. Martin Kulldorff:** *What helps the elderly is if the young take this very minimal risk and live normal life until there's herd immunity, and then, when we have herd immunity, then the older people can also live more normal lives.*
>
> **Dr. Jay Bhattacharya:** *Checking asymptomatic kids, the main purpose of it is essentially to close the school, to create a panic and close the school down I think.*

These themes were reiterated during a roundtable discussion from March 2021,[2] along with copious disinformation about COVID's risk to young people, the durability of "natural immunity," and the "risks" of masks. Some representative quotes include:

> **Dr. Martin Kulldorff:** *So for old people have to be very careful because this is more dangerous than the annual influenza. But for children, this is less dangerous than the influenza. So we should have utilized that feature of COVID to protect the old with focus protection while letting a younger people live normal life to avoid all the collateral public health damage from lockdown, which are enormous.*
>
> *It's not dangerous for children to be in school and it's not dangerous for teachers either. The only exception is that if you're a teacher and you're above 60, maybe you should be allowed to do online teaching until you have the vaccine. But other than that, there's no reason to do that. [...]*

Children should not wear face masks. No. They don't need it for their own protection and they don't need it for protecting other people either. [...]

Yeah. So we know, I mean, there'd be very few reinfection, so we know that there's good immunity from national infection for at least a year now will that last five years, or 10 years, or 20 years, we obviously do not know that, but also for vaccines, we have good immunity, but it's not quite as good because we've seen numbers of 95% and we know that still after a number of months. So at this point, it's very clear that naturally infection, there's much more evidence that naturally infection provide immunity than it is from vaccines.

Dr. Scott Atlas: *The reality is that the kids have extremely low risk from COVID-19...It happens to be icing on the cake, as we say, that children are not significant spreaders to adults. But that's really just icing on the cake.* [...]

It's bad to wear a mask during exercise, yet where I'm from in California, the gyms that are open, they require you to wear a mask during exercise. It's not just unnecessary, it's harmful. And people have not really been explained this kind of negative harms. [...]

There's zero reason to prioritize or insist the teachers get to the front of the line for vaccination.

The overwhelming majority of people do not have a problem with this virus. And so this idea, this panic driven fear of getting this infection if you're under 70, your infection fatality rate is very low. [...] *There's a moral, ethical question here if you're going to start saying that young children should be vaccinated for an infection that they have essentially no problem with.*

Dr. Jay Bhattacharya: *We should instead have adopted a policy, and most places, should have adopted a policy that got rid of lockdowns and instead focused on people we knew to be truly vulnerable to disease, older populations, people with certain chronic diseases, adopted policies, actually much more similar to what Florida has done, rather than the state where I live, California, which has relied on lockdowns to a disastrous effect.*

I think masks, in fact, in some ways they've been harmful because people believe that masks protect them, vulnerable people, and they end up taking more risks than they ought because they feel like they're protected by something that actually does not protect them. So I think on net, I think the masks not only have not been effective, but have been harmful. [...]

There's a vast array of evidence in the scientific literature that shows definitively that if you've had COVID and recovered, the vast, vast majority of people have a durable immunity that it's very unlikely that you'll be reinfected and you'll be protected from, from reinfection. [...] I think a very large fraction of the population is already been infected and are immune the evidence from the trials don't demonstrate any efficacy of vaccinating that population. In fact, the vast majority of cases are relatively mild, asymptomatic, or with mild symptoms.

On July 26, 2021, Dr. Jay Bhattacharya had more good news for the governor and citizens of Florida:

We have protected the vulnerable—by vaccinating the older population, we have provided them with enormous protection against severe disease and death. That's why you see, even as the cases have risen in Sweden in the past wave, or in the UK in this past wave, and in Florida in this past wave, the number of deaths have not risen proportionally. Why? Because we protected the vulnerable.

The key thing to me is hospitalizations and deaths from COVID. While we've done an incredible job at decoupling the cases from the deaths, the public focus on cases at this point, I think, only serves to panic people without actually serving any other public health purpose. […] I don't think the delta variant changes the calculus or the evidence in any fundamental way.[3]

On August 1, 2021, Gov. DeSantis blasted Dr. Bhattacharya's optimistic message on both Twitter and Facebook. He quoted Dr. Bhattacharya as saying:

We have protected the vulnerable by vaccinating the older population.

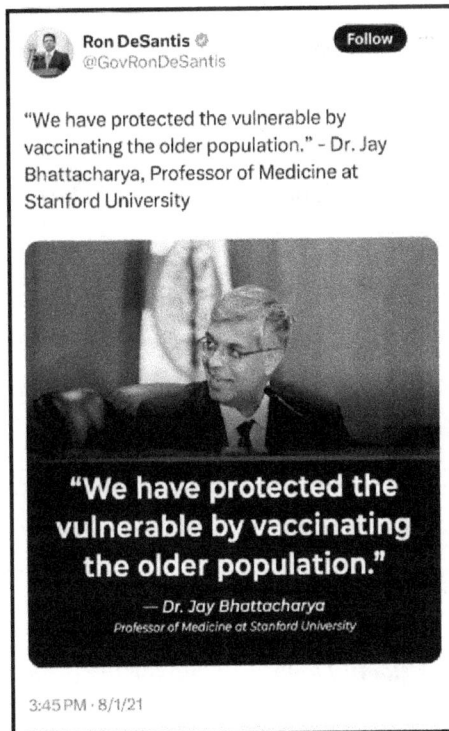

Ron DeSantis
@GovRonDeSantis

Follow

"We have protected the vulnerable by vaccinating the older population." - Dr. Jay Bhattacharya, Professor of Medicine at Stanford University

"We have protected the vulnerable by vaccinating the older population."

— *Dr. Jay Bhattacharya*
Professor of Medicine at Stanford University

3:45 PM · 8/1/21

Tweet by Florida Governor Ron DeSantis on August 1, 2021

**Florida Delta Wave Cases Plunge, Leaving Record Deaths In Its
Wake.**
— News Headline October 2021

Reality would soon prove otherwise. That same day—August
1, 2021—the headline read, "Florida Reports A Record Number Of
COVID-19 Cases."[4] Despite Dr. Bhattacharya's claim that Florida had
"protected the vulnerable," the fact was fewer than 50% of Floridians
were fully vaccinated at the time.[5] Florida ranked 44th in vaccinating 18-
to 64-year-olds and 46th for vaccinating those between 12- to 17-years
and those older than 65-years.[6] Anyone actually concerned with protecting rather than pacifying the vulnerable would have recognized that
Florida was a disaster waiting to happen.

A disaster is exactly what happened.

Despite Dr. Bhattacharya's casual dismissal of the Delta variant, it
changed the calculus in a very fundamental way. In August and September 2021, Delta ripped through the state, causing unprecedented death
and suffering. Just four days after Floridians were told the vulnerable had
been protected, Dr. Marc Napp, the chief medical officer for Memorial
Healthcare System in Hollywood, Florida, made the following statement:

> *We are seeing a surge like we've not seen before in terms of the
> patients coming. It's the sheer number coming in at the same
> time. There are only so many beds, so many doctors, only so
> many nurses.*[7]

Florida fared well during the pandemic's first year, and Gov. DeSantis initially embraced COVID vaccines when they first came out in 2021.
According to one article:

> *Early in the pandemic, Florida Gov. Ron DeSantis repeatedly
> praised President Donald Trump for the expedited development*

and rollout of a coronavirus vaccine. The governor's office
pushed for $480 million in pandemic resources, including me-
dia campaigns promoting the shots, according to state budget
documents. And DeSantis, a Republican, even lauded the Biden
administration for helping to expand access to vaccines.
"We're having more vaccine because of this, which is great,"
DeSantis said of a federal program shipping shots to pharmacies
in February 2021.[8]

However, since April 2021, when vaccines became available to those 16-years-old and older, Florida has shown the highest COVID death rate among the country's six most populated states, double the rate of New York and California.[6] More Floridians died of COVID *after* Dr. Bhattacharya's "we protected the vulnerable" comment than they did before it, and 20,000 people died in August and September 2021 alone.[9]

As with New York City during its initial wave, mobile morgues were needed to store the corpses.[10] During the August 2021 peak, 17,200 Floridians were hospitalized with COVID.[11] The mayor of Orlando asked citizens to conserve water to help maintain liquid oxygen supplies. Just three weeks after Dr. Bhattacharya assured Floridians that the vulnerable had been protected, AARP reported that "Florida led the nation in nursing home resident and staff deaths [...] in the four weeks ending August 22, 2021."[12] Fifteen educators in the Miami-Dade County Public Schools District died in a 10-day period.[13] Overwhelmed healthcare workers suffered too. "We are exhausted," said Dr. Rupesh Dharia,[11] an internist. "Our patience and resources are running low." Months later the headlines would read, "Florida Delta Wave Cases Plunge, Leaving Record Deaths in Its Wake."[14] It quoted Dr. Jason Salemi, a University of South Florida professor, as saying:

The fact we had record numbers of hospitalizations, record numbers of deaths, even in younger populations -- that was just so astonishing to me, it showed you just how bad the delta wave was.

Much of this suffering was avoidable. According to the article, "Most COVID Deaths in Florida Happened After Vaccines Were Readily Available":

Floridians died at a higher rate, adjusted for age, than people in almost any other state during the Delta wave. Florida made up 14% of deaths between July and October 2021, despite representing less than 7% of the country, according to The Times. Twenty-three-thousand Floridians died during the Delta wave, and 9,000 of them were younger than 65 — a majority of whom were either unvaccinated or had not finished their two-dose regimen. [15]

One study from October 2021 estimated that if Florida had vaccinated 74% of its citizens, as many other states had done, by the end of August that year, it would have had 61,327 fewer hospitalizations and 16,235 fewer deaths. [16]

Tragically, not all of Delta's victims were elderly people with multiple medical comorbidities only days away from dying of these diseases when they happened to contract COVID. According to one news report:

Dr. Chirag Patel, assistant chief medical officer of UF Health Jacksonville, said the patients hospitalized with the virus during this latest surge tend to be younger and had fewer other health issues, but were nearly all unvaccinated. Of those who have died, including patients ranging in age from their 20s to their 40s, more than 90 percent were not immunized. [11]

"We've had more patients this time around that have passed away at a younger age with very few, if any, medical problems," Dr. Patel said. "They simply come in with COVID, and they don't make it out of the hospital."

Delta did not spare children either, many of whom were old enough to be vaccinated. During the peak of the Delta wave, 68 children were being hospitalized daily in Florida.[17] Some of them were sick enough to need mechanical ventilation in the ICU, and several died.[18] A headline from September 2021 declared "Child COVID Deaths More Than Doubled in Florida as Kids Returned to the Classroom."[19] Doctors on the ground spoke of the suffering. Dr. Mobeen Rathore, a Florida pediatrician, stated:

> Kids do get sick. Kids do get hospitalized. Kids do get sick and go to the ICU, get intubated, be on a ventilator and even be on ECMO which is a heart lung machine, sort of a last ditch effort to support these children. Unfortunately children do die. In fact many of you probably heard the news, there's a 17-year-old who died in St. Johns County just in the last few days so I think we have to be very sure and understand that kids can get serious illness. And I can tell you that in the almost 18 months ending in June we had three deaths in our area in children. That's one death every six months. And just in July and August we had four deaths in children so that's two deaths a month.[20]

As the Delta wave receded, the *Tampa Bay Times* reported, "4 Kids Among Florida's COVID Death Toll as State Sets Another Record for Fatalities."[21] The article quoted a pediatric ICU nurse manager who said:

> The delta variant really kind of changed the game for us, because we weren't seeing that many children — now we're starting to see them in the ICU. Families are just reeling from this. These

*are normal healthy children who are suddenly just really struck
down with this disease.*

It also quoted a neuropsychologist who described the virus's impact
on children as "relentless, unforgiving and terrifying. [...] You have patients who are air hungry – they're struggling for breath. As scary as that
is for adults, imagine what that is like for kids to go through that."

Predictably, parents expressed their regret for not vaccinating their
children. One headline from September 2021 read:

> *Victoria tested positive for COVID-19 almost two weeks ago. She
> had a fever and body aches. Later she was sent home from the
> hospital, but then her dad, Hector, had to take her back. "With-
> in four or five days, her breathing started getting worse and
> worse," he said. Doctors told Hector she had COVID pneumo-
> nia. Just after she started to get better, she stopped breathing.
> Hector had to leave the room while they tried to resuscitate her.
> "About 15, 20 minutes later, they couldn't bring her back," Hec-
> tor said as he held back tears.* [22]

"She was so beautiful and so smart," her father said.

> *Hector Ramirez says he's now thinking of getting vaccinated. He
> didn't get the shot for his daughter, and he regrets it. "It's some-
> thing that's going to be stuck with me for my whole life, think-
> ing maybe I should have done that sooner," he said. "Maybe I
> could've done something to help prevent this." He says Victoria
> was healthy, but that changed quickly.*

The sad truth is that Mr. Ramirez absolutely could have done something to prevent this. Victoria should still be alive.

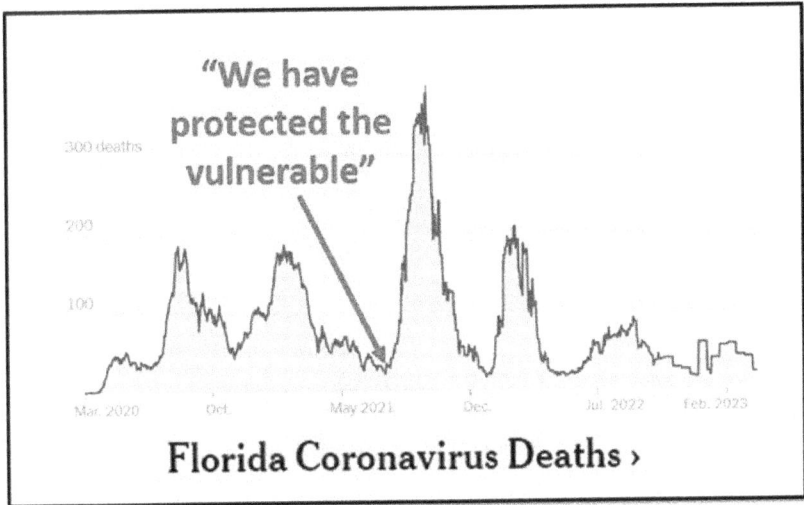

"We have protected the vulnerable"

300 deaths

200

100

Mar. 2020   Oct.   May 2021   Dec.   Jul. 2022   Feb. 2023

Florida Coronavirus Deaths ›

COVID Deaths in Florida. Source: Our World In Data

These vaccines are honestly—they're the Antichrist of all products.
— Dr. Joseph Ladapo

Doubt and anti-vaccine disinformation are now state policy in Florida, and leading the way is Dr. Joseph Ladapo. Like all WWTI doctors, he has impeccable credentials. His biography reads:

> *Joseph A. Ladapo, MD, PhD, is the State Surgeon General of Florida. He also serves as Professor of Medicine at the University of Florida, where his research examines behavioral economic strategies to reduce cardiovascular risk in low-income and disadvantaged populations. Clinically, he has cared primarily for hospitalized patients. His research program has been supported by the National Institutes of Health and Robert Wood Johnson Foundation, and includes clinical trials of interventions for*

weight loss, smoking cessation, and cardiovascular disease pre-
vention among people with HIV. Dr. Ladapo's studies have been
published in leading medical journals, including The Journal
of the American Medical Association, Journal of the American
College of Cardiology, and Annals of Internal Medicine. His
writings about health policy and public health have appeared in
the Washington Post, Wall Street Journal, and USA Today. Prior
to joining the faculty of University of Florida, he was a tenured
Associate Professor at David Geffen School of Medicine at the
University of California, Los Angeles (UCLA).

Dr. Ladapo graduated from Wake Forest University and received
his medical degree from Harvard and PhD in Health Policy from
Harvard Graduate School of Arts and Sciences. He completed his
clinical training in internal medicine at the Beth Israel Dea-
coness Medical Center, where he received the Harvard Medical
School Class of 2012 Resident Teaching Award and the Daniel
E. Ford Award in Health Services and Outcomes Research from
John Hopkins University.[23]

Despite this impressive background, Dr. Ladapo was a firehose of
disinformation regarding COVID. By March and April of 2020, Dr. Ladapo had already formed firm, unalterable opinions, writing articles titled
"Coronavirus Pandemic: We Were Caught Unprepared. It Is Too Late for
Lockdowns to Save Us"[24] and "Lockdowns Won't Stop the Spread."[25]
In these articles, he warned against "fear and hysteria." He said leaders
should "focus on the economy" and that it was pointless to try to limit the
virus:

Tragically, over the coming weeks, as the numbers of people
sickened and killed by COVID-19 increase — and they will — the

resulting fear and the hysteria will be used to try to prolong the
shutdowns. This move might work in some states that lean left,
but states that lean right will resist. Short of a miracle, expect to
see a tragedy unlike anything we've seen in generations. Heart-
breakingly, people you know will die. Celebrities and politicians
we all know will die. Hospitals will be overwhelmed and help-
less.[24]

He said he derived his views from his experience "taking care of
patients with COVID-19 at UCLA's flagship hospital," although there is
no record of him treating COVID patients at UCLA.[26]

Dr. Ladapo befriended other opponents of mitigation measures, such
as Drs. Scott Atlas, Martin Kulldorff, and Bhattacharya, joining them in
an Oval Office meeting with President Trump in August 2020. He would
later sign the Great Barrington Declaration (GBD). As the pandemic
progressed, he continued to disparage mitigation measures and promote
quack treatments in articles such as "Are Covid Vaccines Riskier than
Advertised?"[27] "Too Much Caution Is Killing Covid Patients,"[28] "Vaccine
Mandates Can't Stop Covid's Spread,"[29] and "Masks Are a Distraction
from the Pandemic Reality."[30]

His work appealed to Gov. DeSantis, and in September 2021, Dr.
Ladapo was appointed Surgeon General of Florida and an associate
professor at the University of Florida, despite allegations that information
about his views was suppressed during the hiring process. During a news
conference at his hiring, Dr. Ladapo said:

Florida will completely reject fear as a way of making policies
in public health. So we're done with fear. [...] That's something
that, unfortunately, has been a centerpiece of health policy in the
United States ever since the beginning of the pandemic.[31]

Once in office, Dr. Ladapo continued to dismantle any attempts to limit the virus. His first executive action was to repeal quarantine rules for children exposed to COVID, and he refused to wear a mask during a meeting with a State Senator who was undergoing cancer treatment, claiming that masks prevent effective communication.[32]

Dr, Ladapo also does not seem to be doing much at the University of Florida. According to an article titled "'Ladapo's a Charlatan': Florida Surgeon General's Tenure at UF is Lackluster, Colleagues Say":

> *Now, more than three years into his tenure, internal records and interviews with more than a dozen professors and administrators raise questions about whether Ladapo is meeting UF's expectations.*
>
> *Ladapo's work calendar shows monthslong stretches with little to no activity. Instead of attaining grants and conducting research, he spent his first year revising manuscripts and writing his memoir, "Transcend Fear," which details his skepticism of vaccines.[33]*

Indeed, spreading disinformation about vaccines seems to be Dr. Ladapo's primary mission, and his rhetoric often took on disturbing, mystical overtones. According to an article titled "DeSantis' Anti-Vax Surgeon General Calls COVID shots 'the Antichrist'" about Dr. Ladapo's appearance on Steve Bannon's podcast:

> *"I think it probably does have some integration at some levels with the human genome," Ladapo said on the War Room podcast, "because these vaccines are honestly—they're the Antichrist of all products. So I think it probably does. But I'm not saying it does."*
>
> *"I'm saying that they themselves have said you should test for*

it," he said of the Food and Drug Administration. "And that hasn't happened, and they've provided no proof that it's happened. And that's so wrong. You know, it's just complete disrespect to the human genome and the importance of protecting it and preserving it. And that is our connection to God." [34]

During an interview on Fox News in 2023, Dr. Ladapo said he would not recommend COVID vaccines "to any living being on this planet" [35] and castigated the CDC and FDA, saying, "They're pushing the product on human beings. That is an anti-human approach … an anti-human policy." The idea that vaccines rob people of their humanity is an old anti-vaccine talking point. Anti-vaxxers, such as Sayer Ji from Green-MedInfo, wrote articles titled "Vaccination Agenda: An Implicit Transhumanism / Dehumanism" [36] long before the pandemic.

Dr. Ladapo also spread a deluge of doubt on social media. Some examples include:

- *While the feds push false narratives, we assessed the data & here's the truth: Over 70% of CDC's so-called "COVID hospitalizations" in FL are not hospitalized FOR COVID. They may be in the ER with a broken leg, have no respiratory symptoms, but happen to test positive.* [37]
- *@CDCgov & @US_FDA are gaslighting Americans with their new, unproven COVID-19 boosters, and recommend them for 6 month-old babies! We say bring data, acknowledge serious safety concerns & acknowledge the many people who believe they've been injured by these vaccines.* [38]
- *CDC & FDA continue to push COVID vaccines that are not backed by clinical evidence, but blind faith alone with ZERO regard for widespread immunity. The American people deserve the truth, but the Biden admin only wants to control your behavior.* [39]
- *Florida data and a new Swiss study show it. CDC and FDA*

are silent. mRNA COVID-19 vaccines are ruining trust in scientists and public health.[40]

- *The most consistent thing the CDC and FDA have done is deny the truth. As State Surgeon General, I am grateful for @GovRonDeSantis' leadership and for choosing facts and reason over fear in response to COVID-19 in Florida.*[41]

- *Don't let the CDC and their minions confuse you with spin. In Florida, total vaccines administered increased by 400% after mRNA COVID-19 vax was introduced, while adverse events increased by 1700%.*[42]

- *Thank you, @SenRonJohnson_, for your dedication. Adverse effects of mRNA COVID-19 vaccines should be addressed with scientifically appropriate attention, rather than the see-no-evil attitude from the FDA and CDC. Pure propaganda.*[43]

- *Parents, don't hold your breath... CDC & FDA abandoned their posts. Keep sticking with your intuition and keep those COVID jabs away from your kids.*[44]

- *"[CDC's] papers are uniquely timed to further political goals and objectives; as such, these papers appear more as propaganda than as science." Great piece by @VPrasadMDMPH.*[45]

Florida Surgeon General Altered Key Findings in Study on Covid-19 Vaccine Safety
— News Headline, April 2023

Unsurprisingly, the state of Florida is now officially anti-vaccine. In 2022, Gov. DeSantis said:

I would say we are affirmatively against the Covid vaccine for young kids. These are the people who have zero risk of getting anything.[46]

Gov. DeSantis made anti-vaccine ideology a centerpiece of his failed presidential bid. According to one article:

DeSantis again tried to rally vaccine-skeptic voters to his side,

headlining a "Medical Freedom" town hall at a ski area in Man-
chester, N.H., alongside Florida's Surgeon General, Dr. Joseph
Ladapo. During the event, which was hosted by Mr. DeSantis's
super PAC, the Florida governor insisted that federal public
health agencies had spewed "nonsense" throughout the pandem-
ic and needed a complete overhaul.

He claimed that the Covid shots have been rolled out without
proper clinical studies and that federal officials had either lied
or were flatly wrong about the benefits and risks — a view that
has been roundly condemned by a wide array of public health
experts, academics and scientists.

"We know the federal government muffed this in many different
ways and we need a reckoning," the governor said.[47]

Indeed, Dr. Ladapo has been Gov. DeSantis's partner in this anti-vaccine campaign, turning his office into a fountain of disinformation. One
article stated:

Florida Surgeon General Joe Ladapo's campaign against
COVID-19 vaccines has intensified in the past few weeks before
Gov. Ron DeSantis' crucial tests in the Iowa presidential cau-
cuses and New Hampshire primary. And experts say that's not a
coincidence.

"It's one thing for a large state's leading health officer to be an
advocate for shared values," said Kenneth Goodman, the direc-
tor of the University of Miami Institute for Bioethics and Health
Policy. "It's another to weaponize medical misinformation to
trick citizens into voting for his boss."[48]

No one has made vaccines a political issue more than this, and Dr.
Ladapo had a few tricks up his sleeve.

The Florida Department of Health issued a statement from 2022, titled "State Surgeon General Dr. Joseph A. Ladapo Issues New mRNA COVID-19 Vaccine Guidance," that stated:

> Today, State Surgeon General Dr. Joseph A. Ladapo has announced new guidance regarding mRNA vaccines. The Florida Department of Health conducted an analysis through a self-controlled case series, which is a technique originally developed to evaluate vaccine safety.
>
> This analysis found that there is an 84% increase in the relative incidence of cardiac-related death among males 18-39 years old within 28 days following mRNA vaccination. With a high level of global immunity to COVID-19, the benefit of vaccination is likely outweighed by this abnormally high risk of cardiac-related death among men in this age group. Non-mRNA vaccines were not found to have these increased risks.
>
> As such, the State Surgeon General recommends against males aged 18 to 39 from receiving mRNA COVID-19 vaccines. Those with preexisting cardiac conditions, such as myocarditis and pericarditis, should take particular caution when making this decision.
>
> "Studying the safety and efficacy of any medications, including vaccines, is an important component of public health," said Surgeon General Dr. Joseph Ladapo. "Far less attention has been paid to safety and the concerns of many individuals have been dismissed – these are important findings that should be communicated to Floridians."[49]

That sounds bad. However, later documents revealed several problems with this "analysis." According to the article "Florida Surgeon

General Altered Key Findings in Study on Covid-19 Vaccine Safety":

Florida Surgeon General Joseph Ladapo personally altered a state-driven study about Covid-19 vaccines last year to suggest that some doses pose a significantly higher health risk for young men than had been established by the broader medical community, according to a newly obtained document.

The newly released draft of the eight-page study, provided by the Florida Department of Health, indicates that it initially stated that there was no significant risk associated with the Covid-19 vaccines for young men. But "Dr. L's Edits," as the document is titled, reveal that Ladapo replaced that language to say that men between 18 and 39 years old are at high risk of heart illness from two Covid vaccines that use mRNA technology.

"Results from the stratified analysis for cardiac related death following vaccination suggests mRNA vaccination may be driving the increased risk in males, especially among males aged 18-39," Ladapo wrote in the draft. "The risk associated with mRNA vaccination should be weighed against the risk associated with COVID-19 infection."[50]

The article quoted Dr. Matt Hitchings, a biostatistician at the University of Florida, as saying:

I think it's a lie. To say this — based on what we've seen, and how this analysis was made — it's a lie.

Another article titled "Florida Health Officials Removed Key Data from Covid Vaccine Report" reported that Dr. Ladapo had removed data showing what every other study shows: COVID is more dangerous than the COVID vaccine. It said:

Now, draft versions of the analysis obtained by the Tampa Bay

> *Times show that this recommendation was made despite the state having contradictory data. It showed that catching COVID-19 could increase the chances of a cardiac-related death much more than getting the vaccine.*
>
> *That data was included in an earlier version of the state's analysis but was missing from the final version compiled and posted online by the Florida Department of Health. Ladapo did not reference the contradictory data in a release posted by the state.*[51]

Dr. Hitchings was also quoted, stating:

> *This is a grave violation of research integrity. (The vaccine) has done a lot to advance the health of people of Florida and he's encouraging people to mistrust it.*

Elsewhere, Dr. David Gorski said:

> *This is the first time that we've seen a state government weaponize bad science to spread anti-vaccine disinformation as official policy.*[52]

Ladapo is much closer to being correct than the FDA and CDC.
— *Dr. Vinay Prasad*

Unsurprisingly, WWTI doctors rallied to Dr. Ladapo's defense. They weren't bothered by his data fraud or articles such as "Joseph Ladapo Says Anti-Vaccine Crusade Was God's Plan. It Cost Him His Peers' Trust."[53] Because they shared his anti-vaccine sentiments and opposition to public health, they overlooked his fraud and mysticism. Dr. Vinay Prasad, for example, described a report on Dr. Ladapo's flawed analysis as "a stupid news story" and that:

> *Ladapo is much closer to being correct than the FDA and CDC. Fascinating that the media does not cover that.*[54]

Dr. Tracy Beth Høeg similarly said:

> *Attempts to quantify exact amount of harm aside, FDA & CDC continuing to approve & recommend young people be exposed to known risks for unknown benefits (>95% already infected!) *is* the real scandal.*[55]

Dr. Bhattacharya hosted Dr. Ladapo on one of his podcasts and promoted the episode on social media by quoting him as saying:

> *I have such trouble… personally with the degree of contempt for honesty that the FDA and CDC demonstrate. They're not interested in informed decision-making.*[56]

In the mirror world, data manipulation and overtly religious anti-vaccine beliefs are acceptable so long as they spread SARS-CoV-2 and undermine trust in public health.

Predictably, Dr. Ladapo expanded his "warning" about COVID vaccines in 2024. He issued a statement that extolled the virtues of "transparency and scientific integrity"[57] and said:

> *The Surgeon General outlined concerns regarding nucleic acid contaminants in the approved Pfizer and Moderna COVID-19 mRNA vaccines, particularly in the presence of lipid nanoparticle complexes, and Simian Virus 40 (SV40) promoter/enhancer DNA. Lipid nanoparticles are an efficient vehicle for delivery of the mRNA in the COVID-19 vaccines into human cells and may therefore be an equally efficient vehicle for delivering contaminant DNA into human cells. The presence of SV40 promoter/enhancer DNA may also pose a unique and heightened risk of DNA integration into human cells.*
>
> *In 2007, the FDA published guidance on regulatory limits for DNA vaccines in the Guidance for Industry: Considerations*

*for Plasmid DNA Vaccines for Infectious Disease Indications
(Guidance for Industry). In this Guidance for Industry, the FDA
outlines important considerations for vaccines that use novel
methods of delivery regarding DNA integration, specifically:*

- *DNA integration could theoretically impact a human's
  oncogenes – the genes which can transform a healthy
  cell into a cancerous cell.*
- *DNA integration may result in chromosomal instability.*
- *The Guidance for Industry discusses biodistribution
  of DNA vaccines and how such integration could
  affect unintended parts of the body including blood,
  heart, brain, liver, kidney, bone marrow, ovaries/
  testes, lung, draining lymph nodes, spleen, the site of
  administration and subcutis at injection site.*

Dr. Ladapo concluded:

*If the risks of DNA integration have not been assessed for mRNA
COVID-19 vaccines, these vaccines are not appropriate for use
in human beings.*

This is also an old and well-worn anti-vaccine trope. Anti-vaxxers
have long spread fear about SV40 in vaccines, especially with regards to
polio vaccines.[58]

Dr. Ladapo's anti-vaccine disinformation earned at least well-de-
served rebukes from federal health officials:

- *The challenge we continue to face is the ongoing proliferation
  of misinformation and disinformation about these vaccines
  which results in vaccine hesitancy that lowers vaccine uptake.
  Given the dramatic reduction in the risk of death, hospitalization and serious illness afforded by the vaccines, lower vaccine
  uptake is contributing to the continued death and serious*

illness toll of COVID-19.[59]

- *Unfortunately, the misinformation about COVID-19 vaccine safety has caused some Americans to avoid getting the vaccines they need to be up to date. This has led to unnecessary death, severe illness and hospitalization. These tragic outcomes not only have a devastating effect on individuals and their families, but they also create a tremendous strain on our healthcare systems and clinicians, potentially compromising care for other patients.*[60]

Indeed, unnecessary death, severe illness, and hospitalization is what happened in the real world.

Statewide Grand Jury to investigate crimes and wrongdoing committed against Floridians related to the COVID-19 vaccine.
— *Governor Ron DeSantis*

Beyond encouraging unvaccinated Floridians to repeatedly catch COVID, the state took a dark turn in 2022 with a press release titled "Governor Ron DeSantis Petitions Florida Supreme Court for Statewide Grand Jury on COVID-19 Vaccines and Announces Creation of the Public Health Integrity Committee"[61] that planned to "investigate crimes and wrongdoing committed against Floridians related to the COVID-19 vaccine." The press release said:

Today, Governor Ron DeSantis held a roundtable discussion joined by Surgeon General Dr. Joseph Ladapo and world-renowned physicians, researchers, and public health experts to discuss adverse events of the mRNA COVID-19 vaccines and announce new, aggressive actions to hold the federal government and Big Pharma accountable, including:

- *Establishing the Public Health Integrity Committee. The*

*Committee will be overseen by the Surgeon General to assess
federal public health recommendations and guidance to ensure
that Florida's public health policies are tailored for Florida's
communities and priorities.*

- *Filing a petition for a Statewide Grand Jury to investigate
crimes and wrongdoing committed against Floridians related
to the COVID-19 vaccine.*

- *Leading further surveillance into sudden deaths of individuals that received the COVID-19 vaccine in Florida, based on
autopsy results. The state will collaborate with the University
of Florida to compare research with studies done in other
countries.*

*The Biden Administration and pharmaceutical corporations
continue to push widespread distribution of mRNA vaccines on
the public, including children as young as 6 months old, through
relentless propaganda while ignoring real-life adverse events.*

*At today's roundtable the Governor and health experts discussed
data covering serious adverse events. These risks include coagu-
lation disorders, acute cardiac injuries, Bell's palsy, encephalitis,
appendicitis, and shingles.*

In addition to Dr. Ladapo, several WWTI doctors were named to the
"Public Health Integrity Committee," including Drs. Bhattacharya, Kulldorff, Høeg, and Joseph Fraiman. In their statements about the committee, WWTI centered themselves and spread doubt. They said:

*"This has been a tremendously difficult time for everybody, but
we are near the tail end of it and it is time to start taking stock
of what went wrong and make reforms so this doesn't happen
again," **Dr. Jay Bhattacharya, M.D., Ph.D., Professor of
Health Policy, Stanford University Medical School.** "I think
the centrally important issue that caused the problems is that we*

silenced qualified people from expressing their thinking, and as a result the decision making at the top of the country was absolutely abysmal. When you have censorship, the kinds of suppression of voices that is essentially a social credit system demeaning people who disagree with the CDC, you're going to get bad decisions that don't get checked. I am looking forward to working in coming years to reform American public health so that when there is another pandemic we do a much better job than we did during this one."

*"It is clear we urgently need updated and fully transparent vaccines risk-benefit analyses for all age groups for physicians to make informed recommendations and patients to make informed decisions," said **Dr. Tracey** [sic] Høeg, M.D., Ph.D., Physician **Epidemiologist and Clinical Researcher at Department of Epidemiology & Biostatistics, University of California San Francisco, Acumen, LLC.** "Blanket mandates or requirements for COVID-19 vaccines are both unscientific and unethical given the vaccines' ineffectiveness at providing lasting protection from infection or transmission and the uncertainty surrounding the current vaccines' benefits and risks."*

*"It is always important to balance benefits and risks. For older high-risk people who have not vet [sic] had Covid, vaccine benefits outweigh potential risks for an adverse reaction," said **Dr. Martin Kulldorff, Ph.D., Scientific Director, Brownstone Institute; Fellow, Hillsdale College's Academy for Science & Freedom.** "For children, young adults and those who have had COVID, the risk of dying from COVID is miniscule, so even a small risk of a serious vaccine adverse reaction, such as myocar-*

ditis, will tip the balance against the vaccine."

In reality, death from COVID is worse than vaccine myocarditis.

In 2024, the Grand Jury released its first report.[62] Dr. Mallory Harris summarized its "findings" as follows:

> *A 33-page document that includes 'vaccine' and related words*
> *exactly 29 times.*
>
> - *21 times in the introduction, to explain the charge of the grand*
>   *jury and how it examined whether there was "criminal activity*
>   *or wrongdoing" with respect to COVID-19 vaccines*
> - *2 times to explain assumptions underlying mathematical SIR*
>   *models of disease transmission and note that COVID-19 vac-*
>   *cines may be assumed to both reduce susceptibility and risk of*
>   *severe disease*
> - *2 times to highlight how some nonpharmaceutical interven-*
>   *tions disrupted administration of international vaccination*
>   *programs against diseases like measles*
> - *3 times to discuss the CDC's changing guidelines about mask-*
>   *ing (in response to new data about infection and transmission*
>   *amongst vaccinated people as the delta variant began to*
>   *spread)*
> - *1 time in the conclusion, to note that "[t]here is a case to be*
>   *made that…lockdowns enabled others in high-risk groups to*
>   *'bridge the gap' until 2021 when they had access to vaccines."*
>   *Notably, this claim (which the report suggests the Grand Jury*
>   *may follow up on at a later date) would mean that both lock-*
>   *downs and vaccines helped to save lives in Florida.*
>
> *Everything else in this report is pointedly not about vaccines: It*
> *rehashes old grievances about shelter-in-place orders, masks,*
> *and other nonpharmaceutical interventions. Even those who*
> *agree with the gist of this report (that COVID-19 wasn't as*
> *deadly as they said and that the measures implemented to prevent*
> *its spread were not worth their costs) should agree that it doesn't*

remotely address the particular concerns that Governor DeSantis seemed to think it would.[63]

However, Dr. Harris also added:

The grand jury is expected to make multiple reports and has requested an extension through the end of this year to complete their investigation, so they may just be waiting on those to get to the alleged mass criminal conspiracy.

When the verdict arrived, no criminality was found. However, that wasn't the point. The point was to spread doubt and mistrust about vaccines and the companies that make them. According to one article on the final jury report:

A statewide grand jury convened at the request of Florida Gov. Ron DeSantis to investigate "any and all wrongdoing" concerning COVID-19 vaccines did not find any evidence of criminal activity, according to a report unsealed on Tuesday.

"(N)ot finding any indictable criminal activity does not mean we did not find any problems. On the contrary, there are profound and serious issues involving the process of vaccine development and safety surveillance in the United States," the grand jury wrote in its final report.[64]

No one is going to jail for producing lifesaving COVID vaccines, fortunately. However, the damage was done and the mission was accomplished.

The vaccination rate of Florida kindergarteners has fallen to 90.6% [...] and concerned pediatricians say they are exhausted trying to combat anti-vax information – including from the state government.
— *News Report September 2024*

Florida's anti-vaccine disinformation isn't limited to only COVID. An article from 2024 titled "Pediatricians 'Exhausted' as Vaccinations Drop in DeSantis' Florida"[65] spoke of the challenges faced by doctors operating in the real world. It said:

> *The vaccination rate of Florida kindergarteners has fallen to 90.6%, the lowest in over a decade, and concerned pediatricians say they are exhausted trying to combat anti-vax information – including from the state government. "It's gotten difficult to manage," said Dr. Lisa Gwynn, a Miami pediatrician and medical director for a mobile clinic that serves uninsured children. [...] Since the pandemic, vaccine hesitancy over the mRNA "jab" spread to other vaccines, pediatricians say, who add that it's becoming difficult to practice in the state.*

In 2024, pediatricians are "exhausted trying to combat anti-vax information – including from the state government."

The article linked to the minutes of a Florida pediatric society, which reported:

> *Dr. Mirza said that the drop in immunization rates is appalling and creates problems for the residency program when assigning residents for their primary care experiences since we want them to work in clinics where immunizations are being recommended and they see that as a major role for pediatricians besides advocacy. She wished that those at the State government level had an opportunity to visit a developing country and see people afflicted by polio or see someone with SSPE* [subacute sclerosing panencephalitis] *because they had measles as a child, to really understand the power of vaccination.*[66]

Dr. Mirza is absolutely right. Dr. Ladapo also opposed standard infectious control policy during a measles outbreak in 2024. In a statement,

Dr. Ladapo mentioned that measles is highly contagious, and that the vaccine is highly effective at preventing the disease.[67] However, it did not actually suggest the MMR vaccine, nor did it suggest that unvaccinated children stay home until the outbreak ended, as is recommended practice. Dr. Ladapo said the Department of Health "is deferring to parents or guardians to make decisions about school attendance." Dr. Ali Khan, Dean of Public Health at the University of Nebraska, said in an interview about this outbreak:

> *I'm flummoxed about this. I've never heard of a surgeon general who didn't at least advocate for best public health practice. If you're undermining confidence in public health, including vaccination and public health measures, you are putting an increasing number of people at risk of these diseases that we no longer see anymore.*[68]

While that measles outbreak didn't spiral out of control—fortunately—Florida has already helped spread measles in 2024. According to one article:

> *Measles cases that turned up in at least three states this year were linked to visits to Florida, federal and state investigators concluded, shedding light on some of the early infections that have fueled an uptick of the highly contagious virus.*
>
> *Florida's health department thinks families of the cases earlier this year from Indiana and Louisiana may have crossed paths in the state, according to messages sent between local investigators and the Centers for Disease Control and Prevention through late February.*[69]

From spreading disinformation about COVID vaccines to yawning at measles, WWTI doctors view Florida as a model and test-run for to the entire country, and that has the potential to be really bad.

Chapter 9: Let the Kids Work

If kids were allowed to work and compulsory school attendance was abolished, the jobs of choice would be at Chick-Fil-A and Walmart.
— Jeffrey Tucker

Here are some headlines most people find disturbing:
- Hyundai Under Scrutiny for Child Labor Violations in Alabama, Georgia[1]
- Chipotle Pays Over $300K to Settle Child Labor Allegations in DC[2]
- 2 Florida Bills Could Roll Back Child Labor Laws. What Do They Do?[3]
- Third Teen Worker Killed in Industrial Accident as States Try to Loosen Child Labor Laws[4]
- Children Risk Their Lives Building America's Roofs[5]
- Where Migrant Children Are Living, and Often Working, in the U.S.[6]
- Slaughterhouse Children: Child Labor Exposed in America's Food Industry[7]
- 'It Should Never Have Happened': Death of Boy, 16, At Sawmill Highlights Rise of Child Labour in US[8]
- California Poultry Supplier Illegally Employed Kids, Stole Wages: Labor Department[9]
- Feds Probe Child Labor Issues in New Bedford Seafood Plants[10]
- They're Paid Billions to Root Out Child Labor in the U.S. Why Do They Fail?[11]

These are all from 2023.

One person who may not be perturbed by these headlines is Mr. Jeffrey Tucker, the former editorial director for the American Institute for Economic Research (AIER) and the chief organizer of the Great Barrington Declaration (GBD), which promised that herd immunity would arrive in under 6 months if only 230 million unvaccinated Americans contracted COVID by the end of 2020. Mr. Tucker assembled epidemiologists, journalists, and camera crew at the signing of the GBD. It was a giant spectacle.

Mr. Tucker explained the origins of the GBD by saying:

> *What happened was that, you know, most scientists—serious scientists—are not political people. And they never expected, they're in science and epidemiology and immunology and public health because they want to help people and minimize the social damage of infectious diseases and pathogens. They're scientific people, not political people. Unfortunately, because of lockdowns, suddenly disease became highly political. It never should have happened, but it happened. And they found themselves in an awkward position.*
>
> *So after months, […] some of them began to speak out. I noticed one in particular, Martin Kulldorff. And then also I noticed Sunetra Gupta, who's, you know, a godlike figure within epidemiology. And then also Jay Bhattacharya, who's similarly highly credentialed, indeed PhD, you name it, at Stanford. Sunetra is over at Oxford, and Kulldorff is [at] Harvard. I noticed that they started to speak out a little bit.[12]*

However, AEIR may have been interested in more than just public health when they sponsored the GBD. AEIR is a libertarian organization that worries about the "new collectivists (DEI/Critical Theory/Marxism)" and claims to value "personal freedom, free enterprise, property rights, limited government, and sound money." Drs. Gavin Yamey and David Gorski wrote about AEIR in their article, "Covid-19 and the New Merchants of Doubt":

This declaration arose out of a conference hosted by the American Institute for Economic Research (AIER), and has been heavily promoted by the AIER, a libertarian, climate-denialist, free market think tank that receives "a large bulk of its funding from its own investment activities, not least in fossil fuels, energy utilities, tobacco, technology and consumer goods." The AIER's American Investment Services Inc. runs a private fund that is valued at $284,492,000, with holdings in a wide range of fossil fuel companies (e.g. Chevron, ExxonMobil) and in the tobacco giant Philip Morris International. The AIER has also received funding from the Charles Koch Foundation, which was founded and is chaired by the right-wing billionaire industrialist known for promoting climate change denial and opposing regulations on business. Koch linked organisations have also opposed public health measures to curb the spread of covid-19.[13]

Mr. Tucker is open about his political leanings. According to his Wikipedia page, he:

Is an American libertarian writer, publisher, entrepreneur and advocate of anarcho-capitalism and Bitcoin. For many years he worked for Ron Paul, the Mises Institute, and Lew Rockwell. With the American Institute for Economic Research (AIER) he organized efforts against COVID-19 restrictions starting in 2020, and he founded the Brownstone Institute think tank in 2021 to continue such efforts.[14]

Mr. Tucker has some views that most people, especially those concerned about the well-being of children, would find disturbing. A report by the Southern Poverty Law Center from 2000 titled "The Neo-Confederates" noted that Mr. Tucker was listed as a founding member of the racist League of the South and that he had written for their publication.[15]

Prior to the pandemic, Mr. Tucker wrote an article that encouraged children to smoke. He said:

> *The time to smoke is when you are a teen. It's when your lungs are strong, and your body is prepared to fight back the ill effects. It's also when you can gain the maximum advantage of the fact that smoking is very cool and enjoyable. I see no reason why parents shouldn't encourage it, while warning that they will probably have to stop after graduating college. And of course this is opposite of what the government says! The anti-smoking campaigns for young people are based on its supposed addictive quality. The fear is that once you start as a teen, you will never stop. But I've never understood what is meant by addictive. It's not like cigarettes take away your free will.*[16]

In addition to extolling the benefits of cigarettes for teens, Mr. Tucker also encouraged them to drop out of school and start working. In an article from 2016, titled "Let the Kids Work," he wrote:

> *The* Washington Post *ran a beautiful photo montage of children at work from 100 years ago. I get it. It's not supposed to be beautiful. It's supposed to be horrifying. I'm looking at these kids. They are scruffy, dirty, and tired. No question.*
>
> *But I also think about their inner lives. They are working in the adult world, surrounded by cool bustling things and new technology. They are on the streets, in the factories, in the mines, with adults and with peers, learning and doing. They are being valued for what they do, which is to say being valued as people. They are earning money.*
>
> *Whatever else you want to say about this, it's an exciting life. You*

*can talk about the dangers of coal mining or selling newspapers
on the street. But let's not pretend that danger is something that
every young teen wants to avoid. If you doubt it, head over the
stadium for the middle school football game in your local community, or have a look at the wrestling or gymnastic team's antics
at the gym.*[17]

Mr. Tucker further explained how he felt public schools damaged
children and that working in fast food would be an improvement for
them. He said:

*And I compare it to any scene you can observe today at the local
public school, with 30 kids sitting in desks bored out of their
minds, creativity and imagination beaten out of their brains, for-
bidden from earning money and providing value to others, learning no skills, and knowing full well that they are supposed to do
this until they are 22 years old if they have the slightest chance of
being a success in life: desk after desk, class after class, lecture
after lecture, test after test, a confined world without end. [...]
If kids were allowed to work and compulsory school attendance
was abolished, the jobs of choice would be at Chick-Fil-A and
WalMart. And they would be fantastic jobs too, instilling in
young people a work ethic, which is the inner drive to succeed,
and an awareness of attitudes that make enterprise work for all.
It would give them skills and discipline that build character, and
help them become part of a professional network.*

Mr. Tucker was careful to criticize only the "local public school." In
Mr. Tucker's vision, parents who can afford private schools should not
encourage their children to drop out and work stocking shelves. Chick-
Fil-A and Walmart need CEOs after all.

Mr. Tucker concluded his article, saying:

> Then we look at pictures of newspaper boys from 1905 and say,
> "Oh how sad that these kids had jobs. We are so much more
> humane now!"
>
> It's time we stop congratulating ourselves for taking away oppor-
> tunity from kids. It's time to let the kids work again.

Mr. Tucker remains proud of this article. After I shared a screen-shot of it on social media, he said his article was "very compelling"[18] and chastised me for not linking to the entire article. Journalist Walker Bragman further revealed Mr. Tucker's enthusiasm for getting kids out of the classroom and into the workforce in his article "Leaked Brownstone Institute Emails Reveal Support for Child Labor, Underage Smoking." In one email, Mr. Tucker says:

> I would fully repeal the 1936 "child labor" law. It's cruel and
> robs kids of a good life.[19]

In another email, Mr. Tucker shared an old picture of smoking adolescents and declared, "These kids seem happier than kids today." Reflecting this philosophy, the Brownstone Institute has published articles defending the vaping industry, such as "The Attack on Juul Is a Scandal."[20]

Many WWTI doctors were fine with all this.

I was there while it was being drafted. I was very moved. I made a couple suggestions here and there.
— Jeffrey Tucker

There is no question that the GBD aligns with Mr. Tucker's philosophy. Days after the GBD was signed in October 2020, he stated in an interview, "I was there while it was being drafted. I was very moved. I made a couple suggestions here and there."[12]

Despite being an avowed child-labor advocate, Mr. Tucker claimed that he was motivated by education and the "well-being of society." He said:

> Basically, what's striking about it is it's a basic statement of public health. We need to think about not just one disease, but all diseases. We need to think about not just physical health, but psychological health and the well-being of people to make choices and that sort of thing. That's all that's suffering, and the closing of the schools has been catastrophic.
>
> Public health, in the sense of the well-being of society, that's what the document is really about. What they say is that these lockdowns have not achieved their aims. In fact, it led to a public health catastrophe.

Mr. Tucker, a bow-tied avatar of the laptop class, said mitigation measures were "a public health catastrophe."

Despite having no expertise in epidemiology or infectious diseases, Mr. Tucker shared his vision that "natural immunity" would lead to herd immunity. As early as July 2020, he declared that New York had reached herd immunity "because the virus got there early and it swept through before the lockdowns,"[21] and in October 2020, he spoke about "the magic of science or mathematics," saying:

> And then they end by talking about an epidemiological truth that everybody has known for at least 70 years, which is that all viruses are mitigated through herd immunity. And they brought up that phrase, which has become a strange taboo. [...]
> You need to upgrade your immune system. That's been the advice, and even my mother knew this [...] but her mother's mother

didn't. And so on. It's the way that societies have learned to deal with disease, not through massive disruption, much less lock-down, but through normal social functioning and intelligence— intelligent protection of the vulnerable population.

And the key to public health and the presence of a new pathogen is to discover who is vulnerable […] and to make sure that those populations are protected while the rest of us develop immunities. And then through the magic of science or mathematics, whatever you want to call it, once a certain number have encoded the new viral information into the immune system, the virus comes under control, at least temporarily, or when I say temporarily, maybe for a full generation.[12]

Immunity did not last a full generation.

After the signing of the GBD, Mr. Tucker founded the Brownstone Institute, which has become a major source of conspiracies and anti-vaccine disinformation, not just with regards to COVID. Some examples are:

- Are There Vaccines in our Food Supply?[22]
- Covid Vaccines: Savior or Killer Shot?[23]
- Illusions in Vaccine Effectiveness[24]
- Mainstream Measles Mongers[25]
- Landmark Victory for the Vaccine-Injured[26]
- Questioning Modern Injection Norms[27]
- Government Investment into Vaccines Hasn't Paid Off[28]
- Vermont Supreme Court Sacrifices Children to Big Pharma[29]
- Biden and the Media's 'Anti-Disinformation Campaign'[30]
- Pandemic Preparedness: Arsonists Run the Fire Department[31]
- What Really Happened: Lockdown Until Vaccination[32]

This is just standard anti-vaccine content that existed decades before the pandemic.

The Brownstone Institute is also a leader of the deliberate COVID amnesia project. Dr. Jessica Hockett, an educational psychologist, published an article that claimed that "New York City's hospital emergency departments were not at a breaking point in spring 2020. In fact, they were relatively empty and saw a 50% drop in visits."[33] This startling conclusion was based on five "observations":

1.   *NYC Emergency Departments weren't overrun by people with COVID-19*

2.   *NYC Emergency Room respiratory visit spike may have been panic-driven*

3.   *Most people who visited NYC emergency rooms between March 2020 and June 2021 for respiratory symptoms were not admitted to the hospital*

4.   *Many patients counted as COVID hospitalizations in spring 2020 were not admitted with COVID-like illness*

5.   *The relationship between hospital inpatient deaths with COVID on the death certificate and people who were hospitalized because they had COVID is unclear*

Only someone who did not work in a New York City hospital could have written this article. It falsely concluded that doctors may have been deadlier than the virus. It said:

> *It's no wonder Michael Senger, Ethical Skeptic, and other analysts (including me) have said it was misuse of ventilators, protocol-induced staffing shortages, isolation, failure to treat, similar factors that resulted in thousands of Spring 2020 iatrogenic deaths in New York City and elsewhere.*

It's sobering to realize that someone with Mr. Tucker's worldview had a profound influence on our pandemic response, especially regarding children and young people.

It's also revealing that many WWTI doctors, who claimed to be *very concerned* about education and routine vaccines when it came to COVID mitigations, were willing to partner with and legitimize a man who wants my son to drop out of school so he can smoke with his friends after his shift at Chick-Fil-A. However, WWTI doctors shared Mr. Tucker's larger goal of spreading doubt about public health and were therefore willing to overlook his pro-tobacco and child labor advocacy, even as child labor laws are rolled back across the country. If high-school dropouts working at Chick-Fil-A bothered them, they kept it to themselves.

Dr. Vinay Prasad, for example, published the following articles at the Brownstone Institute:

- Why are Standards So Lax on Covid Drug Approvals?[34]
- The Fragmented Trust in Public Health[35]
- Who Among the Fringe Is Dangerous?[36]
- Things the CDC Does Not Know[37]
- The Hypocrisy of Medical Experts[38]
- Covid Zero Transitions to Covid Everyone[39]
- The White House is Now Your Doctor![40]
- The 4th Shot: The Flawed Research[41]
- What Happens When Cases Rise?[42]
- How the Flu and Covid Shots Are Different[43]
- Most Academics Went Silent. Why?[44]
- Mask Studies Reach a New Scientific Low Point[45]
- CDC Director Almost Admits Failure[46]
- CNN Loves Weathervane Pandemic Pundits[47]
- Testing Will Not Save Us[48]
- It Is Time to Face Reality about the Vaccines[49]
- Myocarditis Under Age 40: An Update[50]
- The Case against Vaccine Mandates for Domestic Flights[51]
- UK Does Not Advise Vaccines for 5-11 Year Olds, While the

US Starts to Mandate Them[52]
- It's Madness What Is Happening to College Kids[53]
- How Could They Have Done This to the Children?[54]
- Boosters for Men 16-40: A Regulatory Gamble[55]
- A Six-Year-Old Child Should Not Be Forced to Get the Covid Shot to Eat in a Restaurant[56]
- Is Anthony Fauci the Same Thing as 'Science'?[57]
- Well-Structured German Study Shows No Deaths among Healthy German Kids Ages 5 to 11[58]
- Should Fauci Resign?[59]
- New Variant, New Travel Restrictions, New Lockdowns[60]
- Do Masks Reduce Risk of COVID19 by 53%? How About 80%?[61]
- Should Every American Older than 18 Get a Booster?[62]
- Aaron Rodgers and the Absurdity of Media Coverage of Covid Policy[63]
- Germany and France Suspend Moderna Vaccination for People < 30 years Old[64]
- For Whom Do the Covid "Fact Checkers" Really Work?[65]
- The Cause of Myocarditis: COVID19 or COVID19 Vaccination?[66]

In one article, Dr. Prasad appointed himself as a spokesman for "poor, minority children from public education."[54] He said:

After we approved vaccines for adolescents (12-15) under the auspices of the EUA (emergency use authorization), school districts like Los Angeles, which were closed for a year, decided to exclude any child who did not comply in a short period of time. This coercion risked excluding poor, minority children from public education, or required them to receive 2 doses in short time interval, which increased their risk of myocarditis. The policy was needlessly cruel and regressive.

I doubt that vaccine mandates were a top concern of the parents of poor, minority children in school districts like Los Angeles. Rather, Dr. Prasad was using them to push his own agenda.

Dr. Jay Bhattacharya also published many articles at the Brownstone Institute, some with others like Dr. Martin Kulldorff as co-author, such as:

- Anthony Fauci: The Man Who Thought He Was Science[67]
- SCOTUS Versus Free Speech[68]
- The Plan: Lock You Down for 130 Days[69]
- The Dangers of the Biden Pandemic Plan[70]
- Democrats are Big Fans of Trump's Early Covid Response[71]
- Does Fauci Bear Any Responsibility? He Says No[72]
- Vaccine Fanaticism Fuels Vaccine Skepticism[73]
- The Emergency Must Be Ended, Now[74]
- The Collins and Fauci Attack on Traditional Public Health[75]
- Straight Talk about the Precautionary Principle[76]
- We Cannot Stop the Spread of COVID, But We Can End the Pandemic[77]
- A Medical News Site and Its Misinformation[78]
- Vaccine Mandates are Unethical[79]
- Misinformation and the Ministry of Truth: Testimony to U.S. House of Representatives Select Subcommittee on the Coronavirus Crisis[80]
- The Six Major Fails of Anthony Fauci[81]
- The Silence of Economists about Lockdowns[82]
- The Dangerous Fantasy of Zero Covid[83]
- The Strange Neglect of Natural Immunity[84]
- The UK Plot to Silence Lockdown Critics[85]
- What a Real Covid Commission Would Achieve[86]
- A Sensible and Compassionate Anti-Covid Strategy[87]
- The Power of Public Health Agencies Must Be Curbed[88]

In that last article, Dr. Bhattacharya said:

Contrary to what you hear these days from those making poor decisions throughout the pandemic, many of the errors were not honest mistakes. Public health embraced positions at odds with the scientific evidence throughout the pandemic, for instance, by pretending that immunity after COVID recovery does not exist, and by overstating the ability of the vaccine to stop COVID infection and transmission. Despite many getting vaccinated, COVID spread and people died anyway, with tremendous collateral harm—both economic and in terms of public health—deriving from the favored policies of our public health institutions. It is time to adopt laws to limit the powers of public health.

Another article at the Brownstone Institute by Josh Stevenson, titled "Trust in Doctors and Hospitals Plummets," bemoaned the lack of trust in medicine. It said:

A new paper in JAMA analyzes survey respondents in the US over the period of time right after the Covid pandemic started in April 2020 and through early 2024. It reveals a significant decline in trust in physicians and hospitals, dropping from 71.5% in April 2020, to 40.1% in January 2024. Lower trust levels were strongly associated with reduced likelihood of receiving Covid-19 vaccinations and boosters. [...]

As we witnessed firsthand in 2020 and 2021, and even today, the condescension, overt political motivations, and outright derision directed at those who were rationally skeptical of a brand-new vaccine, masks, and the extreme and harmful lockdown policies by medical practitioners and hospital systems have finally led to an inevitable consequence: the public simply does not trust them anymore. And not by a small margin—there has been a massive swing from majority trust to majority distrust. For anyone who was paying attention, this is not shocking.[89]

I've been paying attention, and this is not shocking.

Who is Funding the Brownstone Institute?
— *Walker Bragman*

No one has done more to reveal the financial networks supporting these COVID disinformation groups than Mr. Bragman. Because I cannot improve on his work, I will share a couple of his articles with his permission.

"Who is Funding the Brownstone Institute?"[90]
Big Money

The donations to Brownstone we were able to identify came through donor-advised funds—passthrough organizations that manage charitable contributions for clients—and private foundations.

How donor-advised funds work: A client will open an account with the fund, depositing money and transferring legal control to the fund managers, who then dispense the cash to charitable causes with input from the client. There are several key benefits of using these funds, but the main draw for political donors is anonymity. Donations appear under the name of the fund itself rather than the client, enabling secretive giving.

The largest donation to the COVID misinformation dark money operation with a source we were able to identify was $100,000 from the Morgan Stanley Global Impact Funding Trust, a donor-advised fund affiliated with banking giant Morgan Stanley. Sometime between July 2021 and June 2022 Fidelity Investments Charitable Gift Fund, another donor-advised fund, which is affiliated with Fidelity Investments, gave $64,000.

Brownstone also received $50,000 from the Bluebell Foundation, *a Florida-based nonprofit that has funded a number of charitable causes from universities to public broadcasting. In addition to Brownstone, the foundation funded another group with a particular focus on COVID: U.S. Right To Know, which describes itself as "a nonprofit investigative public health research and journalism group working globally to expose corporate wrongdoing and government failures that threaten our health, environment and food system." The group's website features a section "COVID-19 origins." It is possible that the virus escaped from a laboratory. Two U.S. intelligence agencies lean in favor of that theory as do a majority of Americans. However, available evidence has consistently pointed to natural origins.*

Another $50,000 came from the Crary Social Ecology Fund, a California-based 501(c)(3) charitable foundation that Cause IQ notes "primarily funds charitable activities." The foundation is overseen by two trustees: John L. Crary, who is listed on the Walker's Research business directory as president of the financial advisory and investment firm Juniper Capital LLC and a director of the Salinas-based Scheid Vineyards, and Barbara W. Crary. Brownstone was just one of several groups that promote anti-vaccine misinformation to receive Crary money. For example, Front Line COVID-19 Critical Care Alliance (FLCCC), a group that promotes quack COVID treatments like ivermectin and hypes up concerns about the safety of the mRNA vaccines, got $55,000. Last week, the group's founder, critical care physician Dr. Pierre Kory, invited his Twitter followers to join him in celebrating "the millions of lives saved by ivermectin in Covid," calling it "an uplifting story as well as a tragic one due to one of

History's most massive global Disinformation campaigns." Kory, an ally of anti-vaccine activist and Democratic 2024 presidential candidate Robert Kennedy Jr., also retweeted notorious anti-vaccine entrepreneur Steve Kirsch, who asked his followers, "Is the CDC totally blind to all the adverse events from the COVID vaccines?"

"I think they are," Kirsch wrote. "What do you think? Kory has frequently amplified Kirsch's anti-vaccine posts, including another tweet from July 7 in declaring, "We are throwing down the gauntlet on whether vaccines can trigger autism," asking, "Will anyone qualified pick it up?"

Kirsch announced he was "assembling a panel of experts (some with h-index over 100 such as Peter McCullough and Paul Marik) who claim vaccines cause autism," and "would like to know if there is any licensed doctor or academic ... or scientist at CDC, FDA, or NIH in America who disagrees with this position would like to question the panel in a live public 'grand rounds.'"

"This is important to get right," Kirsch wrote. "Their side refuses to be questioned, but our side is open to respectful public challenges from our scientific peers." Crary money also went to Informed Consent Action Network ($100,000) and Kennedy's Children's Health Defense ($50,000).

The last large Brownstone donor we were able to identify is the Woodshouse Foundation, which gave $50,000. Among the range of groups the foundation gave to are two Koch-backed libertarian groups. Woodshouse gave $75,000 to AIER, and $30,000 to the Reason Foundation, which publishes Reason Magazine.

Smaller Donations

Important Context *was able to put names to smaller donations as well. The Schwab Charitable Fund, for example, a donor-advised fund operated by financial titan Charles Schwab and Co., gave Brownstone roughly $6,000. Another $4,000 to the institute came from the Nebraska-based Creigh Family Foundation, which is overseen by corporate and securities attorney James C. Creigh. Creigh is a partner at the national law firm Kutak Rock LLP. According to his profile, he is "a nationally recognized lawyer with extensive experience in corporate finance, mergers and acquisitions (M&A) and other transactional matters" and "has led more than 250 financing and acquisition transactions in both legal and business capacities."*

Another $3,500 came from the Quest Family Foundation, a well-funded nonprofit that gives to a number of right-wing groups including fundamentalist Christian organizations and hate groups. In 2021, Quest gave $6,000 to Billy Graham Evangelistic Association. The foundation also gave $10,000 to the Family Research Council and $5,000 to the American Family Association, both of which are designated as anti-LGBTQIA+ hate groups by the Southern Poverty Law Center.

Quest gave $16,000 to the influential Council for National Policy (CNP), a secretive group that provides networking for right-wing donors and operatives, and $2,500 to the Leadership Institute, a dark money group that trains young conservatives to get involved in politics. CNP co-founder Morton Blackwell is the institute's president. Quest also gave $5,000 to Judicial Watch and $1,000 to Turning Point USA.

Questions Remain

The donations we identified amount to roughly half of the nine donations that comprise most of Brownstone's 2021 revenue. Much remains shrouded, including the largest donation to the group: $600,000.

As more tax records become available, it is possible questions surrounding Brownstone's funding will be answered.

Mr. Bragman also published the following regarding Brownstone Institute funding:

"New Scientist Group Calling for Pandemic Answers Has Ties to Right-Wing Dark Money"[91]

A new medical group behind an 80-page "blueprint" for a potential congressional commission to investigate the harms of the U.S. government's COVID-19 response has ties to the political right and dark money.

The Norfolk Group purports to be eight independent scientists from different political backgrounds who are not working "on behalf of any institution, public or private" but are rather seeking answers to explain how the U.S. has fared so poorly throughout the pandemic.

"Certainly, deaths are unavoidable during a pandemic," the group declares. "However, too many U.S. policy makers concentrated efforts on ineffective or actively harmful and divisive measures such as school closures that generated enormous societal damage without significantly lowering COVID-19 mortality, while failing to protect high-risk Americans. As a result, Americans were hard hit both by the disease and by collateral damage generated by misguided pandemic strategies and decisions that

ignored years of pandemic preparation guidance crafted by numerous public health agencies, nationally and internationally." Benign as the Norfolk Group may appear at first blush—an ABC News affiliate called it "a small group of renowned infectious disease experts"—the reality is murkier. The group represents the latest volley in an ongoing war on public health measures waged by the business-aligned right wing. With Republicans in control of the House of Representatives, it may well prove highly influential.

Dark Money Origins

On the third page of the Norfolk Group white paper is an acknowledgment that the authors came together through a meeting organized by the Brownstone Institute, a shadowy COVID misinformation nonprofit. Important Context *and the OptOut Media Foundation previously reported that Brownstone received most of its funding from just nine anonymous large donations in 2021.*

"Seven of us started the work at an in-person meeting in Norfolk, Connecticut, organized by the Brownstone Institute in May of 2022," the document reads. "We wrote and edited the bulk of this document during the subsequent six months. In honor of the place where we met, we call ourselves the Norfolk Group."

Since it was first established in May 2021, Brownstone has promoted a number of extreme positions including advocacy for child labor and an end to public education. Its main purpose, however, has always been opposing public health mandates. Brownstone was founded by anarcho-capitalist Jeffrey Tucker, who has ties to neo-Confederate groups and is a longtime veteran of billionaire industrialist Charles Koch's political influence network, as the "spiritual child" of the Great Barrington Declaration (GBD).

The GBD was an influential open letter that arose out of an October 2020 conference hosted by the American Institute for Economic Research, a libertarian think tank on the edges of Koch's network where Tucker worked—he was instrumental in organizing the effort. The document, which was rejected by the mainstream scientific community, called on governments and scientists to eschew broad public health measures in favor of embracing mass infection as a quick path to herd immunity.

Brownstone has become a hub of COVID-related misinformation, including anti-vaccine narratives, downplaying the seriousness of the pandemic. As we have previously reported, the institute has even tacitly encouraged violence against public health officials. Brownstone gave a fellowship to former Trump Health and Human Services science adviser Paul Alexander, who had previously called for hanging public health officials who tried to limit the spread of COVID. Brownstone founder, Tucker published an article on the group's website with a guillotine image suggesting "consequences" for such officials.

Right-Wing Ties

The scientists involved in the Norfolk Group have all been vocal opponents of public health measures—the group is a combination of GBD alums and signatories and organizers of the error-ridden Urgency of Normal toolkit, which aimed at getting children back into schools without COVID mitigation measures in place. Some have connections to the political right beyond Brownstone and are favorites of conservative institutions.

Norfolk Group members and GBD co-authors Drs. Jay Bhat-

tacharya and Martin Kulldorff, for example, are darlings in the world of right-wing dark money. They have been interviewed, promoted, imbued with various honors, and booked for speaking gigs by various business-aligned right-wing groups and institutions.

Bhattacharya, the more prolific of the two scientists, is a senior fellow at the conservative public policy think tank, the Hoover Institution, which is housed at Stanford University where he is a professor of health policy and economics. Hoover has received funding from Koch and other wealthy conservatives including the Walton Family. In 2021, it got more than $500,000 from DonorsTrust, a preferred funding conduit of the Koch network and even more extremist funders.

At some point since mid-December, Bhattacharya's profile page on Hoover's website was altered. His role is now listed as "courtesy." He was previously a research fellow at the institution. Bhattacharya has been a featured speaker at conferences hosted by Hoover, Council For National Policy, and the American Institute for Economic Research. He helped the American Commitment Foundation, a dark money group co-founded by a former vice president of the Koch flagship political operation, Americans For Prosperity, with its Supreme Court amicus brief supporting a challenge to the Occupational Safety and Health Administration's vaccine-or-test mandate for large businesses. Just this week, he was hosted by the University of Chicago chapter of the Federalist Society, the infamously well-funded conservative legal group dedicated to stacking the judiciary with extreme right-wing judges. The group got $3.7 million from DonorsTrust in 2021.

The university is also famous as a hub of laissez-faire economic thought, which provided much of the intellectual framework behind the modern conservative movement.

The Stanford professor and Kulldorff are teaching fellows at Hillsdale College's Academy of Science and Freedom. Hillsdale received $55,000 from the Charles Koch Foundation and another $17,000 from DonorsTrust in 2021. The scientists are being represented pro bono by Koch-funded litigation outfit New Civil Liberties Alliance (NCLA) in a lawsuit against the Biden administration for allegedly coercing social media and technology companies to 'censor' them. NCLA, which is headed up by a former in-house counsel for Koch Industries, received $1 million from Stand Together Fellowships—formerly the Charles Koch Institute—in 2021, as well as $15,000 from the Charles Koch Foundation and another $1 million from DonorsTrust.

Bhattacharya and Kulldorff have helped Republican lawmakers craft COVID policy at the federal and state level and have been called to testify as experts before Congress. They directly advised the Trump White House and Florida Gov. Ron DeSantis' administration and currently serve on DeSantis' new Public Health Integrity Committee to investigate federal pandemic response measures.

Another Norfolk scientist, Dr. Tracy Beth Høeg, is similarly connected on the right. Høeg is a consultant epidemiologist for Florida's Department of Health. Like Bhattacharya and Kulldorff, she is a member of DeSantis' Public Health Integrity Committee. Along with fellow Norfolk Group and Urgency of Normal member, Dr. Ram Duriseti, Høeg is being represented pro bono by

NCLA in a lawsuit against California over a new misinformation law, which empowers the state's medical board to punish doctors who promote COVID-related misinformation.

Meanwhile, Dr. Marty Makary, a surgical oncologist, Johns Hopkins professor, and Norfolk Group member, made the rounds on conservative media as a critic of the federal pandemic response and a COVID minimizer before being tapped by Republican Gov. Glenn Youngkin of Virginia as a COVID adviser last January.

Last month, in its "post-pandemic" roadmap, the Heritage Foundation, a prominent conservative think tank, highlighted Bhattacharya, Kulldorff, Høeg, and Makary. Like Hoover, the foundation has gotten funding from many prominent conservatives over the years including Kochs and the Waltons. In 2021, it received $15,000 from the Charles Koch Foundation, $8,000 from Stand Together Fellowships, and $361,000 from DonorsTrust.

Dubious Narratives

Implicit, dubious, and unproven assumptions underlie the Norfolk Group's document. The inquiries begin with the perspective that the Great Barrington Declaration and Urgency of Normal were fundamentally correct; that government officials censored their ideas to the detriment of the national pandemic response; that mitigation efforts such as lockdowns, school closures, widespread testing, vaccine mandates, and masking—particularly masking of children—did more harm than good.

There is an entire section, for example, dedicated to "collateral lockdown harms," beginning with a declaration that "the collateral damage associated with pandemic lockdown policies is enormous, cutting across multiple areas of physical and mental health, education, culture, religion, the economy, and the social fabric of society." Among the harms listed is an increase in 2020 in deaths from heart disease and stroke, conditions that have been linked to COVID infection.

"How much of this increase was collateral lockdown damage?" Norfolk Group asks. "Why was this problem not foreseen by the health agencies and politicians implementing lockdowns?"

Despite the fact that none of the scientists involved in the Norfolk Group are credentialed child development experts—Duriseti works in pediatric emergency medicine, has written about pediatric abdominal pain, and researched diagnosing pediatric appendicitis—the group's paper dedicates much ink to exploring the various possible psychological harms to children from COVID mitigation measures.

Straying beyond their field is a problem several of the scientists involved in Norfolk Group have been criticized for in the past, including those behind Urgency of Normal and Bhattacharya. U.S. District Judge Waverly Crenshaw called the latter's testimony in a case over school mask mandates "troubling" and "problematic," explaining that the Stanford professor had "offered opinions" involving "a discipline on which he admitted he was not qualified to speak."

"His demeanor and tone while testifying suggest that he is advancing a personal agenda," Crenshaw noted.

A substantial section of the Norfolk Group document deals with the alleged harms of school closures. The group suggests that the closures may have fueled a mental health crisis in young people. Data from the Centers for Disease Control and Prevention show that suicide rates for young people dropped off during the early months of the pandemic and have not otherwise deviated from pre-pandemic trends. Similarly, there was no spike in mental health emergency room visits for young people.

The Norfolk Group paper also takes issue with masking requirements for children, rehashing familiar, unproven narratives about speech and developmental delays as well as breathing difficulties while demanding randomized, controlled trials to demonstrate efficacy.

"Children face the least risk of COVID-19 and face the highest risk of harm from prolonged masking," the paper states. "Why were the youngest and most vulnerable children in the Head Start programs, overseen by the Department of Health and Human Services, some of the very last to be allowed to remove their masks in the Fall of 2022?"

In August, the American Academy of Pediatrics recommended that children wear masks, explaining that concerns about developmental delays were overblown. Dr. Diane Paul, Senior Director of clinical issues in speech-language pathology at the American Speech-Language-Hearing Association, had a similar assessment.

"At this point, we haven't seen any large-scale, long-term studies related to mask use during the pandemic and speech/language delays or disorders in children, Paul told Important Context/ OptOut *after reviewing the Norfolk Group section on masking children. "What we do know is that research shows that children look at a communication partner's eyes and use voices (tone, inflection) to recognize words and understand emotions. Masks don't interfere with these language learning processes."*

Paul noted that "It's true that typically developing children look at faces during the language learning period," but clarified, "they don't stare at faces all the time."

"We also know that in some cultures, adults regularly wear face coverings without a detrimental effect on their child's speech and language development," she said.

Paul did acknowledge that students with speech and language disorders may have "additional difficulties in educational or social settings communicating with masks," but added that "teachers, speech-language pathologists, and many others who work with children found many ways to improve communication and compensate for such challenges when mask wearing was widespread—at a time when most of us were working under less-than-ideal circumstances."

"And we recognize too that most children, with and without diagnosed speech and language disorders, spent most of their time during the pandemic with their families who did not wear masks at home," Paul said.

Overstating the harms of COVID mitigation efforts while downplaying the harms of the virus is a feature of the Norfolk Group's white paper, just as it was for the Great Barrington Declaration and Urgency of Normal before it. While the document bemoans learning loss from school closures, for example, it fails to address caregiver death. According to an estimate by the Imperial College of London, nearly 280,000 American children have lost a primary or secondary caregiver to the virus. Similarly, the only mentions in the document of long COVID are in a brief section questioning whether or not the condition poses a serious enough concern to warrant current levels of funding allocated to researching it by the National Institutes of Health.

A November report from HHS found that at the time, as many as 23 million Americans were suffering long COVID and that "it can be extremely disruptive, dismantling their ability to work, their sense of self, and their entire existence."

'Officials Have Questions To Answer'

The 80-page Norfolk Group paper actually reads a bit like score-settling for the scientists involved. It takes particular aim at perceived enemies of the Great Barrington Declaration like Dr. Deborah Birx, the former White House Coronavirus Response Coordinator. Birx notably refused to participate in a roundtable discussion with Bhattacharya and Kulldorff back in the summer of 2020, calling them "a fringe group without grounding in epidemics, public health or on the ground common sense experience."

"Did policy experts know about pre and early pandemic statements in which experts cast doubt on the ability of quarantine and lockdown measures to stop community spread without excessive collateral damage?" the document asks. "Why did Dr. Birx purposely avoid meeting with public health experts who had specifically proposed such measures?"

Other targets include Drs. Anthony Fauci and Francis Collins, respectively the former directors of the National Institute for Allergy and Infectious Diseases (NIAID) and the NIH. Both had been dissenting voices in the Trump White House as the administration embraced the Great Barrington Declaration.

Bhattacharya and Kulldorff blame the two public health officials for the widespread rejection of their ideas, highlighting an email exchanged between them in which Collins suggested that the declaration required a "quick and devastating published take-down." The exchange occurred three days after a well-publicized White House meeting between the declaration co-authors and HHS Secretary Alex Azar.

The Norfolk Group paper frames Fauci and Collins as propo-nents of a "lockdown philosophy" and suggests they worked covertly to undermine dissent against COVID mitigation efforts. "Why was so much influence on public health policy accorded to Drs. Collins and Fauci?" Norfolk Group asks. "They control the largest source of infectious disease research funding in the world. How many infectious disease scientists, who should have been strong voices during the pandemic, kept quiet for fear of losing the research funding on which their livelihood depends?"

Fauci, the NIAID, and the NIH are defendants in Bhattacharya and Kulldorff's NCLA lawsuit.

"The pandemic response is the worst assault on the working class since segregation and the Vietnam War and both Trump and Biden officials have questions to answer," Kulldorff told Import-ant Context/OptOut.

The Norfolk Group takes aim at teachers' unions as well, which have fought for safer schools and classrooms throughout the pan-demic. The group blames the unions for "lobbying for school clo-sures" and asks questions like, "What role did teachers unions play in shifting the burden of risk to grandparents and day care workers (who may have been older) to care for children during school days?"

'Hard To Take Anything From The Group Seriously'

Experts Important Context/OptOut *spoke with were critical of the new Norfolk Group. Dr. Robert Morris, for example, an epidemiologist who has advised several federal agencies including the CDC and the NIH, pointed out that only one member of the group—Høeg—has a Ph.D. in epidemiology. Even then, he explained, her only previous work in the field was related to ophthalmological epidemiology. She practiced physical medicine before the pandemic.*

"I'm not suggesting that any of them is not smart," Morris said. "But you can be the best brain surgeon in the world—you would not do well on a heart transplant. There's differences between these fields."

"And somehow, epidemiology looks really easy but again and again, these people prove how hard it is by doing it poorly," he added. Indeed, Bhattacharya was launched into the spotlight by right-wing media early in the pandemic with a deeply flawed seroprevalence study that significantly underestimated the severity of the virus. In May 2020, Buzzfeed revealed that the researchers had accepted money from the founder of JetBlue Airways, David Neeleman, a vocal opponent of business closures, without disclosing it.

Morris noted that his own Ph.D. is in Environmental Engineering; that he has a master's in biostatistics and epidemiology and an MD but clarified "I did epidemiologic research for 15 years and wrote about 50 papers, so I feel I can call myself an epidemiologist. And I taught epidemiology for 15 years."

Dr. Deepti Gurdasani, an epidemiologist and associate professor of artificial intelligence in public health at the Kirby Institute at the University of New South Wales, told Important Context/OptOut, *"It's hard to take anything from the group seriously given the history of the Brownstone Institute and the 'experts' within it, who have a long history of misrepresenting evidence and platforming misinformation."*

Gurdasani has long been a vocal critic of the Great Barrington Declaration, calling it "dangerous pseudoscience." She is a co-founder of a response declaration called the John Snow Memorandum.

Eleanor Murray, an assistant professor of epidemiology at the Boston University School of Public Health, told Important Context/OptOut *that the Norfolk Group document left her with "two initial impressions."*

"First, the fact that they refer to COVID-19 as in the past reflects a lack of understanding about the epidemiology of the disease," Murray said. *"Second, there seems to be a general lack of knowledge that after-action evaluation reports are standard and expected in public health. Once health departments are actually at a place where they are no longer bouncing from crisis moment to crisis moment with COVID-19, after-action reports will of course happen."*

'No Easy Choices'

Dr. Julia Raifman, an assistant professor at Boston University School of Public Health who leads the COVID-19 U.S. State Policy Database, cautioned against taking the wrong lessons from the pandemic.

"The mitigation measures we took were costly but the alternative was even more costly," she said. "There were no easy choices, but I appreciate the leaders who chose temporary setbacks to education and the economy over even greater permanent loss of life."

Raifman explained that "closures helped avoid many more people dying while we learned about how to mitigate spread of the virus, while health care workers learned how to provide better care for people infected, and while scientists developed a vaccine."

Raifman did point out, however, that "economic supports" were "key to any such closures," noting that the assistance provided by Congress and two presidential administrations "during this period actually led to a record decline in poverty."

'A Blueprint'

While the effort may struggle to find mainstream scientific legitimacy, the Norfolk Group has a clearer goal: "[T]o present a blueprint containing key public health questions for a COVID-19 commission." With Republicans in control of Congress, it is likely the group will succeed in this measure—especially now that Fox News has picked up on it.

For months, Republicans in the House and Senate have been promising to investigate various aspects of the pandemic, including COVID's origins and the actions of public health officials—namely Fauci—in responding to the crisis.

Over the summer, in the lead-up to the midterms, House Republican Leader Kevin McCarthy tweeted that "Dr. Fauci lost the trust of the American people when his guidance unnecessarily kept schools closed and businesses shut while obscuring ques-

tions about his knowledge on the origins of COVID."

"He owes the American people answers," McCarthy wrote. "A @HouseGOP majority will hold him accountable."

Last month, following a tumultuous speakership fight, the new GOP House majority took steps to follow through on McCarthy's promise, establishing a select subcommittee with broad powers to investigate the government's pandemic response. Rolling Stone *reported that conspiracy theorist Marjorie Taylor Greene, who has compared masking to the Holocaust, had been appointed to sit on the subcommittee, which is part of the House Oversight and Accountability Committee.*

Already there are indications that the new body will promote the same narratives as the dark money groups fighting against public health measures.

After a so-called Twitter Files thread by writer and COVID contrarian David Zweig, which Important Context *has previously covered, Oversight Committee Chairman James Comer (R-Ky.) tweeted in December, for example, that "Big Tech shouldn't be in the business of hiding facts."*

I am sure there is more work to be done uncovering the networks and financial ties that link WWTI doctors.

Motivating biases need not be considered nefarious, only considered.
— Drs. John Mandrola, Adam Cifu, Vinay Prasad, and Andrew Foy

In their foundational paper, "The Case for Being a Medical Conservative," Drs. John Mandrola, Adam Cifu, Andrew Foy, and Prasad warned of "dualities of interests."[92] They said:

Dualities of interest must be considered in determining the quality of evidence. [...] The medical conservative, therefore, is pragmatic about human nature and the prevailing business model of medical science. To wit, content experts, professional societies, or journal editors who too harshly criticize an industry product jeopardize future funding. Motivating biases need not be considered nefarious, only considered.

These doctors were right to be concerned about "motivating biases." Many studies have demonstrated that, although most doctors believe themselves to be immune from financial incentives, they do influence their practice. I devoted an entire chapter to this in my book on cognitive errors in medicine that concluded:

Beneficence is one of the four core principles of medical ethics. It states that clinicians should strive to always do the most good for their patients. Clinicians who view their patients as an ATM machine by performing unnecessary procedures and tests or selling supplements to them are violating this principle. Their primary duty, the health of their patients, becomes intertwined with the potential for increased income.

Clinicians should not pretend they are immune from unconsciously responding to financial incentives. Jamie Koufman, an otolaryngologist, wrote:

> *Though they would vigorously deny it, entrepreneurial doctors often treat each patient as an opportunity to make money. Research shows that physicians quickly adapt their treatment choices if the fees they get paid change. But the current payment incentives do more than drive up costs—they can kill people.*[93]

In the interests of disclosing my motivating biases, I earned about

$10,000 from *We Want Them Infected* after paying for a voice reader and an editor. This is not a small amount of money, but I could have made more by picking up a handful of weekend moonlighting shifts. Writing dense books about a pandemic most people want to forget isn't the pathway to riches and fortune, it turns out. I lose money on my podcast about the WWTI movement and earn nothing from my writing at *Science-Based Medicine*. Anyone can comment there for free.

I am sure many WWTI doctors had no conflicts of interest and made no money from sharing their pandemic opinions. Others, however, developed more consistent and lucrative revenue streams. Some doctors didn't just interact with business interests; they *became* businesses, and it's worth considering how these motivating biases may have affected their public communications.

According to a news report about Dr. Marty Makary's nomination to lead the FDA:

> *Makary is a director on the board at Harrow, an ophthalmic pharmaceuticals company, and an adviser to Sidecar Health, an insurance provider that aims to lower customer costs by eliminating provider networks and drug formularies. He's also chief medical adviser to Nava, a benefits brokerage, and chief medical officer at Sesame, a cash-pay health service market that offers compounded semaglutide.*[94]

Dr. Makary earned $40,000 in 2023 consulting for Harrow,[95] and at one time he charged $20,000–$30,000 for speaking engagements.[96]

Other doctors found less traditional but potentially more lucrative revenue streams. In their must-read article, "Subscription Science: How Crowdfunding Has Become a Conflict of Interest," Drs. Benjamin Mazer and Michael Rose wrote that "conflicts of interest are an ongoing threat to medical practice."[97] They further noted that:

> *Digital platforms such as Patreon, Substack, YouTube, and*
> *Twitter allow fans to offer recurring payments to healthcare*
> *professionals who produce opinion articles, explanatory videos,*
> *and podcasts. […] Substack, an online newsletter platform, is*
> *increasingly used by physicians to write medical commentary,*
> *with some newsletters reaching 10s of thousands of subscribers.*
> *Substack estimates that 5-10% of readers will upgrade to a paid*
> *tier, and paid subscriptions on the service cost a minimum of $5*
> *per month. Although $5 sounds negligible, consider a newsletter*
> *with 10,000 total subscribers, 1000 of whom pay a $5 monthly*
> *fee. After subtracting Substack's 10% cut, a doctor could expect*
> *$54,000 in annual payments. If physicians accrue 5000 backers,*
> *they can expect $270,000 in revenue. This is greater than the*
> *$265,000 average salary of primary care physicians in the US.*

Indeed, several WWTI doctors had large, monetized YouTube channels, social media feeds, podcasts, and Substacks. Dr. Bhattacharya, for example, made $11,995 from posting on X and $25,772 from giving speeches in 2024.[98] Drs. Mandrola, Prasad, and Cifu founded a Substack named *Sensible Medicine*.[99] As they instructed us to do, it's worth it to wonder what motivating biases this may have produced. *Sensible Medicine* currently has 84,000 subscribers and three payment models. One can become a "founding member" for $250 per year, and unlike *Science-Based Medicine*, only paying customers can comment on *Sensible Medicine* articles.

Drs. Mazer and Rose recognized the potential conflict of interest this might create. They wrote:

> *The political polarisation of the covid-19 pandemic has fuelled*

subscription science and its resulting conflicts of interest. Many physicians and scientists who were sincerely sceptical or supportive of public health measures, for example, have acquired large, paying audiences over the last three years. Members of the public who were outraged by perceived government overreach or apathy sought out professionals who would bolster their political views with scientific justification. Physicians have been encouraged by their devoted admirers to draw assertive conclusions in lieu of exploring epistemic uncertainty. Subscription science can lead to doctors promoting anti-vaccine views at one extreme or fear mongering about SARS-CoV-2 at the other.[97]

Monetized blogs like *Sensible Medicine* don't just have readers; they have paying customers who expect value for their money. These people are paying to get anti-vaccine, anti-mask content dressed up as evidence-based medicine and *Sensible Medicine* produced a steady stream of such material.

- Why We Question the Safety Profile Of mRNA Covid-19 Vaccines[100]
- How Many Covid Vaccines Are Enough?[101]
- The Annual Covid19 Booster[102]
- The CDC Director Just Got Covid. She Got the New Bivalent Booster A Month Ago.[103]
- Before We Push the New Omicron Vaccine, Let's See the Data[104]
- Covid19 Therapeutics & Boosters All Need New Studies[105]
- You Have No Mandate: A Preemptive Argument Against Mandating Bivalent Boosters[106]
- Is It Ok for Internists to Wear Masks Forever?[107]
- *Sensible Medicine* X *Vaccine Curious*: Tracy Beth Høeg and Christine Stabell Benn Compare US & Danish Covid-19 Response and Child Vaccination Policy[108]

- Our New Analysis of Myocarditis after Vaccination[109]
- How Myocarditis Influences Vaccine Mandate Decisions[110]

Dr. Makary published his typical material there. He promoted his article, "The Political Badge of Ignoring Natural Immunity,"[111] by posting:

If you think ignoring natural immunity in vaccine mandates was not a big deal, please read my piece here. It was a catastrophic error, resulting in thousands of lives lost, careers ruined, and a 4-day school week for hundreds of public schools today.[112]

Dr. Makary's article spoke about "public health oligarchs" who didn't say enough nice things about SARS-CoV-2.

Nothing speaks more to the intellectual dishonesty of public health leaders than their complete dismissal of natural immunity. Since the Athenian plague of 430 B.C. it has been known that prior infection is protective against severe disease. Natural immunity works for nearly every other virus. The CDC website tells you not to get the chickenpox vaccine if you had chickenpox. And the only 2 other coronaviruses that cause severe disease in humans other than Covid (SARS & MERS) both resulted in long-term immunity. Oddly, public health oligarchs hypothesized that COVID-19 would break the rule. They got it terribly wrong.[111]

Many *Sensible Medicine* articles contained blatant factual errors and anti-vaccine disinformation. For example, one article from October 2022 said the following:

At the peak of hospitalization from Covid in this age group, 2.1 per 100,000 adolescents were hospitalized with Covid. None died. Pfizer's vaccine data from the NEJM study suggests that just under 9 per 100,000 adolescent boys were hospitalized with myocarditis. None died. So risk of hospitalization from Pfizer's vaccine series may have been over four times as likely to land a young boy in the hospital than Covid over this time period.[113]

Everything about this is wrong. The *Sensible Medicine* article referenced a paper titled "Hospitalization of Adolescents Aged 12–17 Years with Laboratory-Confirmed COVID-19 — COVID-NET, 14 States, March 1, 2020–April 24, 2021"[114] to claim that no adolescents died of COVID. However, COVID-NET is a surveillance network that covers about 10% of the US population.[115] That other 90% matters. The American Academy of Pediatrics, which collected data from 43 states, reported that 296 children had died by the end of April 2021.[116] So yes, some adolescents died of COVID during this time period. Furthermore, the CDC article showed that COVID could make some children very sick. Death is not the only bad outcome from COVID, after all, and most adolescents with vaccine myocarditis recover after a short time, and they do not need mechanical ventilation.

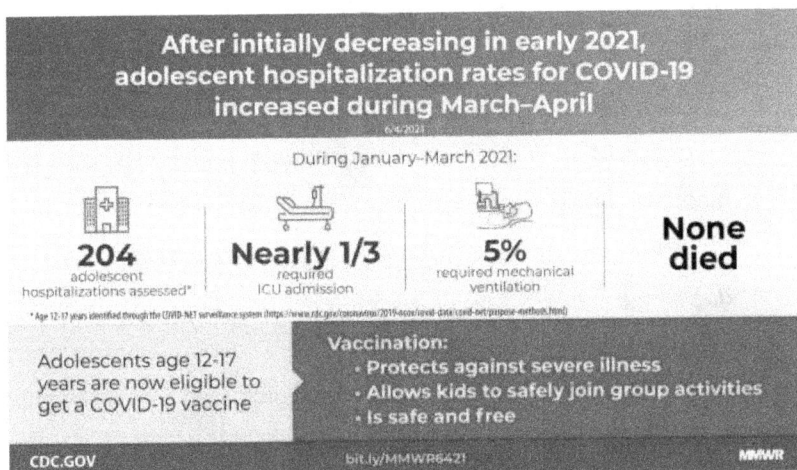

Source: CDC

The *Sensible Medicine* article also made absurd comparisons, claiming that the "risk of hospitalization from Pfizer's vaccine series may have been over four times as likely to land a young boy in the hospital than Covid over this time period."[113] However, the risk of an adolescent being hospitalized during "this time period" was a single week—the week ending January 9th, 2021. This was not their risk of being hospitalized during the entire pandemic. Of course, every vaccine would fail if its risks and benefits were judged this way.

Additionally, the article provided no rationale for choosing the period from March 1, 2020, to April 24, 2021, to evaluate COVID's risk to children. The second year of the pandemic was much worse for children than the first. Mitigation measures vanished, and Delta and Omicron arrived, causing unprecedented illness in children. The period from March 1, 2020, to April 24, 2021, was far from the "worst case scenario" the article claimed. In reality, 20% of pediatric deaths occurred during the Omicron wave.[117] About 180 children died from COVID in January 2022 alone,[118] and the virus hospitalized 6,527 children in one week that month.[119]

The *Sensible Medicine* article also said this:

> *I trusted our public health and medical institutions blindly in the early pandemic, based on my perception of an impressive track record and rigorous peer review. That record is being tarnished and trust betrayed by sloppy science and overly broad mandates.*[113]

That was its real message, and nearly all *Sensible Medicine* articles were designed to create mistrust and doubt. A quick reading of the comments shows their success. For example, the article "How Many Covid Vaccines Are Enough?" predictably concluded:

> *The CDC and FDA are whittling away at public trust by forgoing their duty to protect and inform. Meanwhile, their recent actions are aligned with the financial interests of Pfizer and Moderna.*

Consent to perpetual COVID boosters is not informed, it is manufactured.[101]

Sensible Medicine readers were ready for it. Here are some of the responses the article generated:

- *Lost my previously healthy 60yo uncle to his Pf booster in Aug 2022, the likely connection acknowledged by his doc and the family. Trust in mainstream medicine and all the agencies irreparably broken for me. I see a health freedom ND now and will only go to a hospital in case of a car or similar accident.*[120]
- *mRNA vaccines have demonstrated ZERO efficacy at saving lives OVERALL in the gold-standard randomized clinical trials, even at the height of the pandemic in Winter 2020-2021.*[121]
- *Money truly is the root of so much evil.*[122]
- *The Emperor has no cloths.*[123]
- *"The CDC and FDA are whittling away at public trust by forgoing their duty to protect and inform." Au contraire... there's nothing there to whittle away. It's GONE. Been GONE. You can't whittle on something that's not there.*[124]
- *Why would anyone in their right mind trust companies that are basically criminal enterprises with more criminal fines than any business sector in history.*[125]
- *Every booster increases your chance of infection and is likely damaging your immune system.*[126]
- *The Covid shots do not fit any reasonable definition of "vaccine." Covid is a fictional virus with a genome cobbled together out of a small number of nucleotide strands found in the secretions of a single patient. What we have is ordinary upper respiratory infections, colds and flu, renamed as Covid.*[127]
- *So many issues. The politization of a pandemic response. The capture of the FDA by Big Pharma. The use of relative vs absolute statistics to confound results. The lack of good science and epidemiologic priniciples. The supression of the origin.*

> *In 50 years of medical practice I've never seen anything like this. Doctors have lost all discretionary decision making and creative solutions to challenging conditions. Just follow the guidelines and algorithms. Question nothing. Weed out free thinkers.*[128]

- *Even one is too many. The lipid nanoparticles and the spike protein you are forced to manufacture are inflammatory and cause damage throughout the circulatory system. Denis Rancourts analysis of excess deaths shows that the clotshot is more harmful than the disease which had a less than one percent fatality rate. Finally we are seeing the research necessary to prove the harm of the mrna technology.*[129]

These comments appeared in large numbers on most *Sensible Medicine* articles. However, occasionally a sensible comment emerged. For example, Dr. Michael Ostacher commented:

> *I'm happy to get a booster to avoid getting Covid. I'm really not sure what your point is, because I'm not getting the vaccine to avoid hospitalization or death, I'm getting to avoid missing work. It seems to work fine for that, and $100 is a small price to pay. This is one more piece unnecessarily sowing mistrust in the medical and public health system, something common on this Substack. Even after everything you write, I'm getting my boosters and I'm not sure, as a family practice physician, why you wouldn't encourage the same.*[130]

While Dr. Ostacher was willing to push back on disinformation, the doctors who ran *Sensible Medicine* never corrected disinformation in the comments section.

Here is where I am going to remember their advice: *Motivating biases need not be considered nefarious, only considered.* I think it's worth considering that certain doctors knew what material their paying audience wanted, and they produced this content, Doctors with monetized Substack and YouTube channels had financial incentives to maintain their engagement and not anger their paying customers. For this reason, they refused to honestly enumerate how COVID had hurt children or report on the generally mild course of vaccine side effects.

> **Do pediatricians not care? What's going on here?**
> *— Resist Digital ID [X profile]*

However, this wasn't a one-way street. Doctors didn't just influence their followers; feedback loops existed. For example, consider this claim by Dr. Makary on social media.

> *It appears the FDA no longer requires clinical trial data Pfizer & Moderna's new Omicron vax (tested in 8 mice) was authorized today for children, who are at the highest risk of vaccine-induced myocarditis FDA bypassed their expert advisers The most political FDA&CDC in U.S. history.*[131]

The following day, a company press release included the results of a study from 900 volunteers,[132] but here are some of the replies he received:

- *Evil !*[133]
- *Sounds like we need to abolish the FDA and CDC.*[134]
- *Do pediatricians not care? What's going on here?*[135]
- *Of course. #TheScience dictates someone somewhere needs a new summer home. Trust the Science.*[136]
- *It's DANGEROUS !*[137]
- *As a former pharma rep, it's appalling to see how careless the FDA has become (due to pharma $$$) yet I could have been fired for off-label promotion of a drug?! Follow the $$$*[138]
- *Clinical trial data that can be cherry picked before presenting to the FDA board is hardly valuable at all. Its not really a secret, but just not well known. SciAm did an article about*

this problem a decade ago and that was long before operation warp speed.[139]

"Do pediatricians not care? What's going on here?" is what anti-vaxxers have said for decades, and WWTI doctors were exposed to a constant stream of anti-vax comments in their carefully curated social media feeds. This invariably influenced them to the point where some of them genuinely thought Robert F. Kennedy Jr. was the perfect guy to lead our federal health agencies.

The term for this is *audience capture*, and no one is immune to it. In an article titled "The Perils of Audience Capture: How Influencers Become Brainwashed by Their Audiences," Gurwinder Bhogal warned of its perils:

> *Audience capture is an irresistible force in the world of influencing, because it's not just a conscious process but also an unconscious one. [...] It involves the gradual and unwitting replacement of a person's identity with one custom-made for the audience.*
>
> *When influencers are analyzing audience feedback, they often find that their more outlandish behavior receives the most attention and approval, which leads them to recalibrate their personalities according to far more extreme social cues than those they'd receive in real life. In doing this they exaggerate the more idiosyncratic facets of their personalities, becoming crude caricatures of themselves.*
>
> *The caricature quickly becomes the influencer's distinct brand, and all subsequent attempts by the influencer to remain on-brand and fulfill audience expectations require them to act like the caricature. As the caricature becomes more familiar than the person, both to the audience and to the influencer, it comes to be*

*regarded by both as the only honest expression of the influencer,
so that any deviation from it soon looks and feels inauthentic. At
that point the persona has eclipsed the person, and the audience
has captured the influencer.*[140]

Indeed, any doctor whose audience routinely says things like, "*Do
pediatricians not care?*" should reflect on how this came to be. James
Heathers explained why in his article "Your Fans Are Dicks, And That
Should Matter to You." He wrote:

> *As we have chosen COVID as a topic, although it is equally
> applicable elsewhere, you can easily imagine the kind of swiv-
> el-eyed bile you might see — comments calling for the execution
> of Anthony Fauci for war crimes, accusing politicians of all
> stripes of criminal incompetence, the persistent misunderstand-
> ing of any and all public policy, and so on. Immune to anything
> as petty as details, angry to a fault, with a reflexive bellowing
> pointed at any restrictions to anything anywhere ever, coupled
> with a toddler's understanding of liberty. Pure avatars of selfish-
> ness, BELLOWING, and CRYING, and tearing their clothes.
> And it is not one person, your own little online army of shit-ticks,
> but every rat Jack of them.*
>
> *In other words, there is not so much a comments section as a
> great eructation of savage braying — violent, mean, intemper-
> ate, hideous shit is the modal response. Braying at great length,
> braying by a great many.*
>
> *And, that is your tribe. Alongside your cardigan, and your cu-
> rated television appearances, and your professorship, and your
> papers in The Good Journals, and your overworked graduate
> students, goes this horde of bilious fucks. These are the people*

agree with you, who are actively promoting your opinion, and
exhort you to have more opinions in future.

Would you pause, at this point?[141]

I would absolutely pause. Instead, WWTI doctors fanned the flames and cashed the checks.

Chapter 10: Another Downside of These Forays into Policy Is the Possibility of Reducing Trust—Which Is Already at a Low Level

I think clinicians should try hard to stay apolitical in the public sphere. We owe it to our patients.
— *Dr. John Mandrola*

Although it's impossible to completely separate medicine from politics and business, most people agree that medicine works best when it is as independent of these interests as possible. Everyone agrees that politics should be kept out of the exam room. There is no Republican or Democratic way to treat a stroke, and everyone deserves excellent medical care. Politics should also be excluded from medical research as much as possible. A vaccine doesn't work differently in people of different political parties.

However, this does not mean that doctors must take a vow of silence regarding their political views. Many political issues affect our patients, our jobs, and our lives. Politicians often insert themselves into our exam rooms, and like everyone else, doctors have the right to speak about whatever we want.

Not everyone agrees with this. Dr. John Mandrola, a cardiologist and writer for *Medscape* and *Sensible Medicine*, spread a great deal of COVID disinformation. He frequently declared the pandemic over in the spring of 2021—"The pandemic is essentially done"[1]—and treated temporary vaccine side effects as a fate worse than death. In December 2020, after thousands of young Americans had already died of COVID, he wrote an essay titled "No, Young Adults Should Not Live in Fear from Coronavirus," in which he argued that "fear of death"[2] was not a valid reason for young people to try to avoid the virus. COVID became the leading disease that killed young people in 2021.[3] However, six months later, he wrote an article titled "Vaccine-Induced Myocarditis Concerns Demand Respect." He wrote:

> *Calling myocarditis mild reminds me of the saying about minor surgery. Minor surgery is surgery on someone else; mild myocarditis is something that happens to other folks' kids. Humans have only one heart; inflaming it at a young age is not a small thing.*[4]

Dr. Mandrola wanted young people to "respect" the thing that wouldn't kill them but not to "fear" the thing that might.[5]

Dr. Mandrola also reprimanded *certain* doctors and advised them to engage in self-censorship when it came to *certain* political issues. In his article titled "Politics and Medicine is a Bad Idea," he wrote, "As private citizens, we can and should have ideas on policy. But our medical training provides us no expertise on policy."[6]

Dr. Mandrola provided three examples where he felt doctors should keep their thoughts private: nuclear war, the environment, and gun violence. He wrote:

> *There are many downsides when healthcare professionals overstep our expertise. Spending time on things that have no bearing on learning and practicing the craft of medicine or public health distracts people from their actual job. People who get sick depend on their clinician to be trained in health and disease, not climate or nuclear policy. There is only so much time. Why not spend it on being better at helping sick people. [...]*
>
> *Another downside of these forays into policy is the possibility of reducing trust—which is already at a low level. Climate, gun, and nuclear issues are inherently political. Taking a stand on a*

political matter is fine for persons, but it is not fine for clinicians or scientists.

Though he felt doctors should use their limited time to "get better at helping sick people," Dr. Mandrola used his time to scold *certain* doctors for voicing *certain* political opinions. On the day the Democratic vice-presidential candidate was announced and celebrated, he repeated his calls for physician self-censorship on social media. He said, "It's going to be difficult in the coming weeks but I think clinicians should try hard to stay apolitical in the public sphere. We owe it to our patients."[7] Dr. Mandrola felt that doctors who publicly voiced their political thoughts were harming their patients somehow.

I'll return to Dr. Mandrola at the end of this chapter; however, he was not alone bemoaning the mixture of politics and medicine. At the start of the pandemic, Drs. Vinay Prasad and Jeffrey Flier wrote an essay as a defense of Dr. John Ioannidis. Likening mean words to a virus that was causing overflowing morgues, Drs. Prasad and Flier wrote:

> *Society faces a risk even more toxic and deadly than Covid-19: that the conduct of science becomes indistinguishable from politics. The tensions between the two policy poles of rapidly and systematically reopening society versus maximizing sheltering in place and social isolation must not be reduced to Republican and Democratic talking points, even as many media outlets promote such simplistic narratives. These critical decisions should be influenced by scientific insights independent of political philosophies and party affiliations.*[8]

As the pandemic progressed, Dr. Prasad continued to warn of mixing politics and medicine. He wrote:

> *The upshot is that science and public health have become political. We now face the very real danger that instead of a shared*

method to understand the world, science will split into branches
of our political parties, each a cudgel of Team Red and Team
Blue.

We cannot let that happen.[9]

In his article "When Doctors Become Political – The 2016 Shift," Dr. Prasad warned that "science and medicine must avoid naked partisan politics,"[10] stating:

> *I worry that this problem is larger today than ever before. More*
> *and more questions are becoming political [...] And at top uni-*
> *versities, the politics is uni-directional. Most of the faculty and*
> *students are liberal, and the goals of the left are increasingly*
> *becoming the goals of medicine [...] School closure of course*
> *hurt poor, minority kids. A good liberal should have opposed it.*
> *But because Trump wanted schools open, liberals had to go the*
> *other direction. They have destroyed a generation of kids. Teach-*
> *ers unions and the democratic nominee worked to keep schools*
> *closed in 2020 and beyond. The harms are yet to be fully tallied.*

He concluded:

> *Science and medicine must aspire to be less political and as-*
> *pire for better evidence. If we continue in this direction, we are*
> *doomed. Sadly, many are along for the ride.*

It's hard to argue with that.

Erosion of credibility and trust really harms the ability to persuade people to take sometimes difficult steps that's in our joint collective interest.
— Dr. Martin Cetron, Director of CDC's Division of Global Migration and Quarantine

Indeed, politicians in the Trump administration interfered with CDC and public health guidance, leading to an erosion of public trust with tragic consequences for many people. A damning report from the U.S. House Select Subcommittee on the Coronavirus Crisis, titled "Trump Administration's Assault on CDC and Politicization of Public Health During the Coronavirus Crisis,"[11] detailed how politicians meddled with science in 2020:

- **The Trump White House Blocked CDC from Conveying Accurate Information to the Public in the Early Months of the Pandemic**

  After a February 25, 2020, CDC telebriefing "angered" President Trump, the White House wrested control of coronavirus communications away from CDC and mandated that all media requests related to the pandemic be approved by the Office of the Vice President prior to release. Trump Administration officials blocked CDC from conducting telebriefings on critical public health issues for three months and restricted scientists from participating in interviews at a time that coincided with a rapid explosion in coronavirus cases.

- **The Trump White House Installed Political Operatives Who Sought to Downplay the Risks Posed by the Coronavirus and Retaliated Against CDC Scientists Who Contradicted Trump Administration Talking Points**

  Trump Administration officials repeatedly sought to alter CDC and HHS press materials to downplay coronavirus risks, promote positive news, and attempt to redirect blame away from the Trump Administration for its poor handling of the coronavirus pandemic.

- **Trump Administration Officials "Compromised" Multiple Public Health Guidance Documents**

  Trump Administration political appointees repeatedly interfered in CDC's coronavirus guidance—overruling scientists to weaken CDC's public health recommendations, including its guidance for faith communities, a meatpacking plant, polling locations and voters, restaurants and bars, and testing.

- **Trump Administration Officials Brazenly Interfered with CDC's Public Health Authorities to Achieve Political Goals**
  Trump Administration officials blocked CDC from deploying a mask requirement on public and commercial transportation ahead of the fall and winter 2020 surge, despite calls from airlines and others in the transit industry for federal support for mask requirements at a time before vaccines were available.

- **Trump Administration Officials Sought to Manipulate and Block CDC Scientific Reports**
  The Select Subcommittee's investigation uncovered that Trump Administration appointees sought to influence CDC's scientific reports—attempting to change the publication process, manipulate the content, or block the dissemination of at least 19 different reports that they deemed to be politically harmful to President Trump.

- **The Trump Administration Wasted Millions of Taxpayer Dollars on a Failed Celebrity Vanity Campaign that Raided CDC's Budget in an Attempt to Spin President Trump's Failed Coronavirus Response Ahead of the Presidential Election**
  Trump Administration officials diverted hundreds of millions of dollars from CDC's budget to launch what amounted to a celebrity vanity campaign to "defeat despair and inspire hope" about the state of the pandemic in the direct lead up to the November 2020 presidential election.

- **The Trump Administration's Assault on the Nation's Public Health Institutions Caused Lasting Harm**
  The Trump Administration's politicization of CDC took a significant toll on the career scientists working tirelessly to protect the nation during a once-in-a-century pandemic. In his transcribed interview, Dr. Butler described how Trump Administration officials' "intentional discrediting" of CDC's

integrity adversely impacted agency morale: "when people have committed to public service, it's really demoralizing to be characterized as a villain in the public health response, or even in the future of our country."

The degree of control and hostility that the Trump Administration exerted on CDC has fundamentally undermined Americans' trust in public health. Dr. Cetron explained that this "erosion of credibility and trust really harms the ability to persuade people to take sometimes difficult steps that's in our joint collective interest."

When asked if she believed that allowing CDC to convey accurate scientific advice to the public would have resulted in fewer Americans dying during the early months of the pandemic, Dr. Anne Schuchat, CDC Principal Deputy Director, told the Select Subcommittee: "Yes, I do." Echoing Dr. Schuchat, Dr. Cetron said that "there are people, you know, who are no longer with us that would have benefited from that kind of very clear messaging."

WWTI doctors never complained about any of this, even though politicization of our pandemic response had tragic real-world consequences. One study comparing Florida and Ohio reported that:

Excess mortality was significantly higher for Republican voters than Democratic voters after COVID-19 vaccines were available to all adults, but not before. These differences were concentrated in counties with lower vaccination rates, and primarily noted in voters residing in Ohio.[12]

Wrong: Dems/ Newsom/ Teachers Unions/ TV pundits/ Fauci/ John Snow signatories Correct: Trump/ Desantis/ GBD
— *Dr. Vinay Prasad*

While WWTI doctors demanded that other doctors censor their political beliefs, most of them made no secret of their political leanings and
whom they blamed for our poor pandemic response. In one article from
December 2022 titled "The Tragedy of COVID19," Dr. Prasad claimed to
be a "far left democrat." However, Dr. Prasad didn't express sadness over
lives lost to COVID; rather, he felt sorry for himself:

> *Nearly every single person who expressed skepticism about*
> *prolonged lockdowns, school closure, masking 2 year olds, vacci-*
> *nating children for COVID 19 (despite dubious clinical data &*
> *high seroprevalence), perpetual boosters, paxlovid's efficacy in*
> *vaccinated people, and the COVID19 testing industry complex*
> *was at one time or another labeled a contrarian, a right wing op-*
> *erative, a grifter, a charlatan, a disgrace, a crook, an anti-vaxxer,*
> *anti-masker, or a MAGA republican, etc etc. The truth didn't*
> *matter. I am a far left democrat. I supported Bernie Sanders and*
> *Elizabeth Warren. [...]*
>
> *We should be embarrassed that 'our side' was wrong. Our fellow*
> *progressives were so nakedly partisan and openly ignorant*
> *that they were unable to read the literature on school closure,*
> *or masking kids. It never had good data, and should never*
> *have happened outside of randomized trials. Liberals were so*
> *close-minded, we could not accept the downsides of vaccine*
> *mandates, nor can even begin to understand the tradeoffs of*
> *boosting 20 year men forever. How can a political group that*
> *identifies itself as scientific be so anti-science?*[13]

He's right that liberals did not feel vaccine boosters and mandates
were priority #1 when COVID was killing 1,000 people per week.

Despite his prior pleas to depoliticize science, Dr. Prasad routinely
shared his political beliefs on social media. He had over 50 rageful posts

about teachers' unions, hysterically claiming they "destroyed a generation." He frequently called out "Dems" and Democratic politicians while
praising Republicans, all while saying, "I support Bernie & am a liberal."

- *Dems have become the corporatist party Pfizer basically
  writes EUA orders based on mice data. At the worst moment
  of the pandemic Dems abandoned kids, esp poor minority kids
  to side with teachers unions. Instead of hearing criticism, they
  preferred to censor Twitter & YouTube.*[14]

- *Yes! @ScienceMagazine loves Fauci, Democrats, Masking
  Toddlers & Wet Market origin, hates Trump, Atlas, DeSantis,
  GBD, & Lab Leak Origin @ScienceMagazine is the journal
  for Dems Republicans, submit elsewhere Zero downsides to
  pair science & politics like this!*[15]

- *I don't care about Trump I care that the editor of Science
  magazine is a naked partisan writing and tweeting constant
  support of Biden policies, denying the possibility of lab leak,
  & criticizing DeSantis & Trump. It is so bad for science to be
  nakedly political Will backfire*[16]

- *We have to name names for who was responsible for school
  closure- the worst decision in 25 yrs I support Bernie & am
  a liberal but we need soul searching Wrong: Dems/ Newsom/
  Teachers Unions/ TV pundits/ Fauci/ John Snow signatories
  Correct: Trump/ Desantis/ GBD*[17]

In a "debate" with Dr. Adam Cifu titled "Which US Presidential Can-
didate is More Anti-Science?" Dr. Prasad answered, "Kamala Harris."[18]
In addition to citing gender identity, affirmative action, and censorship,
Dr. Prasad's first reason was "public health policy." He said:

> *Harris will continue approving annual COVID19 boosters,
> including for kids as young as 6 months old, without randomized
> trials. Biden-Harris' CDC recommends boosters even for people
> who have had COVID 4 times before. Under Harris, by 2028,
> some kids will get 12 or more doses. In contrast, nearly all Euro-*

pean Nations restrict boosters to the elderly. There is no evidence to support aggressive boosting, and it may be harmful. Furthermore, this administration just paid for more COVID19 tests without data that these tests improve outcomes. On boosters & tests, Harris will transfer public money to pharmaceutical and testing companies and not know if health is improved.

Even though 800,000 Americans died of COVID under President Biden's watch, Dr. Prasad was only upset about his administration's tepid attempts to limit the disease. He felt the single most pressing scientific issue in the 2024 election was the "overuse" of COVID vaccines and tests.

Dr. Prasad also frequently accused "the left" of trying to stop people from dying of COVID *only* because they were blinded by hatred of President Trump. Some examples include:

- *Also if Trump wore a mask the left would never have masked toddlers. The left is full of 'experts' whose brains just oppose trump.*[19]

- *Masking has become a cult on the political left. Only because Donald Trump didn't wear a mask. The evidence has always been very weak. It was pushed by people who are advocates rather than scientists. This was the largest cluster randomized trial.*[20]

- *Public Health has always leaned to the political left. But only with COVID has the political left become synonymous with irrational policies that are the opposite of whatever Donald Trump once said. Public Health used to be about data and meeting people where they were.*[21]

- *Without Trump, we would have had different policies, and also a different reaction to the policies. The left most progressives would not have been such ardent proponents of restrictions without resources.*[22]

According to Dr. Prasad, only he and other advocates of mass infection could see the world objectively, untainted by political bias.

An elite group of scientists tried to convince President Donald Trump that locking down the country would be the real danger.
— *Stephanie Lee*

However, many WWTI doctors did much more than voice their political opinions. Many of them mixed politics and medicine openly and freely. As Stephanie Lee documented, some scientists—namely Dr. Ioannidis—tried to influence politicians as early as March 2020. She wrote:

Stanford University scientist John Ioannidis has declared in study after study that the coronavirus is not that big of a threat, emboldening opponents of economic shutdowns — and infuriating critics who see fundamental errors in his work.

But even before the epidemiologist had any of that data in hand, he and an elite group of scientists tried to convince President Donald Trump that locking down the country would be the real danger.

In late March, as COVID-19 cases overran hospitals overseas, Ioannidis tried to organize a meeting at the White House where he and a small band of colleagues would caution the president against "shutting down the country for [a] very long time and jeopardizing so many lives in doing this," according to a statement Ioannidis submitted on the group's behalf. Their goal, the statement said, was "to both save more lives and avoid serious damage to the US economy using the most reliable data."

Although the meeting did not happen, Ioannidis believed their message had reached the right people. Within a day of him sending it to the White House, Trump announced that he wanted the

country reopened by Easter. "I think our ideas have infiltrated
[sic] the White House regardless," Ioannidis told his collabora-
tors on March 28, in one of dozens of emails that BuzzFeed News
obtained through public records requests.[23]

In March 2020, Dr. Ioannidis felt the flu was much more dangerous
than COVID. Writing about China's drastic measures to contain it, he
said:

If only part of resources mobilized to implement extreme mea-
sures for COVID-19 had been invested towards enhancing influ-
enza vaccination uptake, tens of thousands of influenza deaths
might have been averted.[24]

While Drs. Prasad and Flier were chastising Dr. Ioannidis' critics
for supposedly mixing politics and medicine, Dr. Ioannidis himself was
directly reaching out to politicians to deliver his minimizing message
and advance his favored policies. Drs. Prasad and Flier never complained
about that.

Dr. Ioannidis was not alone in trying to influence politicians at that
time. According to the House Report, "The Atlas Dogma":

Dr. Scott Atlas began attempting to influence federal pandemic
policy soon after the start of the coronavirus crisis. New evi-
dence obtained by the Select Subcommittee shows that Dr. Atlas
reached out to Centers for Medicare & Medicaid Services (CMS)
Administrator Seema Verma on March 21, 2020, arguing that the
federal government's pandemic response was "a massive over-
reaction" that was "inciting irrational fear" in Americans. Dr.
Atlas estimated that the coronavirus "would cause about 10,000
deaths"—a number he claimed "would be unnoticed" in a nor-
mal flu season—and said, "The panic needs to be stopped."[25]

This outreach was undeniably effective. It paved the way for WWTI
doctors to directly influence political matters at the highest level. Several
of them—Drs. Scott Atlas, Jay Bhattacharya, Martin Kulldorff, Joseph

Ladapo, and Cody Meissner—had a "secret" meeting with President Trump in August 2020, and the next month he credited them by saying:

> *And you'll develop, you'll develop like a herd mentality. It's going to be, it's going to be herd developed and that's going to happen. That will all happen. But with a vaccine, I think it will go away very quickly. But I really believe we're rounding the corner and I believe that's true. As you know, Dr. Fauci disagrees with that. Well, I mean, but a lot of people do this, do agree with me. You look at Scott Atlas, you look at some of the other doctors that are highly, from Stanford, look at some of the other doctors, they think maybe we could have done that from the beginning.*[26]

Dr. Atlas would eventually serve as Trump's COVID advisor in the fall of 2020, where he opposed all measures to control the virus outside of nursing homes.

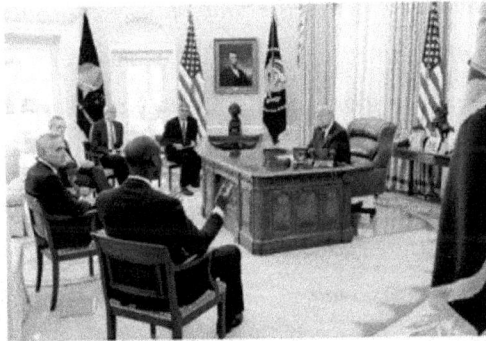

In our secret meeting with expert physicians and scientists in the Oval Office, President Trump listened intently to Dr. Joe Ladapo. I looked on next to Dr. Ladapo, while to my left, Drs. Cody Meissner, Martin Kulldorff, and Jay Bhattacharya (far side) also listened. *(Credit: Official White House photographers)*

In October 2020, several WWTI doctors teamed up with Mr. Jeffrey Tucker, the libertarian, pro-tobacco, child-labor advocate, to promote herd immunity via mass infection and advance their political objectives.[27] The result was the Great Barrington Declaration (GBD), which earned its authors more meetings with top politicians. According to an article titled "Trump Advisors Consult Scientists Pushing Disputed Herd Immunity Strategy" from October 6, 2020, just two days after the publication of the GBD:

> *The Trump administration's health chief met Monday with a trio of scientists who back the controversial theory that the United States can quickly and safely achieve widespread immunity to the coronavirus by allowing it to spread unfettered among healthy people.*
>
> *The meeting with Health and Human Services Secretary Alex Azar, which also included Trump adviser Scott Atlas, is the latest example of administration officials — including the president himself — seeking out scientists whose contrarian views justify the government's handling of a pandemic that has killed 210,000 people and infected nearly 7.5 million so far in the U.S.*
>
> *"We heard strong reinforcement of the Trump Administration's strategy of aggressively protecting the vulnerable while opening schools and the workplace," Azar tweeted after his meeting with Harvard medical professor Martin Kulldorff, Stanford medical professor Jay Bhattacharya and Oxford epidemiologist Sunetra Gupta.*
>
> *Mainstream medical and public health experts say that seeking widespread, or herd, immunity in the manner the scientists prescribe could result in the deaths of hundreds of thousands or even*

millions more U.S. residents.

The trio, who Azar described as "three distinguished infectious disease experts," favors moving aggressively to reopen the economy while sidelining broad testing and other fundamental public health measures. "Three months, maybe six is sufficient time for enough immunity to accumulate ... that the vulnerable could resume normal lives," Gupta said Monday night in an appearance on Laura Ingraham's Fox News show.

That aligns with the "herd-immunity" strategy endorsed by Atlas, who Bhattacharya said was their "point of contact" for the meeting. Atlas, a neuroradiologist and senior fellow at Stanford University's Hoover Institution, has emerged as a favored adviser to the president despite his lack of expertise in public health, infectious disease or epidemiology.[28]

Despite claiming to be silenced outsiders, these doctors *were* the medical establishment.

As the pandemic progressed, multiple WWTI doctors became advisors to Florida Governor Ron DeSantis, including Drs. Bhattacharya, Atlas, Kulldorff, Tracy Beth Høeg, Joseph Fraiman, and Michael Levitt, as well as Dr. Ladapo, who became the Florida Surgeon General. Several WWTI doctors served on Gov. DeSantis' Public Health Integrity Committee[29] and held multiple "roundtable discussions" where they spread blatant pro-infection disinformation and complained about "censorship."

Dr. Bhattacharya often heaped praise on Gov. DeSantis. According to one article, "Stanford Doctor Jay Bhattacharya Praises Ron DeSantis for COVID Response: 'He's Extraordinary'":

Dr. Jay Bhattacharya, a professor at Stanford University Medical School, has praised Florida Governor Ron DeSantis for his response to the coronavirus pandemic.

*"I mean, I've never met a politician like him. He's extraordi-
nary," Bhattacharya said during an interview on The Tom Woods
Show. The podcast, hosted by libertarian Tom Woods, aired April
17.*

*Bhattacharya said he didn't know DeSantis well before they had
a "remarkable" conversation about COVID-19 in the fall of last
year. The governor, he said, had read lots of papers on the subject and "knew all of the details."*[30]

In collaboration with right-wing tech moguls, Dr. Bhattacharya later
endorsed and openly campaigned for Gov. DeSantis during his failed
presidential run. An article titled "Stanford Professor Jay Bhattacharya
Joins Ron DeSantis' 2024 Presidential Campaign Kickoff" stated:

*Florida governor Ron DeSantis announced his 2024 presidential
campaign bid through Twitter earlier today on May 24, garner-
ing more than 1.3 million views on his 2-hour Twitter Space live.
Stanford professor of health policy Jayanta Bhattacharya A.M,
A.B '90, MD '97, Ph.D. '00, was featured as a speaker on the
live stream alongside figures like Twitter CEO Elon Musk and
PayPal founding COO David Sacks.*

*Bhattacharya and DeSantis have worked together in the past
on COVID-related issues, with both figures having historically
supported the easing of pandemic restrictions.*[31]

When Gov. DeSantis' campaign fizzled out, Dr. Bhattacharya moved
on to that of Robert F. Kennedy Jr. He spoke at one of his campaign rallies and introduced himself by saying, "I am Professor Jay Bhattacharya,
and I am a scientific dissident." Though he was speaking at a political
rally, he said:

Since I work in public health, I am not here to endorse anyone for president. In public health, we are supposed to be beyond politics, and what we say should be equally suitable and just for Democrats, Republicans, and independents alike.[32]

Dr. Marty Makary served as an advisor to Virginia Governor Glen Youngkin. According to the article, "Youngkin Pick for Medical Adviser Bucks Trends on Covid":

Gov. Glenn Youngkin has named a respected physician who opposes blanket vaccine mandates and downplayed the threat of the coronavirus to children as his lead adviser on pandemic response. [...]

While Makary serves Youngkin's political needs and is compatible with the views the governor has shared, Rozell (Mark Rozell, the dean of the Schar School of Policy and Government at George Mason University) wondered whether the appointment is in the best interests of public health and science.[33]

Knowing which politicians WWTI doctors praised, you can probably guess which politicians they lambasted and the reasons why. There was literally no action any government official could take to limit the virus that would not infuriate WWTI doctors. In a pandemic where 1.2 million Americans died, "*COVID19 tests without data that these tests improve outcomes*"[18] was the single most important scientific issue for the country according to Dr. Prasad. Trying to slow COVID in any manner was the worst thing a politician could do in his eyes.

By forcing children to have a vaccine that they don't need because they already have the disease, that undermines the trust in other vaccines, like the measles vaccine or the polio vaccine, and that's very, very serious
— Dr. Martin Kulldorff

Several WWTI doctors testified before both branches of Congress. During Senate testimony in December 2020, Dr. Bhattacharya spoke about "how well we've done." He again said that 70 was the age at which COVID became dangerous:

> It's a deadly disease, especially for older people. Under 70, the survival rate is 99.95%. Let me say that again, 99.95%.[34]

Dr. Bhattacharya also testified before the U.S. House of Representatives Select Subcommittee on the Coronavirus Crisis in November 2021, where he claimed to be a victim of censorship and bragged about the fact that he "called for" things.[35] He referenced the GBD and said that it merely "Called for focused protection of the vulnerable elderly and an end to lockdown policies, including school closures and other measures which have caused enormous collateral damage to the health and well-being of the population." Dr. Bhattacharya neglected to mention that the GBD also called for "natural immunity" to reach herd immunity.

Dr. Makary testified before the Select Subcommittee the next month, where described himself as a "public health researcher at Johns Hopkins"[36] and issued his familiar complaint that public health officials hadn't said enough nice things about SARS-CoV-2. He said:

> Over 20 scientifically sound studies have demonstrated that natural immunity is as good as or better than vaccinated immunity, yet our public health officials continue to ignore it. In fact, they never talk about it.

Dr. Makary also complained about boosters and said, "Is that what we've come to? Pharma tells people what to do in a press release and the CDC just falls in line?"

During a 2021 discussion with Congressman Jim Jordan, Dr. Makary spread bizarre conspiracies that the CDC was hiding vital information about "natural immunity" from the American public.[37] He said:

> **Rep. Jordan:** *Dr. Makary, do you know how many people work at CDC? 31,000 people between CDC and NIH. 31,000 people spending $58 billion a year. Why hasn't our government done a study on natural immunity?*
>
> **Dr. Makary:** *If I can be honest, Representative Jordan, I don't think they want to know the answer. It would undermine the indiscriminate vaccine vaccination policy for every single human being, including extremely low risk people [...]*
>
> *Most of our learnings come from Israel and other countries. Yes, sir. The Israel study is the largest study done worldwide, and it found that natural immunity adjusted for age and comorbidity is 27 times more effective than vaccinated immunity. The scientists in our government at CDC and NIH, they don't account for that. They don't talk about that. What do they say about that study? They never talk about it, unless asked. But I would say that they are doing worse than being absent on the topic.*
>
> *They are undermining natural immunity through two studies that the CDC did that are so flawed, that are so poorly put together. Honestly, they would not qualify for a seventh grade science fair. We can spend money. Some of that 58 billion and some of the resources at NIH and CDC can be used to fund gain of function research and give a grant to EcoHealth, who then sends some of that money to a lab in Wuhan, China.*
>
> *That's just fine, but we can't find any resources to deal with a fundamental question about natural immunity and so much so that you have to go out and get private funding to do it yourself. It's either they know the answer and don't want the American people*

to know or they do know the answer and are trying to hide it.

Dr. Makary was upset that scientists "in our government at CDC and NIH," who were given all that money after all, were "undermining natural immunity."

Dr. Høeg also testified before the Select Subcommittee on the Coronavirus Pandemic in 2023, where she blended her medical credentials and political opinions. She fretted mightily about academic loss in "those students with the highest poverty levels"[38] and spread fake statistics, claiming that "that kids faced similar risks from COVID-19 as from seasonal influenza."

In 2023, Drs. Bhattacharya, Kulldorff, and Makary participated in a roundtable before the House Committee on Oversight and Accountability in a session titled "Preparing for the Future by Learning from the Past: Examining COVID Policy Decisions."[39] There, they spread predictable disinformation. In his testimony, Dr. Kulldorff invented a fantasy where children were forcibly vaccinated and said that "vaccine fanatics" were to blame for the lack of trust in other vaccines.[40] He said:

> *By forcing children to have a vaccine that they don't need because they already have the disease, that undermines the trust in other vaccines, like the measles vaccine or the polio vaccine, and that's very, very serious. I think during the last several decades, we have the "never vaccinate" people, the anti-vaccine people, [who] have tried to undermine the trust in vaccines, but with very little success. But the vaccine fanatics who want to vaccinate every person in this country, even though they are children with very little risk for it, even though they have already, already had the COVID, that has undermined the trust in other vaccines enormously, creating enormous vaccine hesitancy. So not allowing*

their provider or physician to determine the risk and the benefit.

At that time, zero American children had been killed by measles and polio in the past 30 years.

Dr. Makary also spread doubt, claiming that public health officials lied and weaponized medical research, saying:

> *The greatest perpetrator of misinformation during the pandemic has been the United States government. Misinformation that COVID was spread through surface transmission, that vaccinated immunity was far greater than natural immunity, that masks were effective.* […]
>
> *We've seen something which is unforgivable and that is the weaponization of medical research itself. The CDC putting out their own shoddy studies like their own study on natural immunity looking at one state for two months when they had data for years on all 50 states.*
>
> *Why did they only report that one sliver of data? Why did they salami slice the giant database? Because it gave them the result they wanted. Same with masking study. Well the data has now caught up in giant systematic reviews and the public health officials were intellectually dishonest.*
>
> *They lied to the American people. Thank you.*[41]

Some lawmakers were not pleased that WWTI doctors were given an opportunity to spread their disinformation. Congressman Krishnamoorthi put out a statement that said:

> *Today, Congressman Krishnamoorthi participated in the Select Subcommittee on the Coronavirus Crisis hearing titled, "Combating Coronavirus Cons And The Monetization of Misinformation." The committee hearing noted the danger of pandemic*

misinformation and the importance of educating the public on the science behind COVID-19 and the vaccine. During the hearing, Congressman Krishnamoorthi questioned Dr. Jay Bhattacharya, a professor of medicine at Stanford University known for his opposition to COVID-19-related restrictions as well as his contributions to the Great Barrington Declaration which made the widely-debunked argument that governments should limit pandemic restrictions only to those at high risk of severe outcomes and let the virus spread naturally to achieve herd immunity.

"It is unfortunate and ironic that my Republican colleagues selected Dr. Bhattacharya as a witness for our COVID-19 misinformation hearing when he himself is a purveyor of COVID-19 misinformation," Congressman Krishnamoorthi said. "As Dr. Bhattacharya acknowledged in questioning, he has drawn criticism from multiple judges for misrepresenting scientific studies and the consensus of medical professionals, while even testifying as an expert on matters on which he admitted he was not qualified. The presence of Dr. Bhattacharya as a witness today is a stark example of the challenges of combatting pandemic misinformation. During a pandemic that has taken the lives of over 765,000 Americans, we cannot afford to allow scientific misinformation and conspiracy theories to run rampant either on social media or in-person interactions. We need to make efforts to educate our communities about the necessity of masks and the safety and efficacy of the COVID-19 vaccine."

In an October 2021 ruling that Tennessee Governor Bill Lee's executive order allowing parents to opt their children out of school mask mandates violates federal law, U.S. District Judge Waverly

D. Crenshaw wrote that Dr. Bhattacharya "offered opinions regarding the pediatric effects of masks on children, a discipline on which he admitted he was not qualified to speak," adding "his demeanor and tone while testifying suggest that he is advancing a personal agenda. At this stage of the proceedings, the Court is simply unwilling to trust Dr. Bhattacharya." Judge Crenshaw also added that Dr. Bhattacharya's testimony was "troubling" and "problematic." Similarly, a Manitoba Judge found the same month that Dr. Bhattacharya's testimony public health restrictions was contradicted by a range of evidence, including his own sources. In August 2021, Dr. Bhattacharya was the state of Florida's expert witness defending the state's ban on mask mandates, during which he noted on child death rates from COVID-19 that it was a "question of what is the trade-off."[42]

As Congressman Krishnamoorthi noted, Dr. Bhattacharya also testified in courts. He hit all three branches of government, at both state and federal levels. He also played multiple roles in the court system. He was an "expert witness," seeking to remove mask mandates, and he was also a plaintiff, suing the Biden administration for "censorship."

Doctors blending politics and medicine wasn't just an American phenomenon. Identical stories of doctors, almost none of whom treated COVID patients, freely mixing politics and medicine could be written about many countries. For example, in December 2020, a British newspaper, *The Sunday Times*, published an article that read:

The medical and scientific experts had been summoned the previous day and warned to keep their Sunday evening rendezvous with the prime minister a secret. When they dialled into the Zoom call at 6pm they found Boris Johnson and Rishi Sunak, the chancellor, at the end of the long mahogany cabinet room table in Downing Street. [...]

But Sunak wanted a different strategy. Faced with dire predictions that half a million people could be made redundant in the autumn, he strongly opposed a second lockdown, which some economists were saying would wreak further havoc on Britain's already limping economy.

Which is why three of the four academics who had been invited to speak by No 10 that Sunday evening advocated a less restrictive approach, which avoided lockdowns.

The strategy of allowing the virus to take its course and build up "herd immunity" in the population had been dropped by the government at the start of the first wave because of evidence that it would lead to an unacceptable death toll and potentially overwhelm the NHS.

The speakers that night included Professor Sunetra Gupta and her Oxford University colleague, Professor Carl Heneghan. Gupta says they were each given 15 minutes in which they argued that a lockdown was unnecessary at that point: the virus could be allowed to spread with lighter controls if those most vulnerable to serious illness were protected. Gupta says herd immunity could be achieved "in the order of three to six months".

They were joined by Anders Tegnell, Sweden's leading epidemiologist, who had masterminded his country's controversial policy of avoiding a lockdown to build up immunity from the virus in the hope it would reduce the impact of any second wave. Tegnell refuses to disclose what he said at the meeting.[43]

The article also said:

Just as in the first wave in March, Johnson would delay the lockdown and ignore warnings that the consequences would be disastrous for both the economy and people's lives.

Speak up against us and our political myth making, and we will publicly smear and punish you with the power of the state.
— *Philipp Markolin*

While WWTI doctors were invited to speak at Congressional hearings, prominent vaccine advocates and virologists were dragged there against their will. In her article on the GOP-led House Select Subcommittee on the Coronavirus Pandemic (HSSCP), "Don't Let House Republicans Rewrite Trump's Pandemic History," Dr. Allison Neitzel wrote:

The HSSCP has not only pushed the lab leak theory, but has tried to pin the pandemic on scientists like Fauci via discussion surrounding NIH funding of WIV research. After putting Fauci through 14 hours of behind-closed-doors grilling in February and sitting on that testimony for months, the HSSCP released the transcript and subpoenaed emails ahead of his June hearing before the subcommittee.[44]

During the hearing, Dr. Anthony Fauci spoke about the death threats he and his family received, and Republican legislators were eager to egg on the mob. Congresswoman Marjorie Taylor Greene insulted Dr. Fauci and said he belongs in prison. His experience was not unique, unfortunately. In his article "After Smearing Anthony Fauci, House Republicans Proceed to Defame a Prominent Vaccine Scientist," Michael Hiltzik said the following:

Peter J. Hotez is one of America's most prominent vaccine ex-

perts. A professor at Baylor College of Medicine, he's also co-di-rector of the Texas Children's Center for Vaccine Development, which has developed and licensed a safe and effective COVID-19 vaccine that has been distributed widely in the third world.

He's also among our most prominent critics of the anti-vaccine and anti-science movements that have so thoroughly infected our public discourse.[45]

The HSSCP had previously tweeted about Dr. Hotez, calling him a "friend and potential accomplice to Dr. Fauci's Senior Advisor." As Mr. Hiltzik recognized, "the tweet exposes Hotez to public vituperation on social media and possibly physical harm." Mr. Hiltzik also noted that:

The subcommittee demanded by letter that Hotez turn over all documents and communications between him and six federal agencies and 25 individuals, most of whom are scientists researching COVID's origins.

Indeed, Dr. Hotez has been one of the most prominent critics of the anti-vaccine and anti-science movements, a fact that has earned him a giant target on his back from right-wing politicians. The obvious goal of this government aggression is to silence and intimidate voices like his. Mr. Hiltzik wrote:

The message, observes scientist and science writer Philipp Markolin, is crystal clear. It's "speak up against us and our political myth making, and we will publicly smear and punish you with the power of the state."

This all has the potential to get much worse. Dr. Neitzel concluded her article about the HSSCP by saying:

The historically nonpartisan scientific institutions did not ask to have politics thrust upon them and it is deeply troubling that physicians aligned with right-wing politics — including some of the Republican members of the HSSCP and their "experts" — have aided in this attack over the last four years. But for the sake of the future of public health in America, the overwhelmingly science-based medical community must join those who have taken a stand against the anti-science aggression of Trump World.[44]

Johns Hopkins to Hold "Fringe," Dark Money Heavy COVID Summit
— *Natalie Jonas and Walker Bragman*

While WWTI doctors visited politicians on their home turf, the favor was repaid. In September 2024, Johns Hopkins Business School held a conference called the "2024 Symposium on Health Policy." It described itself by saying:

Join us in the heart of Washington, D.C., for a one-day public conference to discuss health policy in 2025 and beyond. Hear from congressional committee leaders, the Congressional Budget Office health director, federal legislative directors, policy experts, employer purchasers, journalists, philanthropists, and academics as they discuss how to achieve a healthier and more prosperous America.[46]

Drs. Bhattacharya, Atlas, and Makary participated in panels such as "Health Policy 2025 & Beyond," "Free Speech in Medicine," and "Physician Leadership in the Public Square." Several Republican Congressmen were also present: Representative Kevin Hern, Oklahoma District 1; Representative Greg Murphy, North Carolina District 3; and Senator Bill Cassidy, Louisiana. According to one article:

> *The top Republican on the Senate panel in charge of the NIH,*
> *Sen. Bill Cassidy (R-La.), wants to reinvigorate an oversight*
> *panel selected by political appointees.*[47]

Representatives from conservative think tanks, such as the CATO Institute and American Enterprise Institute, were also present.

Investigative journalists Natalie Jonas and Walker Bragman wrote an article documenting how prestigious universities and WWTI doctors seamlessly blended medicine with right-wing politics and business interests titled "Johns Hopkins to Hold 'Fringe,' Dark Money Heavy COVID Summit."[48] It is worth sharing in its entirety.

> *Johns Hopkins is under fire after announcing that it will host*
> *a forum next week with a number of well known public health*
> *contrarians and representatives of right-wing dark money*
> *groups that have worked to politicize public health throughout*
> *the COVID-19 pandemic. A number of those groups have ties to*
> *billionaire industrialist and conservative powerbroker Charles*
> *Koch, who has been a major donor to Hopkins, giving $1.3 mil-*
> *lion to the school through his personal foundation between 2021*
> *and 2022 and an additional $728,000 in 2019.*
>
> *The "2024 Symposium on Health Policy," which is set to take*
> *place on September 11, is being organized by the university's*
> *Carey Business School with no involvement from its school of*
> *public health. The event appears to be another right-wing effort*
> *to rewrite the history of the COVID-19 pandemic in order to cast*
> *government efforts to control the spread of the virus that has*
> *killed roughly 1.2 million Americans in a negative light. A similar*
> *event featuring some of the same speakers is being planned at*
> *Stanford for early October. Koch has also been a major donor*
> *to Stanford, giving $3.3 million through his personal foundation*

between 2020 and 2022.

Like the Stanford summit, the Hopkins symposium is drawing sharp criticism from public health experts who are alarmed by the fringe medical perspectives the prestigious school is amplifying.

"Looks like there is big money behind the far-right COVID caucus as they seem to be able to pay for meetings now on two coasts," Yale epidemiologist Gregg Gonsalves posted on Threads. "This is filled with a few good people, but mostly packed with the crew of folks who got it wrong from day one and spread misinformation for a living on the pandemic. It's convenient that it's hidden away from the public health school at @jhucarey, where those in charge are less familiar with this nonsense."

Virologist John P. Moore, a professor of microbiology and immunology at Weill Cornell Medical College, told Important Context that "This meeting has nothing to do with genuine improvements in public health policy."

"It's all to do with fringe eccentrics meeting each other to preen and posture in front of politicians and a few journalists," he said. "Some of the participants are after positions in the Trump administration... and will no doubt use this meeting to buff up their 'credentials.'"

There is significant overlap between the Hopkins symposium and the Stanford conference in terms of speakers. The organizer of the latter is participating in the former. Health economist and Stanford professor Dr. Jay Bhattacharya, a vocal advocate for a widely rebuked and discredited COVID herd immunity strategy based on the mass infection of young people, will join panel discussions on "physician autonomy and leadership" and "free speech in medicine," which are remarkably similar to in theme to the planned "misinformation, censorship, and academic freedom" Stanford panel. They also mirrored a theme from the GOP House Select Subcommittee's opening hearing in February 2023, at which Bhattacharya was a Republican expert witness.

The discussions seem engineered to provide a prestigious platform to a favorite narrative of Bhattacharya and the political right: that he and other contrarian medical voices were "censored" throughout the pandemic by the U.S. government despite being correct.

Notably, Bhattacharya's false and misleading statements about COVID are too numerous to mention in this article. In May 2020, for example, he said it was highly unlikely that children would spread the virus to their parents or other adults. In January 2021, weeks before the country experienced a devastating COVID surge, he argued that a majority of India had achieved herd immunity and widespread vaccination was unnecessary.

The professor had his day in court to adjudicate his censorship claims. He and a group of private plaintiffs, represented by a legal outfit funded in part by billionaire industrialist and conservative powerbroker Charles Koch, sued the Biden administration for allegedly strong-arming social media companies into removing their content in violation of the First Amendment. The conservative Supreme Court, however, disagreed, finding 6-to-3 that Bhattacharya and his compatriots lacked standing because they had failed to show that they had actually been harmed by *the government.*

Two other contrarians speaking at Stanford next month are join-ing Bhattacharya at Hopkins. Neuroradiologist Dr. Scott Atlas, who helped steer the Trump administration's COVID response and was condemned in 2020 by fellow faculty members over his efforts to "promote a view of COVID-19 that contradicts medical science," will participate in the physician autonomy panel at Hopkins and another about "health policy 2025 and beyond." Meanwhile, Dr. Marty Makary, a surgeon at Hopkins who joined Bhattacharya as a GOP expert witness before the House Select Subcommittee on the Coronavirus Pandemic in February 2023, will also join the Stanford professor for both of his scheduled panels next week.

Many of the Hopkins panelists, including Bhattacharya, Atlas, and Makary, have ties to ideologically right-wing dark money groups. Bhattacharya and Atlas are both senior fellows at the Hoover Institution, a right-wing think tank housed at Stanford. Bhattacharya and Makary are members of the so-called Norfolk Group, which was organized by the opaque Brownstone Institute. Beyond the doctors, there is Leck Shannon, who will speak on a panel about "philanthropy and health policy." Shannon is the healthcare director at Stand Together Trust, a dark money fund-ing vehicle led by Charles Koch's son, Charles Chase Koch, who is also a director and vice chairman of his father's personal foun-dation. Koch's political influence network has been particularly active throughout the pandemic, working to politicize COVID mitigation measures.

Another panelist from the Koch network is Michael F. Can-

non, who will be moderating the health policy 2025 discussion. Cannon is an economist who serves as director of health policy studies at the libertarian Cato Institute and founded the group's "Anti-Universal Coverage Club," which is staunchly against universal healthcare.

Notably, some of the earliest recommendations from the World Health Organization when the pandemic hit included making healthcare free at the point of use and increasing government funding for public health systems.

Cato, which has long been opposed to both of those ideas, has been a recipient of Koch money for years. According to the latest federal tax filings, which are from 2022, the institute got $34,000 from Koch's personal foundation, $47,000 from Stand Together Fellowships (formerly the Charles Koch Institute), and $1.8 million from Stand Together Trust that year.

The institute was also one of the earliest organizations to call for an end to COVID stay-at-home orders. Cannon himself has opposed mask mandates and called for a property tax strike to force schools open in early 2021 before the COVID vaccines were authorized for youths. In February 2022, as deaths from the deadly Omicron surge were skyrocketing, he argued that public health officials were too enticed by their own power to do what was necessary to restore public trust in public health, which he claimed was dialing back recommendations and allowing normal life to resume.

"These folks in these public health agencies—Dr. Fauci, you know, the FDA, the CDC...they're good people who want to save lives and they have power, and they want to use that power to

save lives, but it's very hard to put down that power," he said. "And so it's very hard for them...even to recognize the negative impact they're having on trust in public health officials."

Speaking on the Hopkins health policy 2025 panel will be Joseph Antos, a senior fellow emeritus at the American Enterprise Institute. AEI is a free market think tank backed by some of the most powerful corporate interests in the country. Over the years, it has received significant funding from the Koch family, including $666,000 in 2022, from Stand Together Trust.

Like other Koch-backed groups, AEI opposed government efforts to slow the combat COVID—even though the group's own research in 2021 showed that a national lockdown would have provided broad societal benefit. As early as April 2020, the group's Twitter account was pushing for a timeline for the end of state "lockdown" orders. By May, it had begun pushing to reopen schools. AEI also criticized the novel use of guaranteed income programs arising from economic pandemic response.

Antos himself has been an outspoken critic of single-payer plans and used the pandemic as an opportunity to push for "market-based reforms" to Medicare.

Two other Koch-funded groups that have embraced pandemic revisionism will be represented at Hopkins. A panel on health-care spending will include Theo Merkel, a senior fellow at the Manhattan Institute for Policy Research and a senior research fellow at the healthcare-focused Paragon Health Institute. In 2022 alone, Stand Together Trust gave the Manhattan Institute $495,000 and Paragon Health $2.9 million.

Both groups staked out positions against COVID mitigation

*efforts. The Manhattan Institute adopting anti-lockdown nar-
ratives and false claims about masks to discourage their use.
Paragon Health has promoted the narrative that the costs of
"lockdowns" outweighed the benefits. The director of the group's
Public Health and American Well-Being Initiative argued that
states without them fared better and, in the fall of 2022, came out
against the recommendation by the Centers for Disease Control
and Prevention that young people receive the bivalent booster
on the grounds that there was insufficient evidence backing the
decision.*

*Like Antos, Merkel also opposes government-run healthcare
and recently warned of the "stupendous" costs of Democratic
presidential candidate Kamala Harris' Medicare-for-all proposal
from 2019.*

*Another Manhattan Institute senior fellow, Chris Pope, is also
participating in the symposium. Pope will speak on a panel about
employer-sponsored health insurance. In the past, he has argued
in favor of pushing Medicare enrollees onto privately administered Medicare Advantage plans, further injecting the free market
into the program. Paragon Health's Brian Blase, meanwhile, is
joining the health policy 2025 discussion.*

*Then there is Avik Roy, president of Koch-backed Foundation
for Research on Equal Opportunity (FREOPP), who is slated to
moderate a panel discussion called "views from the Hill." Roy
was previously a senior fellow at the Manhattan Institute and is
the policy editor at Forbes.*

*FREOPP, which received $225,000 from Stand Together Trust in
2022, features a section on its website dedicated to COVID-19*

that reads, "We should learn from excessive economic restrictions and school closures in order to ensure that we protect both lives and livelihoods in future pandemics. Most importantly, we must overhaul the ways in which we make decisions and acquire data about critical public health threats."

Alongside the various panels stacked with right-wing operatives and public health contrarians, the Hopkins symposium will also feature a discussion to field perspectives from prominent, mainstream journalists who write about healthcare and public health, such as moderator Caitlin Owens from Axios *and Dan Diamond from* The Washington Post.

In a post on BlueSky on Tuesday, Diamond wrote that he had been invited weeks earlier to the journalist panel without knowledge of the full agenda. A spokesperson from The Post *confirmed that Diamond's role is limited merely to the journalism panel.*

Clear limits and checks must be placed on the state to prevent this from ever happening again.
— *Dr. Vinay Prasad*

Other WWTI doctors bypassed politicians and spoke directly to parents to advance their political agenda. Drs. Prasad, Høeg, Lucy McBride, and several other doctors formed the Urgency of Normal, which provided an "advocacy toolkit" so parents could lobby for policies that permitted the mass infection of unvaccinated children.[49] It was published in early 2022, at a time when the youngest children—those most vulnerable to COVID—weren't able to be vaccinated and just after the Omicron wave sent a record number of them to the morgue and hospital. It said:

In our original toolkit you will find clear, understandable data on

Everyone Else is Lying to You

vaccine efficacy with Omicron, the state of student mental health, and how to protect the vulnerable while also restoring normalcy to all of our children's lives. Our new "Under 5" toolkit explores the impacts of continued COVID restrictions on our youngest children and contextualizes risk for informed decision-making. We hope our toolkits empower you in discussions with your school, friends, leaders, and everywhere else that COVID continues to impact our children.

The toolkit was full of the usual disinformation, falsely claiming the flu was more dangerous than COVID for young children, for example. For a single year—2022—The Urgency of Normal team was very worried about children's mental health, writing articles such as "Coalition of Scientists, Pediatric Infectious Disease & Mental Health Experts Issue Open Letter to White House & CDC."[50] They used their credentials—*an independent collaboration of diverse voices from the medical community*—to gain credibility for their political beliefs. Indeed, they wrote articles not about science and medicine, but about policies. Examples include: "Urgency of Normal Calls for an End to Covid Vaccine Mandates"[51] and "Urgency of Normal Calls for an End to School Mask Mandates."[52] Dr. Prasad made no secret of its political agenda, writing:

The Urgency of Normal is a group of doctors and scientists—I am one—who have created a toolkit for policy makers, showing the way to return the joys of childhood. Clear limits and checks must be placed on the state to prevent this from ever happening again.[9]

The Urgency of Normal doctors got everything they wanted. It's been years since communities tried to control the virus, and so the Urgency of Normal doctors no longer express concern about the mental health of children.

The failure of public health messaging how it's turned into a political topic as opposed to just simple scientific advice.
— *Dr. Jay Bhattacharya*

There's nothing inherently wrong with doctors advocating for their political beliefs or advising politicians. In fact, politicians need input from doctors, preferably those who actually treat sick people, when dealing with medical issues. However, WWTI doctors and the politicians they advised shared a political agenda, and they made no secret about it.

WWTI doctors were hardly neutral scientists, simply reporting the facts so the people could decide the best policy. They happily took stands on political matters. In fact, for several of them, their political activism dwarfed their miniscule scientific output. These weren't doctors who occasionally dabbled in politics. They were political activists who occasionally dabbled in medicine. While other doctors treated COVID patients, WWTI doctors used their medical credentials and posed as neutral scientists, all while functioning as lobbyists for the virus, defending it against allegations it was dangerous or something to be avoided.

Unsurprisingly, WWTI doctors felt they bore no blame for the politicization of the pandemic. You won't be surprised to learn who they thought was at fault. An article from May 2021 said:

> When it comes to masks, Bhattacharya said it was "very unfortunate" that the issue has become "such a political hot button topic."
>
> "It should not be," he told Newsweek, "and frankly represents the failure of public health messaging how it's turned into a political topic as opposed to just simple scientific advice to the population on how to keep themselves and others safe."[53]

Predictably, Dr. Mandrola, who worried about "the possibility of reducing trust" if doctors entered the political arena, had nothing to say about any of this. It didn't bother him one bit. In fact, after Dr. Bhattacharya was confirmed as NIH Director, Dr. Mandrola berated his critics for being "political":

> *There's plenty to be worried about but the 100% partisan vote on @DrJBhattacharya for NIH ranks high on the list. If you want to heal science, how can 47 thinking humans vote against a proven academic and a Stanford professor? Science should be apolitical. Come on, you all.*[54]

When Dr. Mandrola said "science should be apolitical," he was only talking about doctors who dared to voice their opinions on nuclear war, the environment, and gun violence. He didn't want to hear from them at all.

Chapter 11: We Need to Make Every Effort to Get People Who Disagree, Even Sharply, In Dialogue With One Another

The speakers represent a wide range of views on this issue. We look forward to a civil, informed, and robust debate.
— *Stanford University Pandemic Policy Symposium Statement*

On October 4, 2024—the fourth birthday of the Great Barrington Declaration (GBD)—Stanford University held a conference called "Pandemic Policy: Planning the Future, Assessing the Past." The conference was promoted by saying:

> *Bringing together esteemed academics, public health practitioners, journalists, and policymakers from all sides of the COVID-19 policy debate in conversation with one another with an eye toward reforms in science and public health to better serve the public.*
>
> *With millions of lives lost, the COVID-19 pandemic wrought havoc on the world. Despite decades of planning for the "next" pandemic, public health systems faced tremendous stress and often buckled and failed. Universities served as centers for valuable scientific work, but did they fail to support their academic freedom mission by sponsoring vigorous discussion and debate on matters of pandemic policy? To do better in the next pandemic, we need to learn the lessons of the COVID-19 era.*
>
> *The conference was organized to highlight some of the many important topics that public health officials and policymakers will need to address in preparing for future pandemics. The speakers represent a wide range of views on this issue. We look forward to a civil, informed, and robust debate.*[1]

While that sounds nice, it's worth discussing this conference, its financial backers, and its speakers in detail, as it reveals the culpability and self-inflicted impotence of some of our most prestigious institutions. Several universities were not only unwilling to correct clear disinformation spread by their faculty members, they also promoted and legitimized WWTI doctors.

> **Collateral Global's fight against pandemic mitigation measures has gone international.**
> *— Walker Bragman*

The Stanford conference was sponsored by Collateral Global, a UK "charity" that describes itself by saying:

> Collateral Global is made up of an international and collaborative community of academics, health professionals, and citizens who document, study, and communicate the collateral effects of the measures taken by governments to mitigate the damage of the COVID-19 pandemic.[2]

Despite that bland description, Collateral Global seeks to spread doubt and anger. These are some of the articles featured on its website:

- 'The Costs Are Too High': The Scientist Who Wants Lockdown Lifted Faster[3]
- We Failed Our Children in Lockdown and That Must Never Happen Again, says Ellen Townsend[4]
- Lockdown Loneliness Is Here to Stay[5]
- The Cult of Covid Censorship Is Finally Being Broken[6]
- 'Wrong all along' Covid Death Figures 'May Have Been Completely Wrong Due to Poor Statistics'[7]
- Did Official Figures Overestimate Britain's Covid Death Toll?[8]
- Covid Deaths Impossible to Calculate as Authorities Used 14 Different Ways to Record Them[9]

- The Catastrophe of Zero Covid[10]
- Lockdown Is a Slow-Moving Car Crash for Young People's Brains[11]
- Sunetra Gupta Interview: The Scientist Who Says Herd Immunity Is the Answer[12]

Here are some quotes from that last article, from October 2020:

We must stop assigning blame and guilt to young people: 'You are going to cause Granny to die.' Grannies and grandpas and other people die of flu every year in large numbers, and somebody is giving it to them, but as a society we absorb the blame.

The article concluded with "good news" about how to end the pandemic. Dr. Sunetra Gupta said:

The good news is that actually there is a way out that would also save us from corona deaths, we think. [...] That way out is afforded by natural immunity.

Journalist Walker Bragman wrote an article exploring the funding behind Collateral Global[13] that is worth quoting at length. He wrote:

Collateral Global's fight against pandemic mitigation measures has gone international.

A recent, controversial health policy symposium at Stanford University was made possible in part by funding from a UK-based charity with ties to anti-vaccine groups that is known for opposing COVID-19 mitigation measures.

"Pandemic Policy: Planning the Future, Assessing the Past" was held on October 4. The event drew the ire of prominent public health experts and scientists for its speaker roster stacked with fringe voices, including anti-vaxxers and right-wing political operatives who had advocated against government efforts to control the spread of the SARS-CoV-2 virus. According to the event's

organizer, Stanford professor and health economist Dr. Jay Bhattacharya—a senior fellow at the right-wing Hoover Institution, which is housed on the school's campus—the purpose of the gathering was to model open dialogue with all sides to achieve some greater understanding and mend bridges.

"This is not the last pandemic we as a world will face, and it's in this kind of event; this kind of dialogue—the hit pieces aside—that, really, advances get made," said Bhattacharya, who famously co-authored the widely rebuked Great Barrington Declaration, which advocated for achieving COVID herd immunity through mass infection. "It's almost an act of faith to come here," he said.

But the real goal of Bhattacharya's symposium appeared to be airing out his personal grievances and those of the other contrarian panelists at having had their ideas rejected by the larger scientific community. By design, the event would place fringe perspectives on equal footing with mainstream science. In that sense, it was part of a larger effort by the political right to rewrite the history of COVID—a continuation of a years-long war on public health to which Bhattacharya has proudly lent his voice.

For weeks, the money behind the controversial summit remained a mystery. But shortly after the conference took place, Stanford's health policy department, which hosted the affair, updated the event page with a disclaimer that the proceedings had been "supported in part by contributions" from Dr. George F. Tidmarsh, an adjunct professor of pediatrics and neonatology at Stanford School of Medicine, and a UK charity called Collateral Global.

"Collateral Impacts"

Collateral Global was incorporated on November 4, 2020 as a private limited company by attorney James Bassam Farha of Farha Secretaries Limited and serial entrepreneur Alex Caccia, who was reportedly the partner of Great Barrington Declaration co-author and Stanford symposium panelist Sunetra Gupta as of December 2020. Until last year, Caccia, himself involved in the drafting of the declaration, headed up the now defunct Animal Dynamics Limited, a company that designed and manufactured "autonomous solutions" like drones and received funding from the UK Ministry of Defence.

All three Great Barrington Declaration co-authors—Gupta, Bhattacharya, and biostatistician Dr. Martin Kulldorff, formerly of Harvard Medical School—were involved with Collateral Global as early as December 2020 as part of its supervisory board. Kulldorff no longer appears on the organization's website.

In February 2021, Gupta became a trustee, which is a director position for legal purposes. She also currently serves on Collateral Global's scientific advisory board. Bhattacharya, who was appointed as a trustee at the end of March 2023, is the organization's editor-in-chief and a member not just of its scientific advisory board, but its editorial board as well. Caccia has resigned his trustee position but is listed as the organization's CEO. Collateral Global claims to be "dedicated to researching, understanding, and communicating the effectiveness and collateral impacts of the Mandated Non-Pharmaceutical Interventions... taken by governments worldwide in response to the COVID-19 pandemic." Unsurprisingly, though, given the individuals involved, the organization has staked out contrarian positions against efforts to control the spread of COVID like lockdowns. Collateral Global has also taken aim at the World Health Organization's stalled pandemic preparedness treaty, which seeks to establish a critical framework for the nations of the world to respond to future crises including through the sharing of medical technologies like vaccines. A major goal of the treaty is addressing inequities between wealthy and developing nations and improve access to lifesaving medicines.

Bhattacharya and Collateral Global director and head of research Kevin Bardosh, an applied medical anthropologist and Stanford health policy symposium panelist, penned an editorial excoriating the treaty for "validating" lockdowns and other mitigation measures as well as infringing on national sovereignty and free speech. Collateral Global features the piece on its website in a section called "in the press."

"Validating this treaty is a vote for the disastrous policies of the Covid years," the pair wrote. "Rather than taking time for deep reflection and serious reform, those pushing the pandemic treaty are set on ignoring and institutionalizing the WHO's mistakes." U.S.-based business-aligned, right-wing groups have also come out against the unfinished treaty. The Heritage Foundation, for example, published a commentary in February lambasting an early draft for potentially doing "grave harm to the property rights of U.S. companies" and "disincentivizing future research and development of vaccines and other medical innovations that could be critical in dealing with a future pandemic."

Collateral Global's website suggests that the organization intends to create policy tools and produce academic research in the future, though, as of this writing, the pages for that work are under development. The site indicates that Collateral Global is focused on mainstreaming contrarian public health stances across the developed world. It has formed working groups in Canada and the UK to study the impacts of COVID mitigations in those countries and hold conferences. The page for the U.S. working group has no text.

The main work of Collateral Global, based on its website site, appears to be commentaries by its members. The site features a section called "UK Covid inquiry," which notes that the organization has been tracking the proceedings since June 2023, producing weekly analyses "in UnHerd and other media." The outlet, which is known for platforming "heterodox" thinkers like anti-vaccine conspiracy theorist Robert Kennedy Jr., is hyperlinked. Another page on Collateral Global's site for "global evaluations" simply links to a May 2023 paper by Bardosh on the harms of COVID mitigation measures.

Extreme Connections

Collateral Global has sought to position itself as a mainstream organization, but it has ties to anti-vaccine groups. There are numerous connections, for example, between the organization and the Health Advisory and Recovery Team (HART), a UK-based advocacy group that opposed pandemic lockdowns and the COVID vaccines. HART also notably sought help from former Cambridge Analytica psychologist Patrick Fagan to spread its contrarian messaging.

Two individuals on Collateral Global's editorial board, Univer-

sity of Nottingham professor Ellen Townsend and University of East Anglia professor David Livermore, are former members of HART. According to leaked internal messages from the group, Gupta was in contact with HART members in 2021 and even offered suggestions as to who they might recruit. Bhattacharya, meanwhile, has participated in a panel discussion with HART co-chair Claire Craig, who was revealed to have suggested seeding the false narrative that "vaccines cause COVID" into the mainstream.

The ties run deeper. Both Gupta and Bhattacharya—along with their declaration co-author Kulldorff—were on the scientific advisory board of an anti-vaccine, anti-COVID mitigation group called PANDA, which has overlapping membership with HART. HART co-chair Jonathan Engler is listed on the group's website as part of "The Team."

PANDA is more extreme than either Collateral Global or HART, going so far as to claim "there was no pandemic."

More ties between Collateral Global and HART run through the All-Party Parliamentary Group on Pandemic Response and Recovery, which purportedly aimed to "inform a more focused and flexible approach to government policy" and "reach new solutions in pandemic management to prevent suffering and loss in the future" but really sought to build a case against COVID mitigations.

An October 2021 filing in the parliamentary register of all-party groups indicated that Collateral Global put up money and in-kind services for the informal group, which was comprised of conservative members of Parliament and the House of Lords. The *funding, however, reportedly never materialized and a filing from the following month does not list the donations. Nevertheless, individuals from both Collateral Global and HART were involved in the group's sessions.* [...]

Big Donations

Collateral Global's opposition to economically disruptive public health measures has aligned it with major business interests. Unsurprisingly, the group has boasted some large donations and big name contributors. Among them is German-born Swiss billionaire businessman Georg von Opel and his wife, Emily.

The Von Opels have been major funders of conservative politics in the UK for years. Their foundation, the Georg and Emily Von Opel Foundation, had a relationship with Gupta before Collateral Global was founded. In April 2020, the group bankrolled her research "into the prevalence of COVID-19 in the population" to the tune of roughly £90,000. They subsequently gave Collateral Global £130,000 between December 2020 and November 30, 2021.

Another major Collateral Global funder in the same period was the King Baudouin Foundation, a Belgian charity established in the 1970s in honor of the then-monarch which supports projects related to health, education, climate, and other issues. The group gave Collateral Global £94,000. DonorsTrust, a U.S.-based donor-advised fund that is a preferred funding conduit of right-wing donors like those in billionaire Charles Koch's political network, gave £70,000. Another £10,000 came from businessman and investor Luke Johnson, a vocal opponent of lockdowns, while about £67,000 originated from unidentified sources.

Between December 2021 and November 30, 2022, Collateral Global received £117,000 through RSF Social Finance, a donor-advised fund affiliated with the Rudolf Steiner Foundation. It got another £157,000 from the King Baudouin Foundation, and £5,000 from the UK-based Mackintosh Foundation, which is dedicated to the performing arts and education.

Collateral Global also received £10,000 from RS Furbs Limited, a UK-based investment firm run by Robert Charles Standing, a former director of J.P.Morgan Europe Limited. Standing has been a director of at least 11 other companies—many now defunct. The company was a contributor in 2022 to conservative members of Parliament with contrarian views on COVID as well, including Steve Baker, a now-ex MP who chaired the informal, anti-lockdown COVID Recovery Group, and Miriam Cates, a former member who worked with a group called UsForThem on a campaign against vaccinating children against COVID. UsForThem does not merely oppose the inoculations. It is against the World Health Organization pandemic treaty, lockdowns, and masking.

Finally, Collateral Global received £14,000 from Toby Green, a professor of African history at King's College in London. Green, who sits on the organization's scientific advisory board, joined as a trustee in March 2023. Contributions and grants totaling £84,000 came from "other," unnamed sources. During Collateral Global's next filing period—running December 2022 to November 2023–the organization took in substantially less money. The King Baudouin Foundation gave nearly £81,000, but was the only reported big donor.

Mystery Money

*While Collateral Global's role in funding the October 4 Stanford
health policy symposium is public, the amount it fronted for the
event remains a mystery. This year's financial disclosures will not
be available for months and Stanford's health policy department
was not forthcoming with the dollar figure.*

*Moreover, the original source of the Collateral Global money
used for the conference is not publicly available, and the organization did not respond to our inquiry on the matter.*

On the day of the Stanford conference, The Nation *published an
op-ed by Yale epidemiologist Gregg Gonsalves about the event
and similar symposiums at other top schools. The piece noted
that "the architects of these meetings come with bags and bags of
right-wing funding." Bhattacharya, who was presented with the
$250,000 Bradly Prize in May by the Lynde and Harry Bradley
Foundation, which has been a major funder of right-wing causes,
took to X to request a "retraction."*

*"I donated the award money for my Bradley Prize to a charity,"
he wrote. "They are not providing me 'bags' of money." Bhattacharya, however, did respond to* Important Context*'s inquiry
about which charity he passed the funds to.*

**They also promoted popular conspiracy theories that have served
to undermine public confidence in public health officials and
institutions.**

— *Walker Bragman*

Mr. Bragman also wrote:

The Stanford health policy summit fit neatly into Collateral Glob-

al's larger mission opposing economically disruptive pandemic mitigation measures. Over the course of multiple hours, panelists served up revisionist takes suggesting that the government response to COVID was more harmful than the virus itself, which has killed more than 1.2 million Americans to date. They also promoted popular conspiracy theories that have served to undermine public confidence in public health officials and institutions.

Although Collateral Global's article from August 2021 was titled "Why It's Time to Move on from Covid,"[14] they have been unable to do so. They all speak about COVID constantly. Here is what Collateral Global paid for:

AGENDA[1]

Program Conductor/Emcee: Laura Carstensen, Professor of Psychology, Stanford University

Opening Remarks: Jonathan Levin, President, Stanford University

Welcome and Introduction: Jay Bhattacharya, Professor of Health Policy, Stanford School of Medicine

PANELS

Panel 1: Evidence-Based Decision Making During a Pandemic

The interventions undertaken to control the COVID-19 pandemic—stay-at-home orders, extended school closures, social distancing, mask mandates, vaccine mandates—were unprecedented in their scope and global impact. How well did these policies work to protect the public from COVID-19 and what were their unintended consequences? How can scientists better inform pandemic policy in real time during the next pandemic?

Moderator: *Wilk Wilkinson, Derate the Hate Podcast Creator/Host*

Speakers:

- Monica Gandhi, Professor of Medicine, Division of HIV, Infectious Diseases, and Global Medicine, UCSF
- Charlotte J. Haug, Executive Editor, NEJM AI
- Marty Makary, Professor of Surgery, Johns Hopkins School of Medicine
- Andrew Noymer, Associate Professor of Population Health & Disease Prevention, UC Irvine
- Douglas K. Owens, Professor of Health Policy, Stanford School of Medicine
- Josh Salomon, Professor of Health Policy, Stanford School of Medicine
- Anders Tegnell, Senior Expert, former State Epidemiologist of Sweden, Public Health Agency Sweden

Panel 2: Misinformation, Censorship, and Academic Freedom

During the pandemic, the challenge of balancing public health protection with the preservation of free speech became a focal point of debate. On one side, governments and public health authorities took measures to limit the spread of misinformation, sometimes by restricting certain content on social media and influencing traditional media narratives to align with official guidance. On the other side, some scientists and academics voiced concerns about these restrictions, arguing that they hindered open discourse and the exchange of diverse perspectives. This raises important questions: Does limiting speech during a public health emergency protect the public by reducing harmful misinformation, or does it risk silencing valid dissent and promoting a singular, approved viewpoint?

Moderator: *George Tidmarsh, Adjunct Professor, Pediatrics and Neonatology, Stanford School of Medicine*

Speakers:

- *Scott Atlas, Robert Wesson Senior Fellow in Health Policy, Hoover Institution*
- *Alex Berenson, Journalist and Author*
- *Gardiner Harris, Journalist and Author*
- *Neil Malhotra, Edith M. Cornell Professor of Political Economy, Stanford Graduate School of Business*
- *Michael McConnell, Richard and Frances Mallery Professor of Law, Director of the Constitutional Law Center, Stanford Law School, and Hoover Senior Fellow, Hoover Institution*
- *Jenin Younes, Litigation Counsel at the New Civil Liberties Alliance*

Panel 3: Pandemic Policy from a Global Perspective

Because the world economy is global in scope, pandemic policy decisions made by Western governments had profound impacts on the health and economic prospects of people worldwide, including the collapse of global markets, severe supply chain disruptions, large-scale government borrowing to finance pandemic policies, and global inflation. How can the interests of the world's poor be better represented in the decisions of Western government during the next pandemic?

Moderator: *Eran Bendavid, Professor of Medicine and of Health Policy, Stanford School of Medicine*

Speakers:

- *Kevin Bardosh, Director and Head of Research, Collateral Global, and Evidence Informed Fellow, Kellogg College, University of Oxford*
- *Peter Blair, Associate Professor of Education, Graduate School of Education, Harvard University*
- *Sunetra Gupta, Professor of Theoretical Epidemiology, University of Oxford*
- *Anup Malani, Lee and Brena Freeman Professor, University of Chicago Law School*

- *Yann A. Meunier, MD, Professor in Global Health, International Institute of Medicine and Science, Inc., Rancho Mirage, CA, and CEO, HealthConnect International, LLC*
- *Vinay Prasad, Professor, Department of Epidemiology and Biostatistics, UCSF*

Panel 4: COVID-19 Origins and the Regulation of Virology

The stakes in the debate about the origin of the pandemic could not be higher. If the pandemic started from an inadequately regulated wildlife trade or zoonoses, reforms to reduce the likelihood of human contact with wild species is vital. On the other hand, if the pandemic started due to dangerous laboratory experiments and inadequate protocols to prevent leaks, then more stringent regulation of such experimentation is warranted. What is the evidence on these topics, and what is the path forward?

Moderator: *Jan Jekielek, Senior Editor,* The Epoch Times

Speakers:

- *Sunetra Gupta, Professor of Theoretical Epidemiology, University of Oxford*
- *Laura H. Kahn, Co-Founder, One Health Initiative*
- *Bryce Nickels, Professor of Genetics, Lab Director, Waksman Institute of Microbiology, Rutgers University, and Co-Founder, Biosafety Now*
- *Simon Wain-Hobson, Emeritus Professor, Pasteur Institute, Paris*
- *Alex Washburne, Scientific Consultant, Selva Analytics LLC*

Conference Closing Remarks:

John Ioannidis, Professor of Medicine and of Epidemiology and Population Health, Stanford School of Medicine

I've already discussed several of these doctors, but it's worthwhile reviewing the track record of several others, although, again, these summaries just scratch the surface of their disinformation.

I would say that covid-19 will result in fewer than 40,000 deaths this season in the USA.
— Dr. John Ioannidis

Dr. John Ioannidis is a professor of medicine, epidemiology, population health, and biomedical data science at Stanford University. He is a world-famous, highly published giant of evidence-based medicine who has won countless awards and who was a ubiquitous media presence, especially in 2020. He gave many interviews, made many YouTube videos,[15] and was a guest of Fox News firebrands Mark Levin[16] and Laura Ingraham.[17] According to the article, "A Top Scientist Questioned Virus Lockdowns on Fox News. The Backlash Was Fierce," Dr. Ioannidis "appeared at least 18 times on major cable news networks, repeatedly questioning the severity of the pandemic."[18]

Dr. Ioannidis began minimizing COVID as soon as it hit our shores. In March 2020, he authored an article titled "Coronavirus Disease 2019: The Harms of Exaggerated Information and Non-Evidence-Based Measures" in which he wrote about "exaggerated pandemic estimates," "exaggerated case fatality rate," and "exaggerated exponential community spread."[19] He said a claim that 20%-60% of adults would be infected was "substantially exaggerated." He stated, "China data are more compatible with close contact rather than wide community spread being the main mode of transmission." He claimed China's efforts to contain the SARS-CoV-2 might save lives, but that "most lives saved may actually be due to reduced transmission of influenza rather than coronavirus." He felt this coronavirus was a false alarm, writing:

> *Even if COVID-19 is not a 1918-recap in infection-related deaths, some coronavirus may match the 1918 pandemic in future seasons. Thus, we should learn and be better prepared.*

He shared these sentiments in the mainstream media as well. In March 2020, he published an article in *STAT* that contained the following paragraph:

> *If we assume that the case fatality rate among individuals infected by SARS-CoV-2 is 0.3% in the general population — a mid-range guess from my Diamond Princess analysis — and that 1% of the U.S. population gets infected (about 3.3 million people), this would translate to about 10,000 deaths. This sounds like a huge number, but it is buried within the noise of the estimate of deaths from "influenza-like illness." If we had not known about a new virus out there, and had not checked individuals with PCR tests, the number of total deaths due to "influenza-like illness" would not seem unusual this year. At most, we might have casually noted that flu this season seems to be a bit worse than average. The media coverage would have been less than for an NBA game between the two most indifferent teams.*[20]

While he felt COVID might be as significant as a meaningless basketball game, he worried that measures to contain it might be catastrophic:

> *We don't know how long social distancing measures and lockdowns can be maintained without major consequences to the economy, society, and mental health. Unpredictable evolutions may ensue, including financial crisis, unrest, civil strife, war, and a meltdown of the social fabric.*

This article also contained the first seeds of the WWTI movement, promoting the idea that schools could be useful to infect children. Dr. Ioannidis lamented that "school closures may also diminish the chances of developing herd immunity in an age group that is spared serious disease."

However, just a few weeks later, Dr. Ioannidis would completely reverse his assumption that 1% of the US would contract COVID. He claimed the virus was more common than previously thought based on a flawed antibody study he co-authored with Dr. Jay Bhattacharya.[21] Predictably, he used this study to minimize COVID as well. If large numbers of people had been infected without knowing about it, that meant COVID's impact would be much less severe than feared. Dr. Ioannidis claimed the virus was "very common"[22] and that the number of known COVID cases was merely the "tip of the iceberg."[23] He said in an interview it would mean the "probability of dying if you are infected diminishes by 50-85 fold."[15]

Dr. Ioannidis said most people had no or mild symptoms and that this was a cause for "optimism" about reopening society. He called COVID a "common and mild infection"[22] for most people. If the virus was already widespread, we were closer to the middle, or even the end, of the pandemic than to its start. In another interview from April 2020, he predicted COVID would kill 40,000 Americans "this season."[24] The U.S. would surpass 40,000 deaths 8 days later. However, on that date, Dr. Ioannidis claimed there was a good chance the pandemic was close to over, saying:

> *Acknowledging for the fact that the epidemic is still evolving, and we cannot be sure whether we will hit even higher peaks in the future, although this doesn't seem to be the case, at least for the European countries, and it seems to be that even in the US, in most states we're very close to the peak, if not past the peak, the risk is something that should be manageable as opposed to the panic and horror stories that are circulating about.*[15]

Dr. Ioannidis expressed a similar sentiment in August 2020 in an article ironically titled "Forecasting for COVID-19 has Failed." He spoke as if the pandemic was over and said:

> However, very few hospitals were eventually stressed and only for a couple of weeks. Most hospitals maintained largely empty wards, expecting tsunamis that never came. [...] Tragically, many health systems faced major adverse consequences, not by COVID-19 cases overload, but for very different reasons.[25]

Dr. Ioannidis repeatedly told his audience to distrust other voices. In his appearance with Mr. Levin in April 2020, for example, he said "the evidence we had early in the pandemic was utterly unreliable."[16] He said predictions of mass death were "completely off; it is just an astronomical error." Dr. Ioannidis told viewers he had newer and better data. This data was what most of us wanted to hear: *except for older, vulnerable people, COVID was a nothingburger.* According to Dr. Ioannidis, "the vast majority" of people:

> Don't even realize that they have been infected; they are asymptomatic, they have no symptoms, or they have very mild symptoms that they would not even bother to do anything about.

He said the risk of dying from COVID was high for elderly people, especially those in nursing homes and those with serious underlying diseases, but "most of the population has minimal risk, in the range of dying while you're driving from home to work and back." Dr. Ioannidis told Mr. Levin that the infection fatality rate is "probably in the range of 1 in a thousand." Mr. Levin repeated the good news by saying, "You say one in a thousand. You're saying well under 1%, that one-tenth of 1% of the population that actually has the virus will pass away as a result of the virus or in connection to the virus."

In another interview that month, Dr. Ioannidis said:

> The risk for people who are less than 65 and have no underlying

conditions is extremely, extremely tiny. These people account for less than 1%. [...] For someone who is less than 65 and has no underlying diseases, the risk is completely negligible. [...] It seems that these deaths are extremely exceptional, very unlikely. [...]

Our data suggests that COVID-19 has an infection fatality rate that is in the same ballpark as seasonal influenza. It suggests that even though this is a very serious problem, we should not fear. It suggests that we have solid ground to have optimism about the possibility of eventually reopening our society and gaining back our lives. [...] We have data now that the infection fatality rate is much, much lower compared to our original expectations and fears. I think that there is no reason to fear.[15]

While Dr. Ioannidis did not want us to fear COVID, he wanted everyone to fear efforts to contain it. He said:

It's very, very difficult to fathom the consequences of what is going on and what we are doing, but I really worry that unless we manage to have a viable plan to exit from lockdown and shelter in place and reopen our world, the consequences will be far worse than coronavirus.

In June 2020 he said, "For people younger than 45, the infection fatality rate is almost 0%."[26] Dr. Ioannidis did not consider that people could survive COVID but be injured by it. Although COVID would become a leading cause of death in young adults in 2021, Dr. Ioannidis instead worried about entirely hypothetical deaths from the vaccine. In a vanity documentary called *Out to See*, he said:

If you have, for example, myocarditis, but you don't have some symptoms, even though you may have a problem with your heart muscle, then you don't really report it because you never felt it. And could that person die at some point? Yes. One in, who knows, a million or 100,000. Maybe that will happen, and then that would be the first event that someone would just drop dead on the floor. So the rest will not be captured.[27]

At the start of the pandemic, Dr. Ioannidis spread doubt about COVID's death toll, claiming it was greatly inflated even as morgues overflowed. He claimed that "99% of people" who succumbed to the virus were "people [who] would have died anyhow." He stated:

> *Because for the data that we have more mature and detailed information, like the data from Italy that has already [gone] through the peak of their epidemic wave, we realize that 99% of people who die with this virus have other reasons as well to die. On average, they have close to three other reasons to die. On average they are 80 years old with other comorbidities, as we say, and there's quite some debate on whether these people would have died anyhow, if not immediately; you know, perhaps in a few days or in a few weeks or a few months. In our country, we see a fairly similar picture.*[15]

No one who worked in a COVID unit would have said that, though the idea that COVID only killed elderly people who were on their death-bed anyway became one of the pandemic's harmful myths.

Variants Shmariants.
— Dr. Monica Gandhi

According to her biography:
Monica Gandhi, MD, MPH, is Professor of Medicine and As-

sociate Division Chief (Clinical Operations/ Education) of the
Division of HIV, Infectious Diseases, and Global Medicine at
UCSF/San Francisco General Hospital. She also serves as the
Director of the UCSF Center for AIDS Research (CFAR) and the
Medical director of the HIV Clinic at SFGH ("Ward 86"). Dr.
Gandhi completed her M.D. at Harvard Medical School and then
came to UCSF in 1996 for residency training in Internal Medi-
cine. After her residency, Dr. Gandhi completed a fellowship in
Infectious Diseases and a postdoctoral fellowship at the Center
for AIDS Prevention Studies, both at UCSF. She also obtained a
Masters in Public Health from Berkeley in 2001 with a focus on
Epidemiology and Biostatistics.[28]

Dr. Monica Gandhi was a ubiquitous media presence, writing articles for *The Washington Post*, *The Wall Street Journal*, and *The Atlantic*,
where she published articles such as "It's Time to Contemplate the End of
the Crisis"[29] and "Overcaution Carries Its Own Danger to Children."[30] Dr.
Gandhi has a large social media presence and was frequently sought after
for podcasts and interviews where she relentlessly minimized COVID.
For example, in August 2020, Dr. Gandhi spoke on the positives of asymptomatic infections, saying:

A high rate of asymptomatic infection is a good thing. It's a good
thing for the individual and a good thing for society. It is an
intriguing hypothesis that asymptomatic infection triggering im-
munity may lead us to get more population-level immunity. That
itself will limit spread.[31]

She was a frequent podcast guest of Dr. Zubin Damania (ZDogg-
MD). In October 2020, before anyone was vaccinated, they recorded
"How to Stop Living in Fear of COVID," where listeners heard Dr.

Gandhi say that "you can still see your friends and family while keeping yourself safe, and you're not gonna die of this."[32] Starting in early 2021, Dr. Gandhi declared the pandemic over. In February 2021 they recorded "The End of the Pandemic," and listeners heard that "a UCSF infectious disease doctor is convinced this pandemic is ending, and sooner than you think."[33] Drs. Gandhi and Damania shared a belly laugh then, mocking variants by saying, "Variants shmariants." Both Delta and Omicron would arrive several months later, and Dr. Gandhi would admit to regretting this comment.

However, Dr. Gandhi predictably minimized the risk of variants as well. In February 2021, she gave an interview titled "Pandemic Exit Interviews: Stop Panicking About the COVID-19 Variants, Says UCSF's Monica Gandhi,"[34] and in March 2021, she said:

> *I genuinely with all my heart apologize for anyone who continues to try to scare you about variants.*[35]

When the Delta variant emerged, she predictably minimized this as well. In an interview, she said:

> *Children are not more susceptible to the delta variant, they're threefold less likely to get any infection with any variant with any ancestral strain, and they're half as likely to spread it.*[36]

The opposite was true.

Dr. Gandhi also authored an article titled "The Reassuring Data on the Delta Variant," in which she stated:

> *There's no sign of a surge in hospitalization or severe illness, and the vaccines remain extremely effective. You read the same alarming headlines every few months, now with Greek letters. As the virus that causes Covid-19 evolves and mutates, the same concerns pop up about whether the variant evades vaccines,*

makes people sicker than the old versions, and increases trans-
missibility. What we know about the Delta variant is reassuring.[37]

When Omicron emerged, she gave an interview in December 2021, in which she said:

> *The final thing I'll say is that adult vaccination protects chil-*
> *dren. We saw that with the Delta variant in this country. In*
> *places with high adult vaccination rates we didn't see so many*
> *cases for hospitalizations and children. It could be that adult*
> *vaccination here is going to protect children. There are still a lot*
> *of unknowns.*[38]

Although Dr. Gandhi also said, "There are many places that are doing very well, including New York City," by the end of the month, the headlines read, "Pediatric Hospitalizations Up 395% in NYC Amid Covid-19 Surge."[39]

Her false forecasts in 2020 and 2021 didn't stop her from making similar podcasts with Dr. Damania in 2022. In May, they recorded "Living with COVID," which declared, "We now have all the necessary tools to end the COVID 'emergency phase.' Here's how (and why) we can live with this coronavirus."[40] They recorded another podcast in December titled "A Better Pandemic Playbook," where Dr. Gandhi again made her case for "COVID optimism"[41] and spoke of "how little severe disease there is." She said that, due to high rates of immunity, "since March of 2022 we've seen very little severe disease in the hospital." In reality, 160,000 Americans died of COVID from March to December 2022,[42] and COVID was the third leading cause of death for the third year in a row.[43]

Early in the pandemic, Dr. Gandhi believed that if COVID killed over 100 Americans daily, citizens would band together and prevent this at all costs. Sadly, she was wrong about this too. Despite her near-perfect record of poor predictions—which included her predicting she would stop making predictions on *The Mehdi Hasan Show*[44]—San Mateo County celebrated their reopening with "Dr. Monica Gandhi Day" on June 15, 2021.[45] Although 596,666 Americans had died of COVID by then, Dr. Gandhi cut a ribbon of masks as part of the celebration. Delta arrived immediately after, and before the end of 2022, an additional 500,000 more Americans would die of COVID.[46]

Dr. Gandhi also overhyped vaccines in 2021 on podcasts and social media. Some examples are:

- **January 2021:** *No time in history do we have this extraordinary detection of asymptomatic infection since latter can transmit to others. So, please be assured that YOU ARE SAFE after vaccine from what matters – disease and spreading. Two vaccinated people can be as close as 2 spoons in drawer!*[47]
- **January 11, 2021:** *So, why can two vaccinated people be as close as two spoons in a drawer? Because both are so highly protected from what matters- disease. Even though vaccines reduce asymptomatic infection (I bet much higher reduction after that 2nd dose, this is just before 2nd dose in Moderna)*[48]
- **February 2021:** *Dr. Damania: So Monica, I'm gonna tell something publicly that I have not said. This table is new, right? The last time you were here, I had a six-foot round table. We were six feet apart. This table is now about three feet. And the reason I'm doing that is, I believe with a 95% efficacy that two vaccinated people can hang out.*

  Dr. Gandhi: They could totally hang out. And remember, it's not 95% efficacy against severe disease. It's 100% against severe disease. (Author note: this was false at the time[49]). *And then yeah, maybe one person who got the vaccine will not feel well for a few days, because it was a mild disease. So that's the amazing thing. Keep on focusing on preventing what got us into trouble to begin with.*[33]

- **April 2021:** *It's simple math. We don't need to vaccinate those under 11 to get to herd immunity.*[50]
- **April 2021:** *Don't worry, even the most pessimistic, variant-discussing, doom-steeped people are no match for the vaccines!*[51]
- **May 2021:** *We now have ample data to show that the vaccines also block transmission. The ability of this virus to transmit from individuals who are infected but do not show symptoms (asymptomatic) has been the reason it was previously so difficult to contain. But multiple studies at this point show us that vaccines massively reduce asymptomatic infection.*[52]

Along with Allison Krug and Drs. Tracy Beth Høeg and Lucy McBride, Dr. Gandhi authored an article in May 2021 that argued:

> *As we saw in Israel and Britain, vaccinating adults indirectly protects children. The same trend is evident here in the United States: Adult vaccination has lowered covid-19 incidence among children by 50 percent in the past four weeks.*[53]

The Delta wave peaked three months later.

Despite these false statements, Dr. Gandhi often spoke about the importance of trust in public health. In an interview with *The New York Times* in 2022, she said:

> *Well, yes, I think it's actually really important to change your views with new data. And things do need to update and change as new data comes in. [...] So you must update with time. If you don't update with time, you will lose public health trust, especially over two years.*[54]

Then in 2024, she recorded a podcast titled "Rebuilding Trust in Health Institutions."[55] She promoted it on social media, posting, "After a chaotic COVID-19 response with lots of political agendas in the US, it is time to rebuild trust in public health here."[56]

To her credit, Dr. Gandhi was unique amongst WWTI doctors in that she authored a strong defense of the pediatric COVID vaccine titled "The Childhood Vaccine Debate Ignores a Crucial Point: Kids Aren't Supposed to Die." "Where did we lose our way?"[57] she asked, though the answer was hardly a mystery.

I think flu is much more dangerous actually than COVID.
— Dr. Sunetra Gupta

Dr. Gupta is a Professor of Theoretical Epidemiology at the University of Oxford. According to her webpage:

My main area of interest is the evolution of diversity in pathogens, with particular reference to the infectious disease agents that are responsible for malaria, influenza, and bacterial meningitis. I use simple mathematical models to generate new hypotheses regarding the processes that determine the population structure of these pathogens. I work closely with laboratory and field scientists both to develop these hypotheses and to test them.[58]

Dr. Gupta is well known for being one of the three authors of the GBD. However, well before the GBD was written, she was a prominent media figure, minimizing COVID and encouraging "herd immunity to build up." In an interview from May 2020, she was asked about COVID's infection fatality rate and said:

I think that the epidemic has largely come and is on its way out in this country, so I think it would be definitely less than 1 in 1,000 and probably closer to 1 in 10,000.[59]

This was a mathematical impossibility at the time based on the number of people who had already died.

In July 2020, she gave an interview, in which she said:

The only way we can reduce the risk to the vulnerable people in the population is, for those of us who are able to acquire herd immunity, to do that. [...] In an ideal situation, you would protect the vulnerable as best you can, let people go about their business, allow herd immunity to build up, make sure the economy doesn't crash, make sure the arts are preserved, and make sure qualities of kindness and tolerance remain in place. [...] We are in a better place to fight off this infection than we actually thought.[60]

In another interview that month, Dr. Gupta claimed the flu was worse than COVID and again spoke positively about herd immunity:

I think we will and already have developed herd immunity, and we will continue to manage it through herd immunity or accommodate it through herd immunity as we do [with] many other, you know, lethal pathogens. I think flu is much more dangerous, actually, than COVID, and I think that this particular virus will settle into an endemic state just like flu does with the human population.[61]

Although we did not have herd immunity at that time, Dr. Gupta continued to repeat her calls for mass infection in the fall of 2020, saying:

We need to start to think more carefully about what we really want to achieve, which is to stop people dying. And we feel that the most parsimonious, effective, efficient, kindest way to do this, the most humanitarian approach, given the huge costs of some of these restrictions, and also given that we know that this pathogen has a very, very low risk of death for a substantial proportion of the population, we feel that the best way to achieve the outcome that we really all want is by allowing what we call herd immunity, in other words, levels of population immunity, to build up because that reduces the risk to everybody and allows us to resume a normal life. We feel that that could happen without the attendant deaths that it might otherwise entail if we focus our protection on those who are most likely to have those adverse outcomes of infection.[62]

Predictably, Dr. Gupta relentlessly minimized COVID's risk to everyone except seniors. In an interview from September 2020, she stated:

I mean, herd immunity, in fact, actually maybe, I think, is our way out of this. We're very fortunate, I think, actually, with this virus, that it doesn't do harm to young people. Indeed, if you're under the age of, should I say, 55, it really isn't something to worry about. And I would say, generally, people under 65 shouldn't; you know, it's in line with all sorts of risks that we take anyway.[63]

That same month, she gave another interview:

Professor Sunetra Gupta, who has been a leading critic of the cost of lockdown, says she welcomes the return of schools as children "if anything... would benefit from being exposed to this and other seasonal coronaviruses."

Gupta, who is a professor of theoretical epidemiology at Oxford, told The Londoner that alongside huge social and educational benefits, the "evidence is mounting that early exposure to these various coronaviruses is what enables people to survive them."[64]

The virus was less than a year old when she said this. There was *no* mounting "evidence" that early exposure to SARS-CoV-2 would "benefit" children, though there *was* evidence that it was dangerous for some of them.[65]

Although babies have the highest risk of any children by far, Dr. Gupta minimized their COVID risk as well as the risk of reinfections. In a conversation with Drs. Martin Kulldorff and Bhattacharya from October 2020. She said:

> The people who will be exposed to the virus in the new epidemic will be the young, the newborns who will be exposed to [it for] the first time. And for them, the risk is probably not terribly high from what we're seeing. And for those of us who might be re-exposed, again, it's likely from looking at the other coronaviruses that reinfection will not carry the same risk of severe disease and death. And that's also true for many other pathogens. But the second exposure does not carry the same risks.[66]

In November 2020, she portrayed herself as a victim for suggesting mass infection. She said:

> I was utterly unprepared for the onslaught of insults, personal criticism, intimidation and threats that met our proposal. The level of vitriol and hostility, not just from members of the public online but from journalists and academics, has horrified me. [...] It is perplexing to me that so many refuse even to consider the potential benefits of allowing non-vulnerable citizens, such as the young, to go about their lives and risk infection, when in doing so they would build up herd immunity and thereby protect the lives of vulnerable citizens.[67]

As the pandemic progressed, Dr. Gupta both overhyped vaccines and minimized variants. In May 2021, she said:

> All this fear around variants really mystifies me because within any traditional epidemiological framework, you would say that the most likely attributes of these variants is that they have

*a slight advantage, maybe in transmission, maybe in avoiding
immunity towards infection.*

I would say [with a] *high degree of certainty—something which
we don't normally enjoy—that the vaccines work against these
variants in terms of delivering immunity against severe disease
and infection, and this is something people need to get in their
heads.*

*What we're trying to do is prevent people from dying. Whether
or not infections go up with a new variant is not relevant. It's important that people don't die. We've protected vulnerable people
now. We've had the great good fortune to have these vaccines,
which protect vulnerable people.*

*I'm sure they'll protect vulnerable people against this new vari-
ant from death, maybe not infection, but that's not relevant, and
given the high costs of these mitigation strategies, the suffering
among the poor and the young, you know, I can't understand how
the balance of the debate shifts in favor of the spectre of this new
variant being some monstrous thing.*[68]

Delta and Omicron arrived before the end of that year.

**One point would be to keep schools open to reach herd immunity
faster.**
— Dr. Anders Tegnell

Dr. Anders Tegnell served as Sweden's state epidemiologist during
the first two years of the pandemic. He also massively underestimated the
virus. An article from April 2020 quoted him as saying:

*In major parts of Sweden, around Stockholm, we have reached
a plateau (in new cases) and we're already seeing the effect of*

*herd immunity and in a few weeks' time we'll see even more of
the effects of that. And in the rest of the country, the situation is
stable.*[69]

Another article published that same month said:

*Sweden's state epidemiologist Anders Tegnell said on Friday
that his country would likely be in a better place to withstand a
second wave of coronavirus because so many people in Sweden
have now been exposed to the virus.*

*He told the BBC that the relatively relaxed approach had
"worked in some aspects," since there had always been at
least 20% of intensive care beds empty and able to take care of
Covid-19 patients.*

*"We believe we passed the peak of the transmission a week ago,"
he added.*

*Asked whether Sweden's approach will help it withstand a possi-
ble second wave, Tegnell said he believed it would. "It will definitely affect the reproduction rate and slow down the spread,"
he said, but added that it wouldn't be enough to achieve "herd
immunity."*[70]

In private emails, Dr. Tegnell revealed one motivation for keeping
schools open, saying, "One point would be to keep schools open to reach
herd immunity faster."[71]

Instead of herd immunity, Sweden was rewarded with headlines such
as "Anger in Sweden as Elderly Pay Price for Coronavirus Strategy."[72]
According to a report in *Science*:

*The virus took a shocking toll on the most vulnerable. It had free
rein in nursing homes, where nearly 1000 people died in a matter
of weeks. Stockholm's nursing homes ended up losing 7% of their*

14,000 residents to the virus. The vast majority were not taken to
hospitals.[73]

Sweden suffered many more deaths than its Nordic neighbors at the
start of the pandemic, and a report by the government-appointed, independent Swedish Corona Commission later reported the unsurprising
news that uncontrolled spread of the virus in the community was the
"single most important factor behind the major outbreaks and the high
number of deaths in residential care."[74] According to one damning investigation, "The Swedish people were kept in ignorance of basic facts such
as the airborne SARS-CoV-2 transmission, that asymptomatic individuals
can be contagious and that face masks protect both the carrier and others."[75] Horrifyingly, it also found that:

> *Many elderly people were administered morphine instead of oxy-*
> *gen despite available supplies, effectively ending their lives.*

Children weren't necessarily spared. Dr. Jonas Ludvigsson, a Swedish pediatrician and epidemiologist who was an original signer of the
GBD, claimed that there were "no major school outbreaks in Sweden,"[76]
despite such outbreaks being reported in Swedish media. He also published a letter in *The New England Journal of Medicine* that claimed
there had been no excess mortality in Swedish children in 2020 compared
to 2019.[77] However, in emails to Dr. Tegnell from July 2020, Dr. Ludvigsson wrote, "Unfortunately we see a clear indication of excess mortality among children ages 7-16 old, the ages where 'kids went to school.'"[78]

By June 2020, the headlines read, "We Should Have Done More,
Admits Architect of Sweden's Covid-19 Strategy." That article said:

> *Anders Tegnell, who has previously criticised other countries'*
> *strict lockdowns as not sustainable in the long run, told Swedish*
> *Radio on Wednesday that there was "quite obviously a potential*

for improvement in what we have done" in Sweden.

Asked whether too many people in Sweden had died, he replied: "Yes, absolutely," adding that the country would "have to consider in the future whether there was a way of preventing" such a high toll.

Sweden's death rate per capita was the highest in the world over the seven days to 2 June, figures suggest. This week the government bowed to mounting opposition pressure and promised to set up a commission to look into its Covid-19 strategy.

"If we were to encounter the same disease again knowing exactly what we know about it today, I think we would settle on doing something in between what Sweden did and what the rest of the world has done," Tegnell said. It would be "good to know exactly what to shut down to curb the spread of infection better," he added.[79]

By November 2020, the headlines read, "Swedish Surge in Covid Cases Dashes Immunity Hopes." The article stated:

New infections and hospital admissions have surged in Sweden as the country battles a second wave of the coronavirus pandemic that officials had hoped its light-touch, anti-lockdown approach would mitigate.

"We consider the situation extremely serious," the director of health and medical care services for Stockholm, Björn Eriksson, told the state broadcaster SVT this week. "We can expect noticeably more people needing hospital care over the coming weeks." Swedish hospitals were treating 1,004 patients for Covid-19, SVT said, an increase of 60% over the previous week's 627. Data from the European Centre for Disease Prevention and Control suggests the rise in recent weeks may be Europe's fastest.

New infections are also surging, hitting a seven-day average of more than 4,000 this week against fewer than 500 at the beginning of October. The country recorded 4,635 new infections on Thursday.[80]

Despite this, many people portray Sweden as a pandemic paradise, which never imposed restrictions on its citizens or closed schools and barely noticed the virus. In reality, Sweden took drastic measures to control the virus at times, though it was too late for many of its most vulnerable citizens. Another headline that appeared in November 2020 was "Sweden Limits Public Gatherings to Eight People Amid Covid Surge." The article said:

Sweden has cut its limit on attendance at public gatherings to eight people, as its light-touch approach to the coronavirus pandemic continues to be tested by a surge in new infections and hospitalisations.

Public gatherings have until now had to adhere to limits of between 50 and 300 people depending on the type of event. The prime minister, Stefan Löfven, said the stricter limit would come into force from 24 November.

"This is the new norm for the entire society," Löfven said, adding that Swedes were not observing coronavirus recommendations as well as they had in the spring. "Don't go to gyms, don't go to libraries, don't host dinners. Cancel," he said.[81]

David Steadson, a public health researcher who co-authored the investigation referenced above, noted that Sweden's restrictions on seniors and vulnerable people led to what he called "the longest continuous lockdown in the world."[82] Mr. Steadson told me via personal communication:

There were also many other restrictions put in place that people ignore, including alcohol sales restrictions, all large events and large localities shutdown, including sports events, zoos, theatres, theme parks. Sports activities all shut down or went outdoors. Even "recommendations" (ie technically binding but unenforced) on restricting travel outside your home region.

While Sweden closed high schools during the winter peak in 2020-2021,[83] it never officially closed schools for younger children. That does not mean schools were open, however. Overwhelming COVID outbreaks caused many school closures at the local level, as happened in the U.S.[84] Mr. Steadson also told me:

*Contrary to popular myth, Sweden **did** close schools. In early March 2020, the Government amended the school regulations to allow all schools from preschool and up, to move to remote or hybrid learning in the event of outbreaks of staff issues. On March 27, 2020, on the recommendation of the Swedish Public Health Agency, all high schools (Grade 10 and up) and Universities and adult education moved to remote learning, with 3 months summer holidays beginning a few weeks later.*

Following the 2020 summer break, many schools, predominantly middle school and up (from grade 7) – elected to continue with hybrid and remote classes, however, no statistics on school closures were kept.

Mr. Steadson, who lives in Sweden himself, told me about his experience with his own children. He said, "I had kids in grades 4, 7, and 8 when the pandemic broke out. The latter two were remote for a year and then hybrid for another 6 months or so."

Looking back on Sweden's response, King Carl XVI Gustaf said, "I think we have failed. We have a large number who have died and that is terrible."[85] Prime Minister Stefan Löfven agreed, saying, "Of course the fact that so many have died can't be considered as anything other than a failure."

Sweden would mostly right the ship after 2020, becoming one of the most highly vaccinated countries, though they resisted vaccinating children.

> **Tone deaf to how this kind of rhetoric contributed to the deaths of thousands of Americans during the pandemic by convincing them to shun vaccines or minimize Covid.**
> — *Dr. Peter Hotez*

Incredibly, doctors with those track records joined Drs. Bhattacharya, Vinay Prasad, Scott Atlas, and Marty Makary to speak about *Evidence-Based Decision Making During a Pandemic* and *Misinformation, Censorship, and Academic Freedom*[1]. Other speakers included the overtly anti-vaccine disinformation writer, Alex Berenson, also known as the pandemic's wrongest man for writing articles such as "We Could 'Beat' Covid-19 Before a Vaccine Is Ready" in August 2020.[86] Jan Jekielek, an editor at *The Epoch Times*, a gross disinformation publication with ties to Falun Gong,[87] was also there, as were many supporters of the lab leak "theory."

Predictably, frontline doctors were excluded, as was anyone who might be bold enough to quote WWTI doctors' early pandemic rhetoric. The conference hosts claimed to be in favor of *vigorous discussion and debate,* but they didn't want to discuss whether their plan to achieve herd immunity via mass infection in three to six months was successful and ethical.

Stanford University was presenting the mirror world, and, understandably, this provoked strong feelings from those connected to the real world. In one article titled "'Embarrassing and Disappointing': Stanford Goes All-In on COVID Contrarians," Mr. Bragman and Dr. Allison Neitzel reported:

> *Public health experts and scientists expressed alarm at the prospect of the Stanford conference. Dr. Peter Hotez, chair of the Center for Vaccine Development at Texas Children's Hospital, took to X (formerly Twitter) to criticize the school for platforming "a full on anti-science agenda (and revisionist history)." Hotez called the event "tone deaf to how this kind of rhetoric contributed to the deaths of thousands of Americans during the pandemic by convincing them to shun vaccines or minimize Covid."*
>
> *Molecular biologist and science communicator Philipp Markolin had a similar take, calling the panelists "a who-is-who of rightwing-propped up contrarians" and telling* Important Context *that the summit represents a victory for conservative ideologues who operate through networks of dark money groups.*
>
> *"To maintain their value to these networks, academic contrarians rely on the imprimatur and reputation of the academic institutions that house them, often using the veneer of academic freedom for spreading harmful scientific disinformation for naked political advocacy or profiteering," he said. "This is antithetical to the scientific method, and corrosive to public trust in science and scientific institutions. However, academic institutions are often ill-equipped or unwilling to speak up against their own politically-entwined contrarians (especially ones with a large platform) for fear of political repercussions and perception of anti-conservative bias."*

Mallory Harris, who graduated in May from Stanford with a Ph.D. in biology, told Important Context *that "It's been embarrassing and disappointing to see Stanford University as an institution conflated with the fringe opinions of a few contrarians." Harris, who did her dissertation on infectious diseases and human behavior, including the spread of anti-vaccine misinformation, and led a student group called Scientists Speak Up focused on countering scientific misinformation, argued that the real issue the summit raises is not academic freedom, but academic rigor.*

"Based on the panelists and framing, I expect this summit will repeat the same grievances and misrepresentations without any substantive academic contribution—which is the prerogative of the organizers," she said. "However, it's alarming to me that the Stanford president is choosing to speak and give the university's tacit endorsement to these speakers and their positions."

"Their definition of academic freedom is entitlement to the largest platforms at the university, regardless of the validity or rigor of your work, without any criticism," she added. "This is, of course, nonsense. They can pursue whatever line of *research* they want. They can host whatever conference they want. But the rest of us aren't required to pretend it's worth attending."[88]

In an article titled "Some of Our Top Schools Are Embarrassing Themselves Over Covid," Dr. Gregg Gonsalves said:

The architects of these meetings come with bags and bags of right-wing funding, some of it laundered through think tanks and other institutions. They have met with Trump officials in the White House and guided Florida Governor Ron DeSantis on

Covid-19 policy. Some of them even got a shout-out from Bret
Stephens at The New York Times *last week.*

They whine on and on about how terribly they've been treated,
but, far from being persecuted, they are celebrated on the right,
even if the mainstream members of their professions have, time
and time again, considered their ideas and roundly rejected them
on their merits. [...]

These Covid contrarians—who have found little support for their
views among their peers—have decided that the science has been
turned into "a dogmatic tool of oppression" for rejecting them.
In their minds they are Galileos against the church, and now they
are tilting their fury against the institutions themselves. This tack
is of course reminiscent of the right's attacks on the universities
as bastions of woke, left-wing ideology, which either need to be
reformed (by hiring more conservative faculty) or gutted and
rebuilt to their liking (e.g., New College of Florida).[89]

An Open Letter to the President of Stanford, Jonathan Levin.
— *Dr. Jonathan Howard*

The opening remarks were given by Stanford president, Jonathan
Levin, an economist who authored several papers on health economics
with Dr. Bhattacharya, such as "Consolidation of Primary Care Physicians and Its Impact on Healthcare Utilization"[90] and "Can Health Insurance Competition Work? Evidence from Medicare Advantage."[91]

Because he was giving the conference his personal *imprimatur*, I
published an open letter to him before the conference titled "An Open
Letter to the President of Stanford, Jonathan Levin: Don't Censor Drs.

Scott Atlas, John Ioannidis, Sunetra Gupta, Marty Makary, Monica Gandhi, Jay Bhattacharya, and Vinay Prasad. Amplify Their Voices."[92] It said:

Dear President Levin,

*Your university will soon be hosting a conference titled Pandemic
Policy: Planning the Future, Assessing the Past. The conference claims to value "vigorous discussion and debate on matters of pandemic policy," and says that it is "bringing together
esteemed academics, public health practitioners, journalists,
and government officials from all sides of the COVID-19 policy
debate."*

*Right off the bat, this is obvious misinformation. There will be no
vigorous discussion and debate on matters of pandemic policy.
The conference organizer, Dr. Jay Bhattacharya, carefully curated the speakers to create an echo chamber and foster groupthink.
Unsurprisingly, they agree with him. I've extensively quoted
many of them in my writing, and I know they basically marched
in lockstep. They were mostly united in their belief that young
people should be infected with SARS-CoV-2 instead of vaccinated
against it, and that the pandemic ended years ago. Each of these
articles/podcasts is by or about one of the speakers:*

- *Dr. Eran Bendavid and Dr. Jay Bhattacharya, March 2020:
  "Is the Coronavirus as Deadly as They Say?"[93]*
- *Dr. John Ioannidis, April 2020: "The Bearer of Good Corona-
  virus News"[94]*
- *Dr. Anders Tegnell, April 2020: "Sweden Resisted a Lock-
  down, And Its Capital Stockholm is Expected to Reach 'Herd
  Immunity' In Weeks"[69]*
- *Dr. Scott Atlas, April 2020: "The Data Is In — Stop The Panic
  And End The Total Isolation"[95]*
- *Dr. Sunetra Gupta, July 2020: "We May Already Have Herd*

Immunity"[60]

- Dr. Monica Gandhi, February 2021: "The End of the Pandemic"[96]

- Dr. Marty Makary, February 2021: "We'll Have Herd Immunity by April"[97]

- Dr. Vinay Prasad, April 2021: "The Motivation We Need to Reach the End of the COVID-19 Pandemic with Dr. Monica Gandhi"[98]

A more accurate name for the conference would be "Doctors Who Declared The Pandemic Over Years Ago Meet In the Middle of a COVID Surge to Claim They Were Right."

What could they possibly debate? Perhaps doctors who said we had herd immunity in 2020 will get into it with those who said we didn't have herd immunity until early 2021. Several doctors who said COVID wasn't anything to worry about in the first place will also chime in. This is what is being promoted as "all sides of the COVID-19 policy debate."

If that wasn't enough doublespeak, one of the sessions, Misinformation, Censorship, and Academic Freedom, features Dr. Scott Atlas, a celebrity radiologist who advised a President and predicted COVID would kill 10,000 Americans. However, despite this professed loathing of misinformation and censorship, I fully expect that this conference will censor its speakers' misinformation. I hope you'll read recent articles on the conference as well as my articles on these speakers. I predict the quotes we've collected will be purposefully censored. I am confident the conference will be a giant exercise in deliberate collective amnesia and pandemic revisionism. I expect the plan to infect 250 million unvaccinated Americans to reach herd immunity in 3-6 months will be silenced and suppressed, even though several speakers *were leaders of the We Want Them Infected movement. I predict the speakers will fantasize that they would have opened schools, but will say nothing about how they actually worked to deliberately infect the unvaccinated students and teachers within them. That's unfortunate.*

Doctors who died of COVID were silenced. In contrast, the conference speakers were loud and famous. They advised world leaders and were ubiquitous in the media. They were everywhere, except hospitals. In this video, the former President of the United States specifically credits Dr. Atlas and other Stanford doctors for influencing his thinking on "herd mentality." Not bad access for "censored" doctors.

Though only a few of the speakers treated COVID patients, they greatly influenced our pandemic response, and for this reason, I've worked diligently to preserve their words. I don't want them to be censored or have their voices erased. Quite the opposite. They deserve to have their pandemic pronouncements amplified and remembered for the rest of their careers. Those of us who worked with COVID patients will never forget the consequences. You are giving the introduction to the conference, meaning you are setting the tone and giving your personal stamp of approval to it. I am sure we both agree it's important to have an accurate account of the pandemic and to reject cancel culture. In that spirit, I believe you are obligated to boost these doctors' voices. The attendees and the general public deserve to know what they said and the policies they pushed. The speakers claim to have been "silenced," and you have a unique opportunity to remedy that injustice.

I can help.

While other doctors were treating sick patients, these doctors were in front of cameras. I have collected some clips below and many more are available here.[99] I trust you'll have the intellectual integrity to play many of them. Anything less would be misinformation and censorship, betraying the purported mission of this conference and your university.

Sincerely,

Jonathan Howard

I provided President Levin with multiple videos he could show of these doctors declaring the pandemic over in the spring of 2021 or treating temporary vaccine side effects as a fate worse than death.

Distrust in public health is good.
— *Dr. Vinay Prasad*

The conference went about as expected. Dr. Bhattacharya gave an introduction where he falsely said there would be a "very, very wide range of views."[100] Dr. Tegnell said:

> *We also found trust in societies is incredibly important. At meetings like this we can rebuild trust.[101]*

Dr. Makary reflexively blamed public health officials for the lack of trust in medicine. He said:

> *The medical field says trust in public health is down because some people said there was a microchip in the vaccine, but that's not true. No. Trust in public health is down because people realize they were lied to for three years.[102]*

Dr. Prasad wrote about it in real time, saying:

> *Many people discuss the need to rebuild trust in public health.*

But a conference attendee made a good point to me: distrust in public health is good.[103]

During his speech, Dr. Prasad mocked Dr. Peter Hotez and said:

I would be surprised if there is a resurgence in trust in public health. It deserves to be distrusted.[101]

In his concluding remarks, Dr. Ioannidis declared himself a champion for "poor children" and said:

We let children down, we let poor people down, we let poor children down, we let our future down.[104]

Dr. Atlas, writing about the event later, predictably obscured his pro-infection philosophy and claimed that if only 250 million unvaccinated people contracted COVID in spring 2020, everything would have been just fine. He depicted himself as being only concerned about "the poor and our children."[105] He said:

"Targeted protection"– that meant increasing the protection of the high-risk people, because the lockdowns were <u>not</u> protecting them, and ending the lockdowns and school closures that were destroying the poor and our children, first advised in March 2020, then repeatedly for months… And then formally codified in October 2020 by Jay, Martin, and Sunetra in their Great Barrington Declaration.

Dr. Atlas neglected to mention that *"targeted protection"* also meant mass infection.

We've had more flu deaths among children this year than COVID deaths.
— *Dr. Jay Bhattacharya*

I have no idea if President Levin read my letter, but none of my suggested videos were played at the conference. However, it's worth review-

492Everyone Else is Lying to You

ing one of the videos I would have shown if I had been there, as it shows institutional indifference to obvious disinformation

In November 2020, Dr. Bhattacharya said, "We've had more flu deaths among children this year than COVID deaths, just in terms of mortality."[106] This was false. The first reported COVID death in the U.S. was February 28, 2020. By the time Dr. Bhattacharya recorded that video, COVID had killed at least 133 children, according to the American Academy of Pediatrics.[107] During that same time frame, the flu killed nine children.[108]

Presumably, President Levin would fail a student who said nine was larger than 133. Yet, Dr. Bhattacharya was given a free pass. President Levin didn't feel such errors were even worth mentioning. Instead of honestly informing the conference attendees about the speakers, President Levin sanitized their record and portrayed all disagreements with them as about policy, rather than basic facts. He gave the following speech:

> *Good morning and welcome to everyone. I appreciate the opportunity to be here.*
>
> *Now, you might wonder: Why is Jon Levin opening this conference on pandemic policy? You might say, Jon is no public health expert. And I might say: Well, I did run a business school during the COVID pandemic, so I have some experience making pandemic policy decisions. They also say you learn most by making mistakes. So I think there are probably a thousand Stanford MBAs who are willing to argue that I'm basically a world expert. However, that's not why I'm here.*
>
> *When I was invited to participate in this event a few months ago, it was with the understanding that the goal was to bring together people with different perspectives, engage in a day of discussion,*

and in that way, try to repair some of the rifts that opened during COVID.

That struck me as a valuable goal, and the sort of goal we should aim for at Stanford. So I agreed to give a few brief remarks to that effect.

What followed was disappointing. When I was invited, I asked around and indeed the organizers were talking to some well-known people with quite different views who were likely to speak. However, it was not so straightforward. Some invitees weren't able to make it, or withdrew, or didn't want to participate in an event with other speakers whose views and behavior they found attacking or abhorrent.

When an initial and partial agenda was posted, it was immediately perceived as one-sided, and as I'm sure you all noticed became the subject of op-eds and social media posts. Ironically, instead of repairing rifts as intended and perhaps spurring fresh thinking, the process seemed to reopen old and existing divisions. As an observer and as the leader of this university, I found the episode dispiriting, in a way that goes beyond the specifics of this particular event. We have many issues today at Stanford, and on other campuses, where views are divided, and in some cases, like this one, where feelings are raw.

Yet I believe we need to make every effort to get people who disagree, even sharply, in dialogue with one another. I believe it's essential for us to do that as members of the faculty and university leaders – not just because it's a way to advance knowledge, but because we need to model that behavior if we want to expect it from our students. And in today's world, we absolutely need to ask and expect our students to be able to engage with, listen to, and debate with people with whom they disagree. My view is that we need to err on the side of talking to one another.

So I hope today's conference will come off in a way that involves just that – thoughtful and robust discussion across different perspectives. I hope it yields some important insights about future pandemic policy – we certainly need that. Perhaps it does even bridge a few divides among those in the room.

And I hope even more that all of you will join in the larger project of trying to make Stanford and other campuses forums for the type of robust and thoughtful discussion that is at the heart of universities when we're at our best.[109]

According to the president of Stanford University, the conference just featured *"people who disagree."* This raises an obvious question. What could any of the speakers have possibly said that would have led President Levin to say, *"You are wrong"*? The answer is literally nothing. Several WWTI doctors predicted COVID would kill 10,000 Americans and that we had herd immunity in 2020. President Levin wouldn't even say they were wrong about that. In the mirror world, objective truth doesn't exist; there are only *"different perspectives,"* and what really matters is that no one has their feelings hurt.

Indeed, rather than standing against disinformation, President Levin was only willing to stand against those who criticized the conference in any way. In his worldview, spreading fake statistics during a deadly pandemic was fine. The problem lay with those who corrected those fake statistics. President Levin accused the conference's critics of opposing *fresh thinking and repairing rifts,* which he claimed was the entire point of the conference. He felt we should model excellent behavior for our students.

Meanwhile, after the conference, Dr. Prasad said:

> *I don't believe in forgiveness because in my opinion, these pieces of shit are still lying. I mean, like if you want forgiveness, the first thing you have to say is what you actually did wrong, and they're still fucking lying.*[110]

Dr. Atlas similarly wrote "On Censorship, Academic Freedom, and the Pandemic," about the conference, which said:

> *Remember - Lockdowns were not caused by the virus. Human beings decided to do lockdowns - they OWN the results. Their lockdowns were implemented. Their policies failed - and killed and destroyed millions. That's fact.*[105]

None of this bothered President Levin, though his indifference to basic facts and incendiary accusations is a tradition for Stanford presidents. In September 2020, 98 Stanford faculty members published a public letter that said Dr. Atlas spread "falsehoods and misrepresentations of science."[111] In an article titled "Academic Freedom Questions Arise on Campus Over Covid-19 Strategy Conflicts," Stanford's president at the time, Dr. Marc Tessier-Lavigne, responded by saying:

> *The university must provide a place where faculty can engage in unconstrained, even heated debate. It is central to what we do, and the reason for our policy on academic freedom. That function of the university would be seriously eroded if we were to publicly take sides either to disavow or to support the specific positions of a faculty member engaged in such a debate. What we do support is the right of faculty members to express their views.*[112]

In the mirror world, the *function of the university would be se-riously eroded* if basic factual errors were acknowledged and corrected. If a university ever uttered the words "you are wrong" to one of its faculty members, that would somehow "constrain de-bate," and in the mirror world, these "debates" mattered more than overflowing morgues in the real world.

Journalist Michael Hiltzik wrote about Stanford's refusal to ac-knowledge basic facts in his article, "Can Stanford Tell the Differ-ence Between Scientific Fact and Fiction? Its Pandemic Confer-ence Raises Doubts." He said:

> *The idea that universities such as Stanford should be arenas for airing all opinions in a search for truth is simplistic and historically incorrect. Universities have always had, and even embraced, the duty to draw the line between fact and fiction — to determine when an assertion or opinion falls below the line of intellectual acceptability.*
>
> *"Science and quackery cannot be treated as having scientific and moral equivalence," John P. Moore, a distinguished biol-ogist and epidemiologist at Weill Cornell Medical College who played a part in debunking misinformation about the role of HIV in AIDS during the 1990s, wrote recently. "Do NASA scientists attend conferences by people who believe the moon-landing was faked? Do geographers and geologists attend conferences held by idiots who believe the earth is flat? Of course not."*[113]

Perhaps President Levin feels we need *thoughtful and robust discus-sion across different perspectives* when it comes to the shape of the earth. When Dr. Bhattacharya was nominated to head the NIH, President Levin said:

> *Jay Bhattacharya has been nominated to be the director of the*

National Institutes of Health, which is the most important funder
of biomedical research in the country, in fact in the world. I think
he'll do an exceptional job in that role.[114]

Shortly after this, the headlines read, "Stanford to Lose $160 Million
in NIH Funding Change,"[115] "NIH Funding Cuts Leave Stanford Researchers 'In Limbo',"[116] and "DOGE Claims NIH Cuts Will Save $4B.
Stanford Says It'll Gut Its Ability to Do Research."[117]

This didn't just happen at Stanford. Johns Hopkins, The University
of Chicago,[118] Hillsdale College,[119] and New College[120] all hosted similar
events sponsored by organizations such as the Global Liberty Institute,
the Academy for Science and Freedom, the Chicago Thinker, the Health
Freedom Defense Fund, and No College Mandates.

As we face the future of epidemics both in the U.S. and abroad, it's
people like Dr. Gandhi who we can rely on to show us a clear path
forward.
— *Dr. Jeffrey Flier*

Meanwhile, most "leaders" of American medicine are either silent
about disinformation or they heap praise on the doctors that spread it.
Despite her track record, Dr. Gandhi wrote a book called *Endemic: A*
Post-Pandemic Playbook,[121] which was blurbed by some impressive doctors. They didn't care that she said the pandemic was over in the spring of
2021. They said the following:

"Throughout the COVID-19 pandemic, Dr. Monica Gandhi has
emerged as a unique voice, passionately arguing for an approach
that balances the threat of the virus and the harms of mitigation
strategies. In this timely, lucid, and well-referenced book, Gandhi
lays out the lessons of the pandemic – lessons that should be heed-

ed as we manage the continued threat of Covid and plan for the next pandemic. An essential addition to the Covid lexicon." **—Robert Wachter, M.D., Chair, Department of Medicine, UCSF and New York Times bestselling author of The Digital Doctor.**

*"As a specialist who has been on the forefront of the HIV/AIDS epidemic, Dr. Gandhi is no stranger to the fear, stigma, discrimination, and uncertainty a new disease can create. Her book provides assurance and clarity as she reflects on the lessons learned from the HIV response and discusses what went right and what went wrong in our response to the COVD-19 pandemic and how to prepare for the next public health emergency."–***Carlos del Rio, M.D., Professor of Medicine, Emory University School of Medicine; President, Infectious Diseases Society of America**

*"Dr. Gandhi has been a star presence in the medical community for many years, particularly in the fight against HIV/AIDS. As we face the future of epidemics both in the U.S. and abroad, it's people like Dr. Gandhi who we can rely on to show us a clear path forward. With this book, Dr. Gandhi provides a solid map."–***Jeffrey Flier, M.D., former Dean, Harvard Medical School**

This is how universities reframed blatant disinformation as mere policy disagreements. This is how "leaders" of American medicine normalized disinformation within their faculty. This is how universities collaborated with WWTI doctors to erase the history of the pandemic.

NEJM Posts a Perspective Saying Stanford Should Have Corrected Scott Atlas: Why? To Look Foolish? B/C Atlas Was Correct & His Critics Were Wrong.
— Dr. Vinay Prasad

Academic freedom is vital. Sometimes the lone contrarian voice may turn out to be correct, and academic freedom protects me. I've been able to bluntly criticize members of my profession without the slightest bit of fear or retaliation from my university. However, this means my institution must also tolerate Dr. Marc Siegel, who held the #1 spot in the article, "The Dishonest Doctors Who Were Fox News' Most Frequent Medical Guests in 2021." According to that article:

> In September on America Reports, Siegel fearmongered that migrants and asylum-seekers would be vectors for disease. Siegel said, "they are going to leak into the neighboring communities," and that Haitians are "clearly spreading COVID." (Blaming migrants for disease spread is a longtime racist myth.)[122]

How should universities respond to faculty members who spread disinformation? I don't know the answer to this conundrum; however, some doctors felt it was appropriate for heads of institutions to speak up. In a *NEJM* article titled "Academic Freedom in America — In Support of Institutional Voices," Drs. Evan Mullen, Eric J. Topol, and Abraham Verghese discussed Stanford and Dr. Atlas. They wrote:

> We believe it's reasonable for an institution to speak out publicly when it concludes that a faculty member's opinion could cause public harm. The gulf between Stanford's internal Covid-19 policies regarding masking and infection prevention and Atlas's external assertions suggests that the university believed that lives were at stake. Though Stanford's concerns about Atlas's academic freedom are not without merit, academic freedom is not an absolute right that abrogates all others, nor does it compel a university's silence. Institutions have not always been shy about

speaking out when faculty members make racist or antisemitic
statements, for example, and the bar for speaking out is lowest
when the university would be challenging faculty who make proc-
lamations in domains where they lack expertise. Furthermore,
although institutions cannot reasonably be held responsible for
their professors' opinions, when the reputation of an institution
lends credence to a professor's claims, institutional silence may
be interpreted as tacit approval. If a university does not speak
for itself, the voices of its professors become its voice, and their
reputation its reputation.[123]

That last line is true. Several prestigious universities don't seem as prestigious as they once were.

Predictably, WWTI doctors have strongly discouraged their institutions from correcting their errors. They argued that Stanford had no right to correct Dr. Atlas because he was right about everything. Dr. Kulldorff said:

Public health policy expert @ScottAtlas_IT was correct about
the pandemic while the 98 @Stanford faculty and @EricTopol
were wrong.[124]

Dr. Høeg similarly wrote, "I'm left wondering what exactly @ScottAtlas_IT got wrong."[125] Dr. Atlas agreed. He said that he was "100% correct"[126] about everything and that he was only concerned about the fate of the "children & the poor."

Dr. Prasad even authored a rebuttal to the *NEJM* article titled "*NEJM* Posts a Perspective Saying Stanford Should Have Corrected Scott Atlas: Why? To Look Foolish? B/C Atlas Was Correct & His Critics Were Wrong." Dr. Prasad wrote:

During the COVID19 pandemic, Scott Atlas made many contro-

versial statements. Community cloth masking doesn't slow the spread of COVID19. Kids should be in school. Lockdowns have no evidence of efficacy. In other words, Atlas was pretty smart. Randomized data would later show conclusively cloth masking doesn't work. School closure is now regarded as a catastrophic error, and even Anthony Fauci regrets how long they lasted. [...] According to them Stanford should have issued statements saying that Atlas was wrong. Really? Why? To look foolish later? The idea in the commentary is laughable. [...]

Of course, not all university researchers read or understood the evidence like Atlas, as the NEJM piece correctly notes 98 Stanford faculty (with absolutely no political bias ;) ;)) disagreed with Atlas, who was hired by Trump.[127]

In Dr. Prasad's telling, Dr. Atlas's critics were motivated by politics and couldn't assess the evidence. In contrast, Dr. Atlas was a wise, kind-hearted spirit who cared deeply about scientific evidence and education. Moreover, Dr. Prasad claims time has vindicated Dr. Atlas, and as such, Stanford had no right to say *anything* negative about this saintly man. Dr. Prasad's argument has largely won the day. Universities are mostly silent.

Unsurprisingly, Dr. Prasad's defense of Dr. Atlas was another exercise in revisionist history. No one criticized Dr. Atlas because of his stance on *community cloth masking*. Rather, Dr. Atlas predicted 10,000 Americans would die of COVID and that "natural immunity" would lead to herd immunity.[128] His critics believe he got this wrong, and they said so at the time. After hearing Dr. Atlas repeatedly say that infections in young people were a net positive, here were the core beliefs of those 98 Stanford faculty members in September 2020:

To prevent harm to the public's health, we also have both a moral

Everyone Else is Lying to You

and an ethical responsibility to call attention to the falsehoods and misrepresentations of science recently fostered by Dr. Scott Atlas, a former Stanford Medical School colleague and current senior fellow at the Hoover Institute at Stanford University. Many of his opinions and statements run counter to established science and, by doing so, undermine public-health authorities and the credible science that guides effective public health policy. The preponderance of data, accrued from around the world, currently supports each of the following statements:

- The use of face masks, social distancing, handwashing and hygiene have been shown to substantially reduce the spread of Covid-19. Crowded indoor spaces are settings that significantly increase the risk of community spread of SARS-CoV-2.

- Transmission of SARS-CoV-2 frequently occurs from asymptomatic people, including children and young adults, to family members and others. Therefore, testing asymptomatic individuals, especially those with probable Covid-19 exposure is important to break the chain of ongoing transmission.

- Children of all ages can be infected with SARS-CoV-2. While infection is less common in children than in adults, serious short-term and long-term consequences of Covid-19 are increasingly described in children and young people.

- The pandemic will be controlled when a large proportion of a population has developed immunity (referred to as herd immunity) and that the safest path to herd immunity through deployment of rigorously evaluated, effective vaccines that have been approved by regulatory agencies.

- In contrast, encouraging herd immunity through unchecked community transmission is not a safe public health strategy. In fact, this approach would do the opposite, causing a significant increase in preventable cases, suffering and deaths, especially among vulnerable populations, such as older individuals and *essential workers.*

Commitment to science-based decision-making is a fundamental obligation of public health policy. The rates of SARS-CoV-2 infection in the US, with consequent morbidity and mortality, are among the highest in the world. The policy response to this pandemic must reinforce the science, including that evidence-based prevention and the safe development, testing and delivery of efficacious therapies and preventive measures, including vaccines, represent the safest path forward. Failure to follow the science -- or deliberately misrepresenting the science – will lead to immense avoidable harm.[111]

That all seemed to age pretty well to me, and I applaud them for using their voice.

Chapter 12: The NIH and FDA Nominees Are Surprisingly Strong

For Leonhardt the deaths of those who may not be fully protected is apparently acceptable.
— Dr. Cecilia Tomori

There was no shortage of excellent COVID journalists and writers, including those who specifically tackled disinformation, such as Dr. Allison Neitzel, Max Kozlov, Tara Haelle, Walker Bragman, Karam Bales, Brandy Zadrozny, Lauren Weber, Melody Schreiber, Laura Weiss, Jeff Kunzler, Kiera Butler, Sheryl Gay Stolberg, Anna Merlan, David Corn, Stephanie M. Lee, and Michael Hiltzek, as well as Derek Beres, Matthew Remski, and Julian Walker from the *Conspirituality* podcast and Artie Vierkant and Beatrice Adler-Bolton from the *Death Panel* podcast.

Several mainstream media outlets covered the WWTI movement as well. Dr. Paul Alexander's original "we want them infected" email received press coverage in 2020, as did Dr. Joseph Ladapo's anti-vaccine disinformation. In 2023, *The New York Times* published an article about the "steep cost" of anti-vaccine sentiment in Florida that said:

> Both he (Dr. Scott Atlas) and Dr. Bhattacharya argued that people who were not at risk of severe consequences should not face Covid restrictions. If they were infected, they would develop natural immunity, which would eventually build up in the population and cause the virus to fade away, they said.
>
> Many public health experts were alarmed by this strategy, which was articulated in a document known as the Great Barrington Declaration. They said it would be impossible to ring-fence the vulnerable, or even to clearly communicate to the public

*who they were. Besides older Americans, as many as 41 mil-
lion younger adults were considered to be at high risk of severe
disease if infected because of underlying medical conditions like
obesity.*

*Dr. Atlas, however, argued that the virus was not dangerous to
an overwhelming majority of Americans. Both he and Dr. Bhattacharya said the Covid death rate for everyone under 70 was
very low. Dr. Atlas claimed that children had "virtually zero"
risk of death. Neither man responded to requests for comment.
As of this summer, more than 345,000 Americans under 70 have
died of the virus, and more than 3.5 million have been hospitalized with Covid. The disease has killed nearly 2,300 children and
adolescents, and nearly 200,000 have been hospitalized.*[1]

Other journalists had a less glorious track record, however. In his
article, "Elon Musk's New Twitter Files Reporter Has Ties to Great
Barrington Declaration," Walker Bragman had this to say about journalist
David Zweig:

*In recent years, Zweig has made a name for himself as a COVID
contrarian adopting positions that have brought him into align-
ment with powerful business interests and the political right,
which have been waging a war on public health measures. He
even assisted a libertarian think tank with ties to billionaire
industrialist Charles Koch in the promotion of The Great Barrington Declaration, a controversial open letter proposing a
herd immunity strategy based around mass infection and minimal government intervention. The ideas in the document helped
inform the disastrous U.S. COVID response, which has seen
limited governmental action and staggeringly high death and*

long COVID numbers.[2]

Indeed, Mr. Zweig produced a steady stream of content that repeatedly minimized COVID's risk, especially to children. His articles appeared in *The Atlantic* and *New York* magazine's Intelligencer. Mr. Zweig received coverage from others in the media as well. Some examples are:

- David Zweig on Twitter's Rigging the Covid Debate[3]
- How and Why the Reality of Covid was Censored[4]
- The CDC's Flawed Case for Wearing Masks in School[5]
- Inside the Schools Open Full Time Right Now What the Data Really Tells Us About Covid-19 Transmission and Safety in the Classroom[6]
- Why Spending Time with Kids Might Actually Help Protect You from Covid[7]
- The Science of Masking Kids at School Remains Uncertain[8]
- New Research Suggests Number of Kids Hospitalized for Covid Is Overcounted[9]
- Experts: CDC's Summer-Camp Rules are 'Cruel' and 'Irrational'[10]
- Why Public Schools Shouldn't Offer a Remote Option This Fall[11]
- Putting Students Behind Plexiglass Isn't Making Them Safer[12]
- Our Most Reliable Pandemic Number is Losing Meaning, a New Study Suggests that Almost Half of Those Hospitalized with Covid-19 Have Mild or Asymptomatic Cases.[13]
- Is the Second Shot Giving Young Men a Dangerous Heart Condition?[14]

That last article, from June 2021, discussed cases of vaccine myocarditis from Israel, but didn't link to the actual report, and it neglected to mention that "95% are considered to be mild cases."[15] Even though COVID had killed at least 316 children[16] and the flu 10 children[17] by that point in the pandemic, Mr. Zweig wrote, "Pediatric mortality is on par with or less than that from influenza in recent seasons." Delta and Omicron arrived within six months, spiking pediatric hospitalizations and deaths, especially in unvaccinated children. Mr. Zweig later wrote a book about school closures while continuing to associate with Jeffrey Tucker, the proud child labor advocate who sponsored the Great Barrington Declaration (GBD). Mr. Tucker's Brownstone Institute even had a party to celebrate Mr. Zweig's book.[18]

Unfortunately, he was not alone. David Leonhardt of *The New York Times* also spread fake statistics, claiming that for children, "the virus resembles a typical flu."[19] In one article, he said that he would vaccinate his own children but also said, "An unvaccinated child is at less risk of serious Covid illness than a vaccinated 70-year-old."[20] This data point has no bearing on whether or not children should be vaccinated; however, anti-vaxxers quoted Mr. Leonhardt in their writing.[21]

Mr. Leonhardt gained a reputation for spreading "good news" with articles such as "Omicron is Milder"[22] and "A Positive Covid Milestone."[23] In response to this second article, which was published in July 2023, historian Nate Holdren wrote:

> *Last week, David Leonhardt took to the pages of the* New York Times *to celebrate the latest COVID death figures, which he claims mean the U.S. is no longer in a pandemic, because there are no more "excess deaths."*
>
> *The hunger for good news is, of course, understandable amid this ongoing nightmare. But to respond to death with "smile everyone, it could have been more deaths!" is grotesque because of the disrespect to the dead and those most affected by the deaths.*
> *[…]*
> *We should resist the temptation to respond to death and injury by looking for ways to say the present level of death is better than*

some counterfactual. Unless COVID deaths are genuinely at zero, no level of death is actually good news, it's just the absence of even worse news. It's especially important to not get pulled into calling a number of deaths "better" when we know that the government, employers, and other powerful institutional actors have chosen to let preventable infections, and thus some avoidable COVID deaths, just happen.[24]

Another article about Mr. Leonhardt, "The NYT's Polarizing Pandemic Pundit," said:

Notable doctors and scientists have written to The Times, *individually or in groups, to poke holes in Leonhardt's coverage of the pandemic. They say that he cherry-picks sources and data, giving too much weight to people who may have medical expertise but not on infectious disease; that he argues strenuously for open schools but downplays the Covid risks for kids as well as their role in spreading the virus; that he held out Britain's vaccination strategy as a model (right before the U.K. itself reversed course); that he underestimates how many Americans — not all over age 65 — are at elevated risk or live with people at elevated risk. He tends, they say, to look at the virus' impact on individuals, not the pandemic's impact on society.*[25]

This article linked to a social media thread by Dr. Cecilia Tomori, which said:

What we learn from this episode is not really what Americans think about the pandemic, but rather Leonhardt's flawed interpretations thereof. It's amazing that someone who has consistently minimized the impacts of COVID and has expressed little concern for those dying or suffering, or becoming disabled from

COVID continues to have the opportunity to claim authority
about this topic. To argue that we should just get on with life
because boosted individuals (like himself) face relatively low
personal risk of death from the virus misses so much. [...] For
Leonhardt the deaths of those who may not be fully protected is
apparently acceptable.[26]

The emergency phase of the disease is over. Now, we need to work
very hard to undo the sense of emergency.
— *Dr. Jay Bhattacharya*

In addition to tolerating disinformation from their own reporters, the
mainstream media also provided an outlet for WWTI doctors to minimize
COVID and spread their disinformation. A classic journalism adage says:

If one person says it's raining and another person says it's dry,
it's not your job to simply report what both say. It's your job to
stick your head out the window and find out what's true.[27]

Of course, it's not always so easy. Imagine an asteroid storm heading
towards Earth and two astrophysicists, each with impeccable credentials,
submit dueling proposals to destroy the threat. Each of the scientists
claims their plan will work, while that of their rival will lead to ruin. How
should newspapers cover this? Obviously, there's no right answer; however, if one scientist destroys 100 asteroids and the other says we need to
build up immunity to them, a good newspaper would quickly learn whom
to platform and whom to ignore.

In contrast, many mainstream publications continued to treat WWTI
doctors as reliable sources well after the virus shattered their farcical
forecasts of herd immunity. Consider the article, "The Covid Endgame:
Is the Pandemic Over Already? Or Are There Years to Go?" which was

published in *The Washington Post* in September 2021. The article quoted Dr. Jay Bhattacharya as saying:

> *The emergency phase of the disease is over. Now, we need to work very hard to undo the sense of emergency. We should be treating covid as one of 200 diseases that affect people.*[28]

It also quoted Dr. Monica Gandhi as saying:

> *I truly, truly think we are in the endgame. The cases will start plummeting in mid- to late September and by mid-October, we will be in a manageable place, where the virus is a concern for health professionals, but not really for the general public.*

There was no need to ask Drs. Bhattacharya and Gandhi their opinions, however. No matter what was happening, they were always going to say, "We are in the endgame." Yet readers were not informed of their litany of previous poor predictions. Unfortunately, Omicron arrived several months later, proving them wrong yet again.

However, instead of reminding their readers of WWTI doctors' past predictions, mainstream media continued to publish their articles and turn to them for quotes. Although I have shared several of these articles already, it's important to show how relentlessly WWTI doctors promoted their minimizing message in newspapers and magazines, including "liberal" publications such as *The Atlantic* and *The Washington Post*, as well as "neutral" medical magazines such as Medscape, STAT News, and MedPage Today. WWTI doctors weren't censored or silenced. Their views were widely publicized, and it shows how they inundated the public with their COVID minimization and message of doubt. Excerpts from some of their articles are below:

- **Dr. John Ioannidis, STAT News, March 2020, "A Fiasco in the Making? As the Coronavirus Pandemic Takes Hold, We Are Making Decisions Without Reliable Data":** *A popu-*

lation-wide case fatality rate of 0.05% is lower than seasonal influenza. If that is the true rate, locking down the world with potentially tremendous social and financial consequences may be totally irrational. It's like an elephant being attacked by a house cat. Frustrated and trying to avoid the cat, the elephant accidentally jumps off a cliff and dies.[29]

- **Drs. Jay Bhattacharya and Eran Bendavid, *The Wall Street Journal*, March 2020, "Is the Coronavirus as Deadly as They Say?":** *If it's true that the novel coronavirus would kill millions without shelter-in-place orders and quarantines, then the extraordinary measures being carried out in cities and states around the country are surely justified. But there's little evidence to confirm that premise—and projections of the death toll could plausibly be orders of magnitude too high.*[30]

- **Dr. Scott Atlas, *The Hill*, April 2020, "The Data Is In — Stop the Panic and End the Total Isolation":** *The tragedy of the COVID-19 pandemic appears to be entering the containment phase. Tens of thousands of Americans have died, and Americans are now desperate for sensible policymakers who have the courage to ignore the panic and rely on facts.*[31]

- **Dr. Scott Atlas, *The Hill*, April 2020, "Reentry After the Panic: Paying the Health Price of Extreme Isolation":** *With a world-wide sense of relief, progress continues in containing the COVID-19 pandemic. Projections have been revised downward for virtually every major negative consequence of the disease. Few doubt that the unprecedented isolation policies and near-total economic lockdowns adopted by most countries had a significant impact on reducing deaths from the virus. And aside from New York, where almost half of the entire country's deaths and cases have occurred, the vast majority of American hospitals were not overwhelmed beyond capacity. All of this is terrific news.*[32]

- **Ian Schwartz about Dr. Scott Atlas, Real Clear Politics, April 2020, "Stanford University Scott Atlas: Virus Panic Induced by Overestimation of Fatality Rate of Infected":** *But now we know from data all over the world, including the U.S., that a massive number of people have the virus that were either asymptomatic. In fact, 50 percent of people that are infected have zero symptoms.*[33]

- **Drs. Vinay Prasad and Jeffrey S. Flier, STAT News, April 2020, "Scientists Who Express Different Views on Covid-19 Should Be Heard, Not Demonized":** *Scientific consensus is important, but it isn't uncommon when some of the most important voices turn out to be those of independent thinkers, like John Ioannidis, whose views were initially doubted. That's not an argument for prematurely accepting his contestable views, but it is a sound argument for keeping him, and others like him, at the table.*[34]

- **Allysia Finley about Dr. John Ioannidis, *The Wall Street Journal*, April 2020, "The Bearer of Good Coronavirus News":** *"Compared to almost any other cause of disease that I can think of, it's really sparing young people. I'm not saying that the lives of 80-year-olds do not have value—they do., but there's far, far, far more [...] young people who commit suicide." If the panic and attendant disruption continue, he says, "we will see many young people committing suicide [...] just because we are spreading horror stories with Covid-19. There's far, far more young people who get cancer and will not be treated, because again, they will not go to the hospital to get treated because of Covid-19. There's far, far more people whose mental health will collapse."*[35]

- **Drs. Jay Bhattacharya and Martin Kulldorff, *The Wall Street Journal*, September 2020, "The Case Against Covid Tests for the Young and Healthy":** *There is little purpose in using tests to check asymptomatic children to see if it is safe for them to come to school. When children are infected, most* *are asymptomatic and the mortality risk is lower than for the flu. While adult-to-adult and adult-to-child and transmission is common, child-to-adult transmission isn't common.*[36]

- **Tunku Varadarajan about Drs. Martin Kulldorff and Jay Bhattacharya,** *The Wall Street Journal*, **October 2020, "Epidemiologists Stray From the Covid Herd":** *"As an epidemiologist," says Mr. Kulldorff, "it's weird and stunning to have this discussion about herd immunity—flockimmunitet in Swedish." He likens it to gravity: "You wouldn't have physicists talking about whether we believe in gravity or not. Or two airline pilots saying, 'Should we use the gravity strategy to get the airplane down on the ground?' Whatever way they fly that plane—or not fly it—gravity will ensure eventually that the plane is going to hit the ground."*[37]

- **Dr. Vinay Prasad, MedPage Today, November 2020, "What Does 'Follow the Science' Mean, Anyway?":** *In other words, science can help quantify the increased risk (or lack thereof) of school reopening on SARS-Cov-2 spread, and help quantify the educational losses from continued closure, but science cannot tell you whether to open or close schools. Making the decision requires values, principles, a vision of the type of society we want to be. How much do we care about the kids that rely on public school? Is it enough to offset a theoretical (but unsubstantiated) risk of viral spread? On this topic, I agree with others that we have chosen poorly.*[38]

- **Drs. Jay Bhattacharya and Sunetra Gupta,** *The Wall Street Journal*, **December 2020, "How to End Lockdowns Next Month":** *Authorities like Anthony Fauci and Bill Gates argue that lockdown restrictions may have to continue through the fall and even into 2022, notwithstanding the catastrophic harms the lockdowns have caused, especially to young people, the poor and the working classes.*[39]

- **Dr. Vinay Prasad, MedPage Today, January 2021, "Throw Away Your Mask After COVID Vaccination?":**

COVID-19 will someday no longer be the topic of daily and breathless news coverage. The virus may always circulate, and some people may always get sick, but the real end will be when we stop thinking about it every moment of every day. That's how this pandemic will end. Not with a bang, but a whimper. People need to know that there is light at the end of the tunnel because there is. Vaccination in the absence of viral escape is the way out of this.[40]

• **Dr. Lucy McBride, *The Washington Post*, January 2021, "Stress Caused by Today's Crisis Can Actually Damage Your Health. A Doctor Has Some Suggestions":** *It's normal to be concerned about the new coronavirus variants. But when you are reassured that the current vaccines will probably work against them (which they should) and you continue to ruminate about vaccine efficacy, we've got a problem. Anxiety, when allowed to roam freely through our brains, wastes precious mental and physical energy. Protect your body from being in a constant state of tension by countering your thoughts with facts.[41]*

• **Isabel Vincent about Dr. Marty Makary, *New York Post*, February 2021, "Johns Hopkins Expert Says Covid-19 Pandemic Could End by April":** *"There is reason to think the country is racing toward an extremely low level of infection," Makary wrote. "As more people have been infected, most of whom have mild or no symptoms, there are fewer Americans left to be infected. At the current trajectory, I expect COVID will be mostly gone by April, allowing Americans to resume normal life."[42]*

• **Eric Ting about Dr. Monica Gandhi, SF Gate, February 2021, "Pandemic Exit Interviews: Stop Panicking About the Covid-19 Variants, Says UCSF's Monica Gandhi":** *I'm surprised that the messaging today is all about how the* *vaccines don't cover the variants, which is misleading. We should be spreading more optimism and talking less about mutations.*[43]

- **Dr. Vinay Prasad, STAT News, February 2021, "Kids Don't Need Covid-19 Vaccines to Return to School":** *Kids are less likely to acquire SARS-CoV-2, the virus that causes Covid-19, than adults.*[44]

- **Dr. Monica Gandhi, *The Atlantic*, February 2021, "Over-caution Carries Its Own Danger to Children":** *Incessant pessimism about the coronavirus is hard to kick, but the vaccines are banishing any doubt about reopening schools.*[45]

- **Dr. Marty Makary, *The Wall Street Journal*, February 2021, "We'll Have Herd Immunity by April":** *Experts should level with the public about the good news. Some medical experts privately agreed with my prediction that there may be very little Covid-19 by April but suggested that I not talk publicly about herd immunity because people might become complacent and fail to take precautions or might decline the vaccine.*[46]

- **Dr. Lucy McBride, Huff Post, March 2021, "I'm a Doctor Seeing Patients with Coronophobia. Here's What You Need to Know":** *COVID-19 cases are dropping, but anxiety is everywhere. And even as the vaccines get distributed, no one is immune to the trauma of the pandemic. Protecting our mental and physical health in tandem can help us stay safe — and sane.*[47]

- **Dr. Marty Makary, *The Wall Street Journal*, March 2021, "Covid Prescription: Get the Vaccine, Wait a Month, Return to Normal":** *The Centers for Disease Control and Prevention has lost a lot of credibility during the Covid-19 pandemic by being late or wrong on testing, masks, vaccine allocation and school reopening.*[48]

- **Dr. Lucy McBride, *The Washington Post*, March 2021, "I've Been Yearning for an End to the Pandemic. Now**

That It's Here, I'm a Little Afraid": *The pandemic will end. With dropping case rates and three incredible vaccines robustly protecting us from covid-19, soon we'll be able to relax the restrictions of pandemic life.*[49]

- **Dr. Marty Makary, *The Wall Street Journal*, March 2021, "Herd Immunity is Near, Despite Fauci's Denial":** *Anthony Fauci has been saying that the country needs to vaccinate 70% to 85% of the population to reach herd immunity from Covid-19. But he inexplicably ignores natural immunity. If you account for previous infections, herd immunity is likely close at hand.*[50]

- **Drs. Martin Kulldorff and Jay Bhattacharya, *The Wall Street Journal*, April 2021, "Vaccine Passports Prolong Lockdowns":** *As tens of millions are inoculated against Covid-19, officials in places as diverse as New York state, Israel and China have introduced "vaccine passports," and there's talk of making them universal. […] It sounds like a way of easing coercive lockdown restrictions, but it's the opposite.*[51]

- **Dr. Vinay Prasad, MedPage Today, May 2021, "Will the Real COVID Experts Please Stand Up?":** *Throughout this pandemic, I have grown tired of listening to pundits scold or shame the public for not doing this or that.*[52]

- **Dr. Marty Makary, *New York Post*, May 2021, "Risk of Covid is Now Very Low — It's Time to Stop Living in Fear":** *Yet some people want the pandemic to stretch out longer, insisting on a futile goal of absolute risk eradication. Posturing to be on the side of science, they ignore the science on the effectiveness of vaccinated and natural immunity and dangle variant fears. They wear masks after being fully vaccinated even though there has never been a documented case of a fully vaccinated person who is asymptomatic transmitting the virus.*[53]

- **Stephanie Sierra about Dr. Monica Gandhi, ABC News, May 2021, "California 'Weeks Away' from Reaching Herd**

Immunity, UCSF Doctors Say": *"I am predicting that Gov. Newsom was actually right," said Dr. Monica Gandhi, an infectious disease physician with UCSF. "June 15th is when we're going to be done…get to herd immunity."*[54]

- **Dr. Monica Gandhi, *The Washington Post*, May 2021, "The Science is Clear: Masks Worked, But Vaccinated People Don't Need Them Now":** *We now have ample data to show that the vaccines also block transmission. The ability of this virus to transmit from individuals who are infected but do not show symptoms (asymptomatic) has been the reason it was previously so difficult to contain. But multiple studies at this point show us that vaccines massively reduce asymptomatic infection.*[55]

- **Dr. Marty Makary, *New York Post*, May 2021, "Don't Buy the Fearmongering: The Covid-19 Threat is Waning":** *As the COVID pandemic wanes, Americans are being fed a distorted perception of the risks by the media and some experts. They continue to fuel fear by repeating speculation that variants will evade vaccines. Don't buy it.*[56]

- **Dr. Lucy McBride, CNN, May 2021, "Doctor: The Secret Weapon for Ending the Pandemic":** *The real-world data on the Covid-19 vaccines is clear: they are stunningly effective. The vaccines essentially take death and severe disease off the table. They dramatically reduce the risks of getting Covid and transmitting the virus to other people. They are powerful weapons against all of the circulating variants. In short, they are the clear ticket to normality.*[57]

- **Drs. Tracy Beth Høeg, Lucy McBride, Vinay Prasad, and Monica Gandhi, *The Atlantic*, May 2021, "American Kids Can Wait":** *Allowing the export of doses would be not only effective vaccine diplomacy but also in Americans' own interest. Gaining better control of the disease across the globe would prevent or slow the emergence of worrisome viral variants.*[58]

- **Allison Krug, Drs. Tracy Beth Høeg, Lucy McBride, and Monica Gandhi, *The Washington Post*, May 2021, "It's Time for Children to Finally Get Back to Normal Life":** *This low risk for children nearly vanishes as cases plummet. As we saw in Israel and Britain, vaccinating adults indirectly protects children. The same trend is evident here in the United States: Adult vaccination has lowered covid-19 incidence among children by 50 percent in the past four weeks.*[59]

- **Dr. Marty Makary, MedPage Today, June 2021, "Think Twice Before Giving the COVID Vax to Healthy Kids":** *Given that the risk of a healthy child dying is between zero and infinitesimally rare, it's understandable that many parents are appropriately asking, why vaccinate healthy kids at all?*[60]

- **Drs. Jay Bhattacharya and Martin Kulldorff, *The Hill*, June 2021, "The Ill-Advised Push to Vaccinate the Young":** *The idea that everyone must be vaccinated against COVID-19 is as misguided as the anti-vax idea that no one should. The former is more dangerous for public health. The COVID-19 vaccines have been one of the few bright spots during this pandemic. While anyone can get infected, the old have a thousand-fold higher mortality risk than the young.*[61]

- **Mary Harris interview with Dr. Monica Gandhi, Slate, June 2021, "Why You Shouldn't Worry About the Delta Variant (if You're Vaccinated)":** *Children are not more susceptible to the delta variant, they're threefold less likely to get any infection with any variant with any ancestral strain, and they're half as likely to spread it.*[62]

- **Drs. Martin Kulldorff and Jay Bhattacharya, *The Wall Street Journal*, June 2021, "A Covid Commission Americans Can Trust":** *The pandemic is on its way out, but how many Americans think the U.S. approach succeeded? More than 600,000 Americans died from Covid, and lockdowns have left extensive collateral damage. Trust in science has eroded, and the damage won't be limited to epidemiology, virology and public health. Scientists in other fields will unfortunately also have to deal with the fallout, including oncologists, physicists,* computer scientists, environmental engineers and even economists.[63]

- **Drs. Tracy Beth Høeg, Monica Gandhi, and Daniel Johnson, *The New York Times*, June 2021, "We Must Fully Reopen Schools This Fall. Here's How":** *Since the pandemic began, Covid-19 has affected children less than adults, and the risk the disease poses to youths is diminishing as vaccinations increase. Children are about half as likely as adults to spread the coronavirus, and long Covid appears to be uncommon in children.*[64]

- **Dr. Marty Makary, *The Wall Street Journal*, June 2021, "The Power of Natural Immunity":** *The news about the U.S. Covid pandemic is even better than you've heard. Some 80% to 85% of American adults are immune to the virus: More than 64% have received at least one vaccine dose and, of those who haven't, roughly half have natural immunity from prior infection. There's ample scientific evidence that natural immunity is effective and durable, and public-health leaders should pay it heed.*[65]

- **Dr. Marty Makary, *The Wall Street Journal*, July 2021, "The Flimsy Evidence Behind the CDC's Push to Vaccinate Children":** *The agency overcounts Covid hospitalizations and deaths and won't consider if one shot is sufficient.*[66]

- **Dr. Monica Gandhi, *The Wall Street Journal*, July 2021, "The Reassuring Data on the Delta Variant":** *There's no sign of a surge in hospitalization or severe illness, and the vaccines remain extremely effective. You read the same alarming headlines every few months, now with Greek letters. As the virus that causes Covid-19 evolves and mutates, the same concerns pop up about whether the variant evades vaccines, makes people sicker than the old versions, and increases transmissibility. What we know about the Delta variant is reassuring.*[67]

- **Dr. John Mandrola, Medscape, July 2021, "Vaccine-In-**

duced **Myocarditis Concerns Demand Respect, Not Absolutism"**: *Calling myocarditis mild reminds me of the saying about minor surgery. Minor surgery is surgery on someone else; mild myocarditis is something that happens to other folks' kids. Humans have only one heart; inflaming it at a young age is not a small thing.*[68]

- **Dr. Monica Gandhi, *The Washington Post*, July 2021, "Yes, the Delta Variant is Taking Over. But the Vaccines Still Work"**: *Yes, the variant means there will be isolated outbreaks and some places will ask residents to put their masks back on. But we are moving in the right direction in the United States, and we should not let fear of the new variant discourage us.*[69]

- **Dr. Lucy McBride, *The Atlantic*, August 2021, "Fear of COVID-19 in Kids is Getting Ahead of the Data"**: *Shielding children from danger is a fundamental instinct. Tolerating risk for them is hard—but necessary—emotional work.*[70]

- **Dr. François Balloux, *The Guardian*, August 2021, "The Pandemic has Created a Market for Gloom and Doom"**: *Question: You've often stated that the pandemic will be over by mid to late 2021. Do you stand by this? Dr. Balloux: Depends on how you quantify it. I would say the pandemic is over when Covid-19 doesn't cause significantly more mortality than other respiratory viruses in circulation. This will happen first in places such as the UK that have been privileged to get vaccine coverage – I expect at the latest early next year.*[71]

- **Drs. Marty Makary and H. Cody Meissner, *The Wall Street Journal*, August 2021, "The Case Against Masks for Children"**: *It's abusive to force kids who struggle with them to sacrifice for the sake of unvaccinated adults.*[72]

- **Dr. Monica Gandhi, *The Washington Post*, September 2021, "We Won't Eradicate Covid. The Pandemic Will Still End"**: *In a matter of months, viral circulation in the United States could dwindle to levels so low we will no longer need to require masks, distancing, ventilation, asymptomatic testing or* *contact tracing.*[73]

- **Dr. Vinay Prasad,** *The Atlantic,* **September 2021, "The Downsides of Masking Young Students are Real":** *Scientists have an obligation to strive for honesty. And on the question of whether kids should wear masks in schools—particularly pre-schools and elementary schools—here is what I conclude: The potential educational harms of mandatory-masking policies are much more firmly established, at least at this point, than their possible benefits in stopping the spread of COVID-19 in schools.*[74]

- **Dr. Marty Makary,** *The Washington Post,* **September 2021, "Natural Immunity to Covid is Powerful. Policymakers Seem Afraid to Say So":** *It's okay to have an incorrect scientific hypothesis. But when new data proves it wrong, you have to adapt. Unfortunately, many elected leaders and public health officials have held on far too long to the hypothesis that natural immunity offers unreliable protection against covid-19 — a contention that is being rapidly debunked by science.*[75]

- **Dr. Monica Gandhi,** *The Atlantic,* **November 2021, The New COVID Drugs Are a Bigger Deal Than People Realize":** *These miraculous drugs arrived with minimal fanfare but represent the biggest advance yet in treating patients already infected with COVID-19.*[76]

- **Dr. Monica Gandhi,** *The Atlantic,* **November 2021, "It's Time to Contemplate the End of the Crisis":** *Americans should be asking ourselves what else needs to happen before we can declare an end to the crisis phase of the pandemic. Although the coronavirus's course remains unpredictable—and bad surprises are still possible—the Delta-variant surge that started in early July ushered in what may have been the final major wave of disease in the United States.*[77]

- **Drs. Monica Gandhi and Leslie Bienen,** *The New York Times,* **December 2021, "Why Hospitalizations Are Now a Better Indicator of Covid's Impact":** *America is in the slow*

*process of accepting that Covid-19 will become endemic —
meaning it will always be present in the population at varying
levels. But the United States has effective tools to deal with
that reality when it happens in the future.*[78]

- **Dr. Vinay Prasad, STAT News, December 2021, "At a Time
When the U.S. Needed Covid-19 Dialogue Between Scientists,
Francis Collins Moved to Shut it Down":** *This week,
emails released through a Freedom of Information Act request
filed by the American Institute for Economic Research revealed
what I see as worrisome communication between Francis Collins,
Anthony Fauci, and others within the National Institutes
of Health in the fall of 2020. At issue was the Great Barrington
Declaration, an open letter written in October 2020 and
eventually signed by thousands of scientists. It argues that
Covid-19 policy should focus on protecting the elderly and
vulnerable, and largely re-open society and school for others.*[79]

- **James Walsh interview with Dr. Monica Gandhi, Intelligencer,
December 2021, "The Cautious Case for Omicron
Optimism Dr. Monica Gandhi Says There's Reason to
Trust Preliminary Reports of Mild Illness":** *The final thing
I'll say is that adult vaccination protects children. We saw that
with the Delta variant in this country. In places with high adult
vaccination rates we didn't see so many cases for hospitalizations
and children. It could be that adult vaccination here is
going to protect children. There are still a lot of unknowns.*[80]

- **Dr. Vinay Prasad and Prof. Vladimir Kogan, Slate, January
2022, "COVID Testing of Asymptomatic Students
Doesn't Make Kids Safer":** *As long as omicron or a similarly
lethal strain is dominant, testing asymptomatic school-age
kids, a policy currently widely in use in many school districts,
is ineffective at best and damaging at worst.*[81]

- **Dr. Jay Bhattacharya and Tom Nicholson, *The Wall Street
Journal*, January 2022, "A Deceptive Covid Study, Unmasked":** *"Follow the science," we keep hearing, but some-*

times scientists and the media present findings in a misleading way.[82]

- **Drs. Lucy McBride, Scott Balsitis, Kristen Walsh, and Carol Vidal, *USA Today*, February 2022, "With Vaccines Available Mask Mandates Are Not Necessary in School":** *As scientists and physicians, we are concerned that COVID-19 mitigation measures for children are doing more harm than good.*[83]

- **Kara Grant about Dr. Lucy McBride, MedPage Today, March 2022, "Meet the Primary Care Doc Who Wants the World to Go Back to Normal":** *"I have taken this virus so seriously," she told MedPage Today.*[84]

- **Drs. Monica Gandhi and Aaron E. Carroll, *The New York Times*, March 2022 "The New Phase of the Pandemic is Covid Exhaustion; We're Over Covid. Are We Able to Move on From It for Good?":** *Well, yes, I think it's actually really important to change your views with new data. And things do need to update and change as new data comes in. […] So you must update with time. If you don't update with time, you will lose public health trust, especially over two years.*[85]

- **Dr. Jay Bhattacharya, *The Wall Street Journal*, June 2022, "The White House Keeps Stoking Covid Fears":** *Covid is 'a far greater threat to kids than the flu is,' Ashish Jha claims, citing a flawed study.*[86]

- **Dr. Jay Bhattacharya, *The Wall Street Journal*, September 2022, "The Mistakes Made Responding to Covid-19":** *It just looked like a horrible world ending kind of disease about to spread. And public health systems, public health officials basically panicked.*[87]

- **Dr. Marty Makary, *The Wall Street Journal*, December 2022, "The Exaggeration of Long Covid":** *Public-health officials have massively exaggerated long Covid to scare low-risk Americans as our government gives more than $1 billion* *to a long Covid medical-industrial complex.*[88]

- **Dr. Monica Gandhi, *San Francisco Chronicle*, January 2023, "COVID is Endemic. Here's How Monica Gandhi Says We Keep It That Way":** *On Sept. 18, President Biden famously said "the pandemic is over." He very quickly followed that up by saying: "We are doing a lot of work on it." These notions may sound contradictory, but they are indeed the way to approach the concept of endemicity; combating COVID-19 will take ongoing and hard work.*[89]

- **Dr. Marty Makary, *New York Post*, February 2023, "10 Myths Told by Covid Experts — And Now Debunked":** *In the final analysis, public health officials actively propagated misinformation that ruined lives and forever damaged public trust in the medical profession.*[90]

- **Dr. Jay Bhattacharya, *Newsweek*, May 2023, "It's Time for Laws Limiting the Power of Public Health Institutions":** *Contrary to what you hear these days from those making poor decisions throughout the pandemic, many of the errors were not honest mistakes. Public health embraced positions at odds with the scientific evidence throughout the pandemic, for instance, by pretending that immunity after COVID recovery does not exist, and by overstating the ability of the vaccine to stop COVID infection and transmission.*[91]

- **By Liz Highleyman about Dr. Monica Gandhi, Slate, September 2023, "What COVID's 'Wrongest Woman' Got Right":** *Gandhi's fundamental arguments about the virus have turned out to be sound.*[92]

- **Dr. Marty Makary, *New York Post*, September 2023, "Don't Believe the Feds' Fearmongering About Long Covid":** *In my experience of treating thousands of patients over two decades, people can be very forgiving if you are honest with them. If public-health officials want to regain the public trust, they should show more humility and less absolutism when it comes to the facts around long COVID.*[93]

- **Dr. Martin Kulldorff, *The Wall Street Journal*, March 2024,**

"Four Years Later: The Real Cost of Covid": *I think that you should never try to enforce something in public health. You have to maintain that trust. And public health has not a lot of trust.*[94]

These outlets also published many similar articles from many other writers. *The Wall Street Journal* published Mike Pence's "There Isn't a Coronavirus 'Second Wave'"[95] in June 2020, as well as overt pro-infection articles such as "Slow the Spread? Speeding It May Be Safer" by Vivek Ramaswamy and Dr. Apoorva Ramaswamy. It warned of the dire consequences of trying to stop COVID. It said:

> *Policies designed to slow the spread of Omicron may end up creating a supervariant that is more infectious, more virulent and more resistant to vaccines. That would be a man-made disaster.*[96]

This was not just an American problem. Karam Bales wrote an article about the UK that began by saying:

> *During the COVID Inquiry, Dr. Kevin Fong gave an emotional testimony detailing a [sic] the experience of frontline healthcare workers facing pressures equivalent to a "terrorist attack" every day.*[97]

Mr. Bales felt false declarations of herd immunity were partially to blame for that deadly second wave. He said:

> *After the majority of the media had spent the summer platforming claims the UK had acquired enough herd immunity to avoid a substantial second wave, as transmission increased at the end of summer many outlets promoted claims by Professor Carl Heneghan that increasing cases were an artefact of false positive PCR tests.*

Mr. Bales provided the following examples:

- 20 July, *Spectator*: "How Many Covid Diagnoses Are False Positives?"[98]

- 12 August, *Telegraph*: "The Statistical Quirk That Means the Coronavirus Pandemic May Never End – A Large Number of False Positives Will Creep in Once Case Numbers Drop Very Low and Testing Remains Very High"[99]
- 5 September, *Daily Mail*: "COVID Tests Could Be Picking Up Dead Virus Cells from Weeks' Old Infections And 'False Positives' Could Be Exaggerating the Scale of The Pandemic, Claims Study"[100]
- BBC Website: "Coronavirus: Tests Could Be Picking Up Dead Virus"[101]
- *The Sun*: "Coronavirus Tests Could Be Picking Up Dead Cells from Old Infections"[102]
- 6 September, *Daily Express:* "Thousands May Be in Pointless Lockdown as Major Flaw Found in Coronavirus Test"[103]
- 7 September, *Telegraph:* "Should We Be Worried About the Uptick In Covid Cases? Almost Certainly Not"[104]

These were all articles of doubt, and this wasn't limited to the print media. WWTI doctors deluged the public with these messages on podcasts, social media platforms, and TV.

The Medical Establishment Closes Ranks, and Patients Feel the Effects.
— *Pamela Paul*

Like WWTI doctors themselves, media outlets haven't looked back on their prior publications. Even though *The Washington Post* quoted Dr. Bhattacharya as saying, *"We should be treating covid as one of 200 diseases that affect people,"* reporters haven't called him back to ask him why he still talks about COVID all the time. Even though *The Wall Street Journal* published "We'll Have Herd Immunity by April" by Dr. Marty Makary, they haven't revisited that prediction. The journalists who asked

Dr. Gandhi about her thoughts on variants haven't published an updated interview with her about these predictions.

Of course, a journalist *could* write an article about how advocates of herd immunity through mass infection are having conferences at Stanford and Johns Hopkins. The fact that these universities promote doctors who cozy up to Robert F. Kennedy Jr. seems at least as important as a plagiarism scandal involving Harvard's president, which grabbed front-page headlines for days.

One *New York Times* columnist, Pamela Paul, wrote an article about Dr. Makary, titled "The Medical Establishment Closes Ranks, and Patients Feel the Effects." However, she did not discuss how the medical establishment was largely silent about Dr. Makary's failed predictions of herd immunity or how patients were hurt by anti-vaccine disinformation. She didn't mention the pandemic at all. Instead, Ms. Paul wrote:

> *This avoidable tragedy is one of several episodes of medical authorities sticking to erroneous positions despite countervailing evidence that Marty Makary, a surgeon and professor at Johns Hopkins School of Medicine, examines in his new book,* "Blind Spots: When Medicine Gets It Wrong, and What It Means for Our Health." *[…]*
>
> *While these mistakes are appalling, more worrisome are the enduring root causes of those errors. Medical journals and conferences regularly reject presentations and articles that overturn conventional wisdom, even when that wisdom is based on flimsy underlying data. For political or practical reasons consensus is often prized over dissenting opinions.*
>
> *"We're seeing science used as political propaganda," Makary told me when I spoke to him by phone. But, he argues, mistakes*

> *can't be freely corrected or updated unless researchers are en-*
> *couraged to pursue alternative research.*[105]

This is how mainstream media helped spread doubt, though Ms.
Paul chose to end her article in a way that reminded me of the *"we're all*
trying to find the guy who did this" meme. She said:

> *With trust in science on the wane, conspiracy theories and misin-*
> *formation proliferating and anti-vaxxers like Robert Kennedy Jr.*
> *setting a deranged example, this may not seem like the best time*
> *to criticize the medical profession.*

She did not mention that Dr. Makary, whom she effusively praised,
teamed up with Kennedy.

Unsurprisingly, the normalization of WWTI doctors in the mainstream press continued after the election. *The Wall Street Journal* published editorials titled "Jay Bhattacharya Can Bring Science Back to
NIH,"[106] "Jay Bhattacharya and the Vindication of the 'Fringe' Scientists,"[107] and "The Man Who Fought Fauci—and Won."[108] *The Atlantic*
published an article about Dr. Makary titled "The Health Official Who
Just Might Stand Up to RFK Jr."[109] that said he was "undoubtedly qualified for the job." *The Washington Post* published the editorial "The NIH
and FDA Nominees are Surprisingly Strong" by Dr. Leanna Wen, who
wrote:

> *Watching last week's confirmation hearings for Jay Bhattacharya*
> *and Marty Makary, President Donald Trump's nominees to lead*
> *the National Institutes of Health and the Food and Drug Admin-*
> *istration, respectively, I was struck by how normal the candidates*
> *were. Yes, I said normal — and qualified.*
> *Unlike their future boss, Health and Human Services Secretary*
> *Robert F. Kennedy Jr. — who in his own hearings struggled with*
> *basic questions about Medicaid and Medicare and refused to*

disavow anti-vaccine conspiracy theories — these candidates grounded their answers in facts and science. They were well versed in what their agencies did and had intriguing ideas for how to improve them.

Democrats shouldn't reflexively oppose these candidates. Bhattacharya and Makary can be allies to limit harm from Trump and Kennedy, and they might even reform biomedical innovation for the better.[110]

This is how the mainstream press is helping to erase the history of the pandemic and encourage apathy about the threat posed by medical disinformation.

The Free Press: Think For Yourself

WWTI doctors were celebrities in the right-wing media, such as Fox News, the Cato Institute, *The Washington Times*, and *The Epoch Times*. They were also the darlings of the "heterodox" media, where WWTI doctors blended their medical credentials and political opinions. Though these outlets claim to value diversity of viewpoints and independent thought, they all published the exact same doctors who said the exact same things while refusing to platform anyone who might correct their disinformation.

The Free Press advises its readers to "think for yourself" and describes itself by saying:

The Free Press is a new media company founded by Bari Weiss and built on the ideals that once were the bedrock of great journalism: honesty, doggedness, and fierce independence. We publish investigative stories and provocative commentary about the world as it actually is—with the quality once expected from the legacy press, but the fearlessness of the new.[111]

In reality, The Free Press published *"provocative commentary"* from the mirror world and thus prevented its readers from thinking at all. It produced content like this:

- **Dr. Jay Bhattacharya:** "The Government Censored Me and Other Scientists. We Fought Back—and Won"[112]
- **Dr. Jay Bhattacharya:** "Free Speech on Trial"[113]
- **Dr. Marty Makary:** "Dr. Fauci's Legacy"[114]
- **Drs. Tracy Høeg and Marty Makary:** "U.S. Public Health Agencies Aren't 'Following the Science'"[115]
- **Dr. Marty Makary:** "Officials Say, Universities' Covid Policies Defy Science and Reason"[116]
- **Drs. Vinay Prasad, Stefan Baral, Lucy McBride:** "Bringing Sanity to the Omicron Chaos, Talking to Three Doctors Who Have Been Islands of Reason in a Sea of Confusion"[117]
- **Dr. Vinay Prasad:** "Let Djokovic Play"[118]
- **Dr. Vinay Prasad:** "We Have a Tripledemic. Not of Disease, But of Fear"[119]
- **Drs. Vinay Prasad and John Mandrola:** "The Epidemic of #DiedSuddenly"[120]
- **Dr. Vinay Prasad:** "How to Save Science from Covid Politics"[121]
- **Dr. Vinay Prasad:** "What RFK Jr. Gets Right—and What He Gets Wrong"[122]
- **Dr. Vinay Prasad:** "Vinay Prasad: Why Was My Talk at a Medical Conference Canceled?"[123]
- **Dr. Vinay Prasad:** "Covid Vaccines Shouldn't Be 'Routine' for Kids"[124]

That last article spread obviously fake statistics, claiming that polio, which has killed zero American children in my entire life, was dangerous for children while COVID was not. Ms. Weiss, however, described this as *"the world as it actually is."*

After the election, The Free Press published an article titled "They Were Public Health Heretics. Now They Are America's Public Health Czars" that boasted of having published Drs. Vinay Prasad, Makary, and Bhattacharya since the inception of The Free Press, and said:

> They demanded transparency, reliable data, and common sense in policy making, instead of the fear-mongering, obfuscation, and draconian crackdowns on normal life that characterized the actions of our public health officials. For this, all three were variously disparaged and maligned. Their views were not only attacked, but suppressed by the government and social media.[125]

According to The Free Press, Drs. Prasad, Makary, and Bhattacharya were so "disparaged, maligned, attacked and suppressed," they were elevated to the pinnacle of American medicine.

UnHerd Is for People Who Dare to Think for Themselves

Like The Free Press, UnHerd, run by British journalist Freddie Sayers, also encourages people to "think for themselves." Their motto is:

> When the herd takes off in one direction, what do you do? Un-Herd is for people who dare to think for themselves.[126]

However, by platforming WWTI doctors, UnHerd prevented its audience from thinking at all. Here are some examples:

- **Dr. Jay Bhattacharya**: "Ron DeSantis was the Last Hope of a Covid Reckoning"[127]
- **Dr. Jay Bhattacharya**: "What I Discovered at Twitter HQ"[128]
- **Dr. Jay Bhattacharya**: "Boris Johnson Is Still in Denial About Lockdowns"[129]

- **Dr. Jay Bhattacharya:** "I Stand by the Great Barrington Declaration"[130]
- **Dr. Jay Bhattacharya:** "Study Into mRNA Vaccine Death Rates Sends 'Danger Signals'"[131]
- **Dr. Jay Bhattacharya:** "New Pfizer Data Kills the Case for Universal Child Covid Vaccines"[132]
- **Dr. Jay Bhattacharya:** "Why Have Scientists Stopped Taking Risks? There's a Reason Breakthroughs are Now So Rare"[133]
- **Dr. Martin Kulldorff:** "What Johan Giesecke Missed Out"[134]
- **Dr. Martin Kulldorff:** "Martin Kulldorff: Lessons from Sweden for the Next Pandemic"[135]
- **Dr. Martin Kulldorff:** "Lockdown Sceptic Forced Out of Harvard"[136]
- **Dr. Martin Kulldorff:** "Fired by Harvard for Getting Covid Right"[137]
- **Dr. Vinay Prasad:** "We Need to Talk About the Vaccines. Public Debate on Side-Effects Is Being Censored"[138]
- **Dr. Vinay Prasad:** "Don't Panic About Unvaccinated Kids. It's Time to Get Back to Normal"[139]
- **Allison Krug and Dr. Vinay Prasad:** "Should We Let Children Catch Omicron? Restrictions In Schools Must Never Return"[140]
- **Dr. Sunetra Gupta:** "Covid Experts: There Is Another Way. Three Eminent Epidemiologists Met in Massachusetts to Plan a Better Response to the Pandemic"[141]
- **Dr. Sunetra Gupta:** "Was I Wrong About the Covid Infection Fatality Rate?"[142]
- **Dr. Sunetra Gupta:** "Sunetra Gupta: Covid-19 Is on the Way Out. The Author of the Oxford Model Defends Her View That the Virus has Passed Through the UK's Population"[143]
- **Dr. Sunetra Gupta:** "Sunetra Gupta: Have My Covid Hypotheses Held Up?"[144]
- **Dr. Sunetra Gupta:** "Matt Hancock Is Wrong About Herd Immunity. Confusion About the Covid-19 Science is Hampering

Debate — and Costing Lives"[145]

That last article said:

> *The development of immunity through natural infection is a common feature of many pathogens, and it is reasonable to assume that Covid-19 does not have any tricks up its sleeve to prevent this from happening.*

Persuasion: Determined To Defend Free Speech and Free Inquiry Against All Its Enemies

Persuasion, run by former *The Atlantic* journalist Yasha Mounk, says it is "determined to defend free speech and free inquiry against all its enemies."[146] Of course, free inquiry requires accurate information, and *Persuasion* inhibited free inquiry by promoting the disinformation of several WWTI doctors. In July 2021, it published a conversation with "three public health professionals" titled "What We Got Wrong (and Right) About COVID-19."[147] It contained their usual familiar poor predictions and pro-infection rhetoric. Some excerpts are:

- **Dr. Monica Gandhi**: *I think that the public health emergency is over. And what that means is that hospitals are in no way overwhelmed. [...] Children under 14 years old are threefold less likely to get the virus than adults. If they get exposed, they are one-half as likely as adults to spread it. [...] When there are low case rates in your community, the risk of your unvaccinated child getting COVID-19 is very low, too. Population immunity means children are so much less likely to be exposed to the virus. There's a principle in infectious disease that if you avoid all infections, what's called your microbiome—your degree of diversity of how you respond to other pathogens—is decreased, and it's actually very important to have some exposure to mild pathogens. I personally want to get some colds. So*

> *I won't be wearing a mask unless someone makes me.*
> - **Dr. Stefan Baral**: *I agree that it is important, particularly youth with their developing immune systems, to be exposed to different pathogens when they're young and healthy. It's amazing that this idea has become controversial, but it has. I similarly am not going to wear a mask unless somebody forces me.*
> - **Dr. Vinay Prasad**: *I think the worst is over. [...] I hate to say it, but the moment Donald Trump said he was for schools reopening, I think a lot of people turned their brains off, and they opposed it totally to thwart him. And I think that is one of the worst things that has happened.*

The Delta variant peaked the next month, leading to record deaths in several states and spiking pediatric hospitalizations. The virus also forced schools to close, not just in Democratic states, but throughout the Deep South. However, according to Dr. Prasad, schools only closed because liberals "turned their brains off" to "thwart" Trump.

Mr. Mounk wasn't bothered by the disinformation he had previously shared with his readers. Rather than revisit these doctors' failed predictions, he published an interview in 2024 titled "Vinay Prasad on What Went Wrong With COVID," which quoted Dr. Prasad as saying:

> *Of course, in the United States, we used the power of the police state to enforce lockdowns. And that I think was a bad policy decision that was not in line with prior public health guidance. It was learned from a totalitarian regime.*[148]

At least some of the article commentators were able to think for themselves, with one person saying:

> *I can't understand why, when Prasad repeatedly said there was no justification to close schools because children were not endangered by the virus, Yascha did not point out the obvious fact that*

schools don't only have children; they have many adults: teachers, administrators, and other staff. This leads me to the conclusion that this is a fundamentally unserious conversation.[149]

Reason: Free Minds and Free Markets

Reason magazine is a libertarian magazine whose motto, according to their masthead, is "Free Minds and Free Markets." However, *Reason* inhibited free thinking by publishing disinformation from WWTI doctors. Some examples include:

- Anthony Fauci, the Man Who Thought He Was Science[150]
- Facing Fauci's Fury: Q&A With Dr. Jay Bhattacharya[151]
- Jay Bhattacharya On Covid, Social Media Censorship, And Trump Vs. Biden[152]
- Why Did Harvard Fire Martin Kulldorff?[153]
- Dr. Vinay Prasad: Stop Trusting the Public Health Establishment[154]
- How Politics Corrupted Science: Dr. Vinay Prasad On Covid[155]
- The CDC's Changing Vaccine Story (Vinay Prasad Analyzes Walensky Statements)[156]
- Dr. Vinay Prasad: The Vaccine Mandates Were Medically Unethical[157]
- Dr. Vinay Prasad: You're Right Not to Trust Public Health[158]

"Trust is justified based on how an organization or system performs," Dr. Prasad said in that last interview. "And the truth is, the entire public health apparatus failed."

Tablet: A Jewish Magazine About the World

Tablet magazine describes itself as "a Jewish magazine about the world."[159] However, in reality, it misinformed its readers about the world.

Some examples include:

- **Dr. Vinay Prasad:** "The Cult of Masked Schoolchildren: History Will Not Look Kindly on Our Evidence-Free Decision to Make Kids Suffer Most"[160]
- **Dr. Vinay Prasad:** "How the CDC Abandoned Science. Mass Youth Hospitalizations, COVID-Induced Diabetes, and Other Myths from the Brave New World of Science as Political Propaganda"[161]
- **Dr. Mary Makary:** "Was the COVID Vaccine Safe for Pregnant Women? The CDC Deferred to Big Pharma Instead of Waiting for Evidence. Now the Facts Are In."[162]
- **Dr. Jay Bhattacharya:** "How Stanford Failed the Academic Freedom Test: For America's New Clerisy, Scientific Debate is a Danger to be Suppressed"[163]
- **Drs. Jay Bhattacharya and Martin Kulldorff:** "The COVID Wars"[164]
- **By Clayton Fox, about Drs. Martin Kulldorff, Jay Bhattacharya, Marty Makary, Vinay Prasad, and Sunetra Gupta:** "The Dissidents"[165]
- **Drs. Leslie Bienen and Tracy Beth Høeg:** "The CDC Is Breaking Trust in Childhood Vaccination"[166]

Even though COVID killed and hospitalized more American children than all other vaccine-preventable diseases combined, that last article said:

> *With its unscientific push to vaccinate all infants and toddlers against COVID, the agency will harm vaccine uptake for more significant diseases.*

None of these outlets has ever looked back and reflected on how these articles aged. This is how the "heterodox" press, which claims to be about "free thinking" and "diversity of viewpoints," instead promoted groupthink and conformity while misinforming its readers and preventing them from thinking for themselves.

Chapter 13: The @NIH Will Never Restore Public Trust in Science Until It Comes Clean to The Public About Its Role in Supporting Research That Likely Caused the Pandemic

The Coronavirus Lab Leak Hypothesis is Damaging Science
— Dr. John Moore

I am not a virologist, and I lack expertise on the origins of SARS-CoV-2. As such, I give credence to people who have proven themselves credible in areas where I am knowledgeable, such as vaccines, and who let the evidence speak for itself rather than resorting to taunts and accusations. Similarly, I disregard advocates of herd immunity via mass infection and those who partner with them. Why should I trust someone speculating about the *origins* of a virus if they spread disinformation about the *consequences* of that virus, which is what matters most?

Obviously, the origin of SARS-CoV-2 matters. It's important to know the truth. From my reading, the most likely origin is an animal market. There is much precedent for this. As Dr. John Moore wrote in his article titled "The Coronavirus Lab-Leak Hypothesis is Damaging Science":

> *The zoonosis hypothesis is solidly evidence based. Viruses often spill over from animals to humans, although usually as dead-end events without the sustained human-to-human transmission that sparks a pandemic. Wildlife coronaviruses have long been poised to infect humans. An estimated 66,000 people are infected with SARS coronaviruses each year due to human-bat contact, almost all resulting in asymptomatic infections with little or no further transmission.*
>
> *That said, zoonotic transfer of three different coronaviruses (MERS-CoV, SARS-CoV-1, and SARS-CoV-2) from other animals*

to humans have resulted in epidemics or pandemics in the past
25 years. The 2002-2003 SARS-CoV-1 outbreak started in a Chi-
nese wet market. The influenza pandemic of 1918, which began
from an animal-human cross-over, most likely from a pig in the
U.S. heartland, killed an estimated 50 million people worldwide.[1]

Moreover, there is converging evidence from multiple angles that
SARS-CoV-2 emerged from an animal market. The epidemiological
evidence was published in an article titled "Huanan Seafood Wholesale
Market in Wuhan was the Early Epicenter of the Covid-19 Pandemic,"[2]
and the genetic evidence was published in an article titled "Genetic
Tracing of Market Wildlife and Viruses at the Epicenter of the Covid-19
Pandemic."[3] According to an article about this second paper:

> *"We are seeing the DNA and RNA ghosts of these animals in the*
> *environmental samples, and some are in stalls where [the Covid*
> *virus] was found too," says Prof Florence Débarre, of the French*
> *National Centre for Scientific Research.*
>
> *The results, published in the journal* Cell, *highlight a series of*
> *findings that come together to make their case.*
>
> *Prof Michael Worobey, of the University of Arizona, said: "Rath-*
> *er than being one small branch on this big bushy evolutionary*
> *tree, the market sequences are across all the branches of the*
> *tree, in a way that is consistent with the genetic diversity actually*
> *beginning at the market."*
>
> *He said this study, combined with other data – such as early cas-*
> *es and hospitalisations being linked to the market – all pointed to*
> *an animal origin of Covid. Prof Worobey said: "It's far beyond*
> *reasonable doubt that that* [sic] *this is how it happened", and*
> *that other explanations for the data required "really quite fanci-*
> *ful absurd scenarios."*

"I think there's been a lack of appreciation even up until now about how strong the evidence is."[4]

In contrast, a novel virus has never leaked from a lab, and all of the "evidence" in favor of the lab leak involves secret meetings, hidden funding, and altered documents. It all seems like cloak-and-dagger stuff from a Hollywood movie or a Robin Cook novel to me, not affirmative scientific evidence the virus leaked from a lab. However, many of these documents show that scientists who now reject the lab leak hypothesis were open to it initially. Like proper scientists, they started with an open mind and only rejected the lab leak hypothesis when the evidence pointed away from it. Dr. Anthony Fauci, for example, sent an email in February 2020 encouraging a colleague to convene a group of evolutionary biologists "as soon as possible" and report the findings to the "appropriate authorities" if they found evidence of a lab leak.[5] "It is inconceivable that anyone who reads this email could conclude that I was trying to cover up the possibility of a lab leak," Dr. Fauci said during one grilling in front of Congress.

Regardless, it seems wise to act as if SARS-CoV-2 came from both a lab *and* an animal market. It's absurd to worry about a new virus emerging from only one of these sources. Most people don't want a deadly virus to emerge, period, and ideally, anyone handling viruses in labs or animals in the wild will be very careful. Achieving this vital but challenging goal requires cooperation and good-faith engagement from multiple stakeholders, not performative vitriol and enmity.

I also don't think the origins of SARS-CoV-2 matter *that much*. If a video emerged of Dr. Fauci spreading SARS-CoV-2 from a lab in Wuhan in 2019, that doesn't mean it was a good idea to spread the virus once it arrived here, and it wouldn't affect a single word I've written about it.

Where SARS-CoV-2 came from says nothing about how we should have handled it, and it reveals nothing about the people it harmed. Only someone who never treated COVID patients would say the *origin* of the virus was its most important feature.

Many people take COVID seriously and argue for the lab leak hypothesis in good faith. This chapter is not about them. Rather, my aim here is to show how the lab leak hypothesis served a useful function for WWTI doctors. Many WWTI doctors and their supporters promoted it to *distract* from the virus's impact and to protect those who openly cheered its spread. Every moment spent discussing where SARS-CoV-2 came from was a moment not spent discussing how it hurt people or the doctors who spread disinformation about it.

The core function of the lab leak hypothesis was to spread anger and mistrust. It was an opportunity to blame public health officials for the entire pandemic and eventually justify funding cuts to virology research and the NIH. According to the article "The Harms of Promoting the Lab Leak Hypothesis for SARS-CoV-2 Origins Without Evidence":

> *Despite the absence of evidence for the escape of the virus from a lab, the lab leak hypothesis receives persistent attention in the media, often without acknowledgment of the more solid evidence supporting zoonotic emergence. This discourse has inappropriately led a large portion of the general public to believe that a pandemic virus arose from a Chinese lab. These unfounded assertions are dangerous. As discussed in detail below, they place unfounded blame and responsibility on individual scientists, which drives threats and attacks on virologists. It also stokes the flames of an anti-science, conspiracy-driven agenda, which targets science and scientists even beyond those investigating*

the origins of SARS-CoV-2. The inevitable outcome is an under-mining of the broader missions of science and public health and the misdirecting of resources and effort. The consequence is to leave the world more vulnerable to future pandemics, as well as current infectious disease threats.[6]

Examples of this abound. In one article, the sponsor of the Great Barrington Declaration (GBD), Jeffrey Tucker, concocted an elaborate evidence-free fantasy about the origins of the virus. He said:

First, in late 2019 and perhaps as early as October, higher-ups in the biodefense industry and perhaps people like Anthony Fauci and Jeremy Farrar of the UK became aware of a lab leak at a US-funded bioweapons lab in Wuhan. This is a place that does gain-of-function research to produce both the pathogen and the antidote, just like in the movies. It's gone on for decades in possibly hundreds of labs but this leak looked pretty bad, one with a fast-transmitting virus believed to be of high lethality.[7]

The next part of the plan, according to Mr. Tucker, was when "the antidote labeled a vaccine came into play."

This effort began in January too: the opportunity to deploy mRNA technology. It had been stuck in research for some 20 years but had never gained regulatory approval through conventional means. But with a pandemic declared, and the fix relabelled as a military countermeasure, the entire regulatory apparatus could be bypassed, along with all indemnifications pushed through and even taxpayer funding.

The people behind the lab disaster would become heroes instead of villains.

In Mr. Tucker's fevered imagination, the people who tried to contain the virus are responsible for the whole thing, and they are lying about it. If Dr. Fauci is lying to you about where the virus came from, can you *really* trust him when he tells you to get vaccinated?

Robert F. Kennedy Jr. presented a similar argument in his book, *The Wuhan Cover-Up: And the Terrifying Bioweapons Arms Race.* The book is described thusly on Amazon:

> *"Gain-of-function" experiments are often conducted to deliberately develop highly virulent, easily transmissible pathogens for the stated purpose of developing preemptive vaccines for animal viruses before they jump to humans. More insidious is the "dual use" nature of this research, specifically directed toward bioweapons development.*
>
> *The Wuhan Cover-Up pulls back the curtain on how the US government's increase in biosecurity spending after the 2001 terror attacks set in motion a plan to transform the National Institute of Allergy and Infectious Diseases (NIAID), under the direction of Dr. Anthony Fauci, into a de facto Defense Department agency. While Dr. Fauci zealously funded and pursued gain-of-function research, concern grew among some scientists and government officials about the potential for accidental or deliberate release of weaponized viruses from labs that might trigger worldwide pandemics. A moratorium was placed on this research, but true to form, Dr. Fauci found ways to continue unperturbed—outsourcing some of the most controversial experiments offshore to China and providing federal funding to Wuhan Institute of Virology's (WIV's) leading researchers for gain-of-function studies in partnership with the Chinese military and the Chinese Commu-*

nist Party.[8]

Kennedy believes the entire pandemic was staged, writing:

Everyone has now seen that pandemics are another way for the military, intelligence, and public health services to expand their budgets and their power. In 2020, public health, defense, and intelligence agencies weaponized a [Covid-19] pandemic, resulting in unprecedented profits to Big Pharma and the dramatic expansion of the security/surveillance state, including a systemic abandonment of constitutional rights—effectively a coup d'état against liberal democracy globally.

Several right-wing politicians, such as Senator Rand Paul (R-Ky.) and Representative Marjorie Taylor Greene (R-Ga.), have amplified this theory and used it to attack Dr. Fauci and other public health experts. Rep. Greene said:

The American people deserve to know Dr. Fauci's true role in the COVID-19 pandemic. How much did he know? How involved was he? Why does he not remember the work he did for President Trump or Joe Biden? It's time to investigate Dr. Fauci and the blood on his hands!![9]

Senator Paul said:

I sent a letter to the DOJ. The question is, will the DOJ Act? And frankly, if you were prosecuting this, what you would do is offer [David] *Morens possible immunity, if he'll testify to what Anthony Fauci was doing, since I believe Anthony Fauci was in charge of the entire conspiracy.*[10]

Elon Musk even tweeted, "My pronouns are Prosecute/Fauci."[11]

Kennedy also authored a book titled *The Real Anthony Fauci: Bill Gates, Big Pharma, and the Global War on Democracy and Public*

Health. Though it is from 2021, this book is currently an Amazon #1 bestseller with nearly 26,000 reviews.[12] David Burke wrote a meticulous rebuttal titled *In Defense of Fauci*. It has 1 review and is ranked #2,127,824 on the Amazon sales list.[13] Kennedy's ideas are not "fringe," unfortunately. They have become mainstream.

> **I think trust in science is down bc scientists were dishonest about the**
> **likelihood of lab leak.**
> *— Dr. Vinay Prasad*

Many WWTI doctors agreed that the first COVID infection—and only that first infection—mattered enormously. Doctors who spent the entire pandemic minimizing SARS-CoV-2 or actively encouraging its spread purported to be very *concerned* about its origins. For example, Dr. Jay Bhattacharya identified two core problems with SARS-CoV-2:

1.   *"It looks like it very likely was a lab leak."*[14]
2.   *"The central problem right now I think is the fear that people still feel about COVID."*[15]

Dr. Bhattacharya thought infection #1 was a catastrophe and tweeted about a "bombshell prediction supporting the lab leak theory."[16] However, once the virus arrived on our shores, Dr. Bhattacharya felt the *lack of infections* was the problem. He said that fear of COVID was "the central problem" in April 2021, just before the Delta wave hit.

This raises an obvious question: Why should anyone care about the origins of SARS-CoV-2 when they opposed all measures to contain it? The clear answer is that WWTI doctors saw yet another opportunity to spread anger and doubt about public health. In their telling, the same people who tried to limit SARS-CoV-2 were entirely responsible for it in the first place. In a YouTube interview, "Dr. Bhattacharya: Francis Collins

DESTROYED Scientists Who Favored Covid Lab-Leak Theory," Dr. Bhattacharya said:

> *He abused his power as head of the NIH to create an illusion of consensus that there was no lab leak, that the lockdowns were going to work, [and] that school closures were a good idea, when in fact, none of that was true.*
>
> *And I'll tell you one other thing about Francis Collins's behavior during the pandemic. That abusive power, I think, in part, was motivated by the fact that during the lead-up to the pandemic, Francis Collins authorized the conduct of dangerous gain-of-function research.*
>
> *The abusive power to suppress the idea of a lab leak looks, in retrospect, very much like a CYA kind of idea—to hide the fact that he had supported this research. He supported, he suppressed the lab leak idea.*
>
> *When in fact, it looks like it very likely was a lab leak. And I think it's finally, it's great to finally see some kind of transparency happening on this topic. Yeah, I mean, so you're talking about, you know, Francis Collins's behavior early on in the pandemic.*[14]

Dr. Bhattacharya repeated this message often on social media:

- *A main goal of the @NIH during the covid era was the reputational protection of Tony Fauci and Francis Collins against the accurate charges that they funded dangerous research that likely caused the pandemic and dangerous lockdowns and social distancing without evidence.*[17]
- *Yes, promising the end of all pandemics, Fauci championed dangerous scientific experiments. Given how poorly that turned out, it's not surprising the NIH is trying to hide.*[18]
- *Among the stakes of the lab leak debate is the legacy of Fauci, Collins, and Farrar. They supported dangerous research that*

> *likely caused devastation. They & their praetorian guard fight*
> *dirty to suppress the idea because they fear joining the ranks*
> *of history's great villains.*[19]

In another post, Dr. Bhattacharya said that only an admission of guilt from the NIH would restore public trust:

> *The @NIH will never restore public trust in science until it*
> *comes clean to the public about its role in supporting research*
> *that likely caused the pandemic, and it repudiates the practice of*
> *'devastating takedowns' by NIH leadership of dissident scien-*
> *tists.*[20]

Dr. Bhattacharya even repeated this during his first town hall as NIH director. "It's possible that the pandemic was caused by research conducted by human beings, and it is also possible that the NIH partly sponsored that research,"[21] he said. His primary argument was that the lab leak hypothesis was popular. "If you look at polls of the American people, that's what most people believe," he said, though, of course, he expended great effort to make that the case.

Dr. Bhattacharya also boasted of an executive order Trump signed limiting so-called "gain-of-function" research. Dr. Bhattacharya said this "will allow us to … de-risk our portfolio in a way that potentially could cause a pandemic, and we'll make the American people trust our research again." Appropriately, dozens of NIH employees walked out of the auditorium in protest.

Dr. Vinay Prasad similarly had a "story" to tell about Dr. Fauci and the origin of the pandemic. He said:

> *Here's, I think, my story. We have to think about what his men-*
> *tality was when this happened. So just now we know from a lot*
> *of leaked documents that he actually probably did worry that a*
> *lab leak was the culprit origin of the virus. He had been funding,*

through NIH grants, the EcoHealth Alliance, which was conducting gain-of-function research in Wuhan. I think he's worried that he's on the hook for this thing.[22]

Dr. Prasad also echoed these sentiments on social media:

- *To me it's obvious that the reason Fauci supported lockdown & school closure was a misguided attempt to atone for the fact he funded the work that led to the pandemic. No one acts more irrationally than the guilty. The house subcommittee has damning evidence.*[23]

- *Is Case western giving Fauci an ethics prize because he lied about mask efficacy (repeatedly), refused to discuss school closure with @DrJBhattacharya_and demonized him, used a private Gmail to circumvent FOIA, or perjured himself on gain of function research?*[24]

- *Most doctors I spoke with agree that accidental lab leak was the likely source of the pandemic and Fauci has lied, repeatedly to the American people PS. It is and he has.*[25]

- *I think trust in science is down bc scientists were dishonest about the likelihood of lab leak, the efficacy of Covid vaccines and the evidence to support school closure, lockdowns and masking young children. Trust in scientists should be down, rationally.*[26]

- *Lab leak might have been the source of the pandemic and subject to a coordinated cover up, leading to millions dead & massive obfuscation.*[27]

- *I think it is pretty clear that Vivek Murthy and others in government colluded to promote the false narrative on mask efficacy, hide vaccine myocarditis, vaccine breakthrough, lab leak etc. I hope the Supreme Court obliterates their censorious policies.*[28]

- *Any article about combating misinformation that argues Anthony Fauci is a truth teller is laughable He lied about mask efficacy, threshold of herd immunity, risk of lab leak, and many*

> other issues. He actively censored @DrJBhattacharya_and @MartinKulldorff.[29]

- *Many people fighting misinformation fought for wrong ideas Suppressed lab leak discussion Promoted cloth masks in toddlers Denied myocarditis in young men Fighting misinfo is mostly an online club for failed scientists Meanwhile real misinfo & bad policy grows.*[30]

- *Lab leak Masking School closure Lockdowns Vaccine policy Discussion on all these issues was censored and stiffled and next few years will see serious revisions of the narrative*[31]

- *Big Tech censored lab leak, natural immunity, myocarditis and didn't censor a huge amount of absolute garbage, lies, errors.*[32]

- *We repeatedly see on social media, censorship is misused. From banning Lab leak debate, to silencing early discussion of mRNA induced myocarditis, to preventing honesty about cloth masks, and silencing dissent for boosting the youth.*[33]

- *I agree with Elon and I think much of our misguided pandemic response was Fauci felt guilty and made erratic suggestions for how to help that lacked evidence, and he didn't foster evidence generation No one is worse at cleaning a wine spill than the person who spilt it.* – in response to a video interview of Elon Musk.[34]

Predictably, Dr. Marty Makary's article, "10 Myths Told by Covid Experts -- Now Debunked," argued for the lab leak hypothesis:

Misinformation #7: COVID originating from the Wuhan lab is a conspiracy theory

Google admitted to suppressing searches of "lab leak" during the pandemic. Dr. Francis Collins, head of the National Institutes of Health, claimed (and still does) he didn't believe the virus came from a lab.

Ultimately, overwhelming circumstantial evidence points to a lab leak origin — the same origin suggested to Dr. Anthony Fauci by two very prominent virologists in a January 2020 meeting he assembled at the beginning of the pandemic.

According to documents obtained by Bret Baier of Fox News, they told Fauci and Collins that the virus may have been manipulated and originated in the lab, but then suddenly changed their tune in public comments days after meeting with the NIH officials.

The virologists were later awarded nearly $9 million from Fauci's agency.[35]

Dr. Makary also spread his message of blame and doubt widely on social media:

- *New information out on the lab leak cover up. Emails show Dr. Fauci commissioned the famous Nature paper in Feb. 2020 to disprove Wuhan lab leak theory. Drs. Kristian Andersen & Robert Garry (co-authors of the puff piece in Nature) changed their tune after telling Dr. Fauci in Jan. 2020 that thought it may have come from the lab. The circumstantial evidence that it Covid came from the Wuhan lab is so overwhelming. The only reason there is not uniform consensus is that it's embarrassing that NIH was funding the lab.*[36]
- *New internal NIH documents: scientists believed in a lab leak/manipulated virus but then suddenly changed their views and then awarded millions in NIH funding. Everyone should watch this incredible report by the best journalist in the business.*[37]
- *Evergrande, a company with close ties to the Chinese Communist Party, donated $115M to Harvard Med Sch. Days after the donation, Harvard-linked experts (some who had proposed a lab leak origin) suddenly changed their position, condemning the lab leak idea*[38]
- *Pretty clear to me that Covid-19 came from a lab leak. WSJ reporting today that lab workers at the Wuhan Instit. of Virology*

became sick enough in Nov 2019 to seek hospital care. Keep in mind that doctors at that same hospital were detained by the police![39]

• *Dr. Redfield always thought it was a Wuhan lab leak origin. Dr. Fauci "cut him out of meetings when Redfield said the government needed to investigate whether the pandemic started from a lab accident in Wuhan, China."*[40]

• *The lab leak hypothesis is no longer a hypothesis, in my opinion, it is the default conclusion of the circumstantial evidence. My piece saluting China's physicians who sounded the alarm.*[41]

Dr. Makary repeated this conspiracy during his congressional testimony, saying:

The reason this is even an issue is that it's embarrassing we funded the lab. If we had not funded the lab, a hundred percent of Americans would say this is obvious, this is a no-brainer. The epicenter of the world is five miles from one of the only high-level virology labs in China. The doctors initially were arrested and forced to sign non-non-disclosure gag documents. The lab reports have been destroyed, they've not been turned over.

The sequences reported from the lab to the NIH database were deleted by a request from Chinese scientists that called over early on and said delete those sequences we put in the database. And two leading virologists, maybe the two top virologists in the United States, Dr. Michael Farzon from Scripps and Dr. Robert Gary from Tulane, told Dr. Fauci on his emergency call in January of 2020 when he was scrambling soon after learning that the NIH was funding the lab, they both said that it was likely from the lab. Both scientists changed their tunes days later in the media and then both scientists received nine million dollars subsequent in

funding from the NIH. It's a no -brainer that it from the lab. I
mean at this point it's impossible to acquire any more informa-
tion and if you did it would only be affirmative.[42]

This is how doctors who spent most of the pandemic trying to numb their audience to COVID also tried to infuriate them about its origin.

The first, second, third, and fifth signers of the letter provably are fraudsters.
— *Dr. Richard Ebright*

Unfortunately, this was just a small part of the bad-faith discourse surrounding the lab leak and few scientists behaved more abominably than Richard Ebright and Bryce Nickels. According to an article about them titled "'Lab-leak' Proponents at Rutgers Accused of Defaming and Intimidating COVID-19 Origin Researchers":

> *Fraudsters. Liars. Perjurers. Felons. Grifters. Stooges. Imbe-*
> *ciles. Murderers. When it comes to describing scientists whose*
> *peer-reviewed studies suggest the COVID-19 virus made a nat-*
> *ural jump from animals to humans, molecular biologist Richard*
> *Ebright and microbiologist Bryce Nickels have used some very*
> *harsh language. On X (formerly Twitter), where the two scien-*
> *tists from Rutgers University are a constant presence, they have*
> *even compared fellow researchers to Nazi war criminals and the*
> *genocidal Cambodian dictator Pol Pot.*[43]

A dozen scientists filed a formal complaint with Rutgers,[44] noting that "several of the people Drs. Ebright and Nickels interact with have made direct threats of death and sexual violence" towards the scientists Drs. Ebright and Nickels harassed. Even though public health officials have needed bodyguards,[45] Professor Ebright responded to their pleas to protect their safety with more immature insults:

> *The first, second, third, and fifth signers of the letter provably are*
> *fraudsters; the first and third signers provably are perjurers; and*
> *all signers provably are coauthors of fraudsters and perjurers.*[43]

Dr. Ebright wasn't just blowing off steam online. He celebrated the election of Trump by fantasizing that prominent scientists might go to jail:

> *Very bad night for unindicted felon Fauci... who now is on a fast*
> *track to becoming indicted and convicted felon... Fauci... His*
> *protection from prosecution has... depended on the... DoJ and*
> *the White House. Which now will be in different hands.*[46]

Bhattacharya, Gupta, and Kulldorff are not merely wrong. They are charlatans and quacks who are dispensing deadly advice, and who need to be held accountable for their role in hundreds of thousands of preventable deaths.

— Dr. Richard Ebright

Dr. Ebright also had strong—and more reasonable—feelings when the GBD first proposed their plan to get rid of the virus by spreading the virus in October 2020. At the time, he said:

> *Bhattacharya, Gupta, and Kulldorff are not merely wrong. They*
> *are charlatans and quacks who are dispensing deadly advice,*
> *and who need to be held accountable for their role in hundreds of*
> *thousands of preventable deaths.*[47]

I've never produced such pugnacious prose.

Dr. Ebright laid out his preferred approach at the time, and it could not have been more diametrically opposed to the GBD. Dr. Ebright said:

> *Testing, tracing, quarantine of contacts, isolation of cases, partial lockdown and distancing at all times, full lockdown when transmission is high, masks, and, decisively, when available, vaccines.*[48]

Drs. Nickels and Ebright later founded the organization Biosafety Now, which describes itself by saying:

> *Biosafety Now is a US-based NGO working for a future where scientific research on pathogens supports human life without also threatening it & public trust in science is restored. Biosafety Now believes that research that creates new, non-natural potential pandemic pathogens poses existential risks to humanity and provides few, if any, benefits for science, medicine, public health, or national security. We are convinced that public health and safety require that all such research be subject to independent external controls, rather than be trusted to the oversight of the scientists performing or the organizations funding the research.*[49]

They say elsewhere on the website:

> *The rapidly increasing power and rapidly decreasing cost of advanced biotechnology has made lab-generated pandemics a threat to the survival of the human species.*

Biosafety Now feels the threat is real and the stakes couldn't be higher. Fair enough.

Despite this, it's not clear this organization can point to any real-world example where they *actually* improved biosafety and, as a result, made the world a safer place. They do, however, solicit donations[50] and sell merch.[51]

One of their products is called the Innocent Wildlife Collection. According to Biosafety Now:

> *The Innocent Wildlife collection highlight animals implicated by scientists as the "intermediate host animal" from which SARS-CoV-2 may have entered humans. It also includes some animals that have not yet been accused but are concerned they may be blamed in the future. Although it is theoretically possible that one of these "innocent" animals served as the intermediate host, the evidence provided so far to support these claims is not convincing.*[52]

Members of the Innocent Wildlife Collection include Pete the Pangolin, Sid the Sloth, Alastair the Raccoon Dog, Adeline the Raccoon Dog, Cindy the Civet, and Axel the Raccoon Dog.

The organization that worries non-natural potential pandemic pathogens might obliterate humanity feels *very differently* about natural potential pandemic pathogens. One is the gravest threat imaginable, while the other is an opportunity to make jokes and push products.

In 2024, Biosafety Now welcomed Dr. Makary to their advisory board. They said:

> *Dr. Makary is a surgeon & public policy researcher at Johns Hopkins University, member of the National Academy of Medicine, & author of 3 NYT bestselling books, including his new book "Blind Spots."*[53]

They did not mention that he had also authored the article "We'll Have Herd Immunity by April"[54] in 2021.

Biosafety Now also named Dr. Bhattacharya to its board of directors, and Dr. Nickels teamed up with Dr. Bhattacharya to complain that people hurt their feelings. In an article titled "The Scientific Establishment Is Turning 'Science' Into a Dogmatic Tool of Oppression," they wrote:

The COVID era has been difficult for scientists whose ideas run against the grain of powerful scientific and government bureaucracies. Even for university scientists with unblemished reputations in the before times, the price of speaking up has been vilification by social media companies, the media, and, unfortunately, even scientific journals and our fellow scientists. It is a wonder that any scientists dared to speak out, with only their commitment to the truth as a reason to do so.[55]

A "biosafety" organization partnering with Dr. Bhattacharya to guard against viruses is like a zebra teaming up with a lion to promote vegetarianism. However, Dr. Ebright explained his willingness to abandon his principles and partner with a "charlatan and quack" by saying:

My views on the @gbdeclaration have not changed, but my views on Bhattacharya have changed.[56] His advice was wrong. Dead wrong. But it now is 2024 (not 2020), and the discussion at hand is how to prevent a next lab-generated pandemic (not how to respond to the last one).[57] I will work with any person from any party and any background to prevent a next lab-generated pandemic. The importance and urgency of the objective over-ride partisan differences and ideological differences (as should be clear to any rational person).[58]

Of course, Dr. Bhattacharya's critics don't have partisan differences and ideological differences with him. Rather, Dr. Bhattacharya's critics believe his *repeated* factual errors and farcical forecasts led to unnecessary suffering. They feel his plan of herd immunity through mass infection was both a moral abomination and a total failure, as Professor Ebright wisely recognized it would be in his unflinching statement from 2020.

However, in Dr. Ebright's telling, 2020 is ancient history with no relevance to today. Dr. Ebright implied that, while it's vital to care about the first COVID infection, we should be indifferent to the billions of infections after that. He feels it's inappropriate to remember the "charlatans and quacks" who spread "deadly advice," even though the cost was "hundreds of thousands of preventable deaths," as Dr. Ebright put it in October 2020. Although Dr. Bhattacharya is a health economist who has no expertise in how to make lab research safer, Dr. Ebright generously awarded him a "do-over" button and furiously demanded that others honor his gift. Dr. Ebright unilaterally declared, *The discussion at hand is how to prevent a next lab-generated pandemic (not how to respond to the last one)*," and he expects everyone else to just fall in line.

In dismissing COVID as yesterday's news, Dr. Ebright is joining the deliberate COVID amnesia project and saying that headlines such as "The Delta Variant Is 'Ripping Through the Unvaccinated' and Crowding Hospitals in Florida, Texas"[59] no longer matter.

Why would he do this? Because if that headline still matters, then Dr. Bhattacharya's COVID disinformation still matters, and Biosafety Now would be an organization that promotes dangerous "charlatans and quacks." Of course, that headline still matters, Dr. Bhattacharya's COVID disinformation still matters, and Biosafety Now is an organization that promotes dangerous "charlatans and quacks."

Moreover, Dr. Bhattacharya didn't abruptly stop spreading disinformation in 2020 as Dr. Ebright implied. Dr. Bhattacharya is still spreading COVID disinformation in 2025. Pick a random article of his, and he will say some version of "the pandemic is on its way out."[60] He started saying this in March 2020[61] and has never stopped. Dr. Bhattacharya's *past* COVID disinformation was not a deal-breaker for Dr. Ebright, and Dr.

Bhattacharya's *current* COVID disinformation isn't a deal-breaker either. According to the leaders at Biosafety Now, nothing Dr. Bhattacharya said or ever will say about an *actual* pandemic matters at all.

Although COVID is still killing and injuring people every day, Dr. Ebright claims that to prevent an actual pandemic, we are all *required* to forget the last pandemic. Dr. Ebright believes that anyone who still cares about COVID is impairing his work somehow and that the vital task of biosafety *requires* Dr. Bhattacharya be shielded from criticism, despite the fact that he tried to spread a virus during an *actual* pandemic.

As with doctors who treat *theoretical* harms from the vaccine with more seriousness than *actual* harms from COVID, Drs. Nickels and Ebright make a grand public display of being very concerned about a *hypothetical* non-natural pandemic pathogen while simultaneously encouraging apathy about natural pandemic pathogens and the *current* pandemic pathogen. Indeed, it's not 2020 anymore, but COVID is still killing thousands of Americans every month, though Professors Nickels' and Ebright's partnership with Dr. Bhattacharya reveals these *actual* deaths don't concern them. They've moved on and are only bothered by anyone who still cares about COVID's current impact.

Although Dr. Ebright feels that doctors who spread disinformation about SARS-CoV-2 should be forgiven and revered, he feels that doctors who experienced and *can't forget* the consequences SARS-CoV-2 deserve childish schoolyard taunts. Dr. Ebright, who never treated COVID patients, is done with 2020, and he feels that people who witnessed mass death that year should just get over it already.

This is not the only time advocates of the lab leak hypothesis have teamed up with advocates of herd immunity through mass infection. In 2021, one of the leading advocates of the lab leak, molecular biologist

Dr. Alina Chan, teamed up with Matt Ridley to write a book titled *Viral: The Search for the Origin of COVID-19*.[62] Mr. Ridley, a libertarian with ties to the coal industry, had previously authored articles such as "Whatever Happened to Global Warming?"[63] During the pandemic, Mr. Ridley promoted the GBD on social media, and the month it was published, he authored an article, "Students Who Catch Covid May be Saving Lives," that said:

> *It is counterintuitive but the current spread of Covid may on balance be the least worst thing that could happen now. In the absence of a vaccine, and with no real prospect of eradicating the disease, the virus spreading among younger people, mostly without hitting the vulnerable, is creating immunity that will eventually slow the epidemic. The second wave is real, but it is not like the first. It would be a mistake to tackle it with compulsory lockdowns (even if called 'circuit breakers'), whether national or local. The cure would be worse than the disease. If you cannot extinguish an epidemic at the start, the best strategy is for the healthy to get infected first.*[64]

Mr. Ridley, who wanted to infect unvaccinated children and have them theoretically serve as human shields for more vulnerable adults, is also a member of Biosafety Now.[65] In October 2021, the year after he published his pro-infection article, the headlines read, "Children Drive Britain's Longest-Running Covid Surge."[66]

> **We're gonna lock down again with the next pandemic, guaranteed.**
> **— *Dr. Bhattacharya***

Dr. Bhattacharya also benefits from his partnership with Biosafety

Now. It allows him to portray himself as someone who is *very concerned* about protecting humanity from dangerous viruses.

All of this will impair our ability to handle a future pandemic. When the next virus arrives, whether from a lab or animal, WWTI doctors will invariably spread disinformation about it and resist efforts to contain it. They are open about this. In an interview from 2023, Dr. Bhattacharya had this exchange:

> **QUESTION:** *All right, a few final questions, Jay. Holman Jenkins in "The Wall Street Journal," quote: "The world inevitably will face new respiratory viruses. There seems to be no good reason nature would afflict us with a disease that spreads as easily as the flu or COVID and is significantly more deadly, but neither can that be ruled out." Are we ready for the next pandemic?*
>
> **Dr. Bhattacharya:** *We're gonna lock down again with the next pandemic, guaranteed. If the current configuration of power in public health and politics stands, we will respond by saying, "Look, the lockdown's the only way," and just as happened in 2020, it'll be the laptop class that'll benefit, and the poor and the vulnerable and children who will be harmed.*[67]

Unfortunately, WWTI doctors have unearned legitimacy because seemingly credible organizations with catchy names, like Biosafety Now, vouched for them and deluged their critics with threats and juvenile insults. When Dr. Bhattacharya histrionically claims that mitigation measures were an epic catastrophe and that vaccines for young people were a tragic mistake,[67] more people will trust him thanks to Biosafety Now's stamp of approval.

Thanks to his ceaseless efforts, we are significantly less prepared to handle a pandemic than we were in 2020. If a devastating pandemic pathogen were to escape from a lab, which is a real and immediate danger according to Biosafety Now, public health officials would need drastic measures and buy-in from the public to contain it. Yet, anyone who seeks to enact the mitigation measures Dr. Ebright championed in 2020 will have a much harder time doing so thanks to Dr. Bhattacharya and other WWTI doctors. If COVID-29 arrives, there's no way the public will adhere to mitigation measures as they did in 2020.

By legitimizing Dr. Bhattacharya, Biosafety Now is ensuring we are much less prepared to fight a future pandemic, as well as existing viruses such as COVID and measles. An organization that is supposedly dedicated to protecting us from deadly viruses is making us *much more* vulnerable to them. Either they don't know this, or they don't care.

To again quote from the article "The Harms of Promoting the Lab Leak Hypothesis for SARS-CoV-2 Origins Without Evidence":

> *The lab leak narrative fuels mistrust in science and public health infrastructures. Scientists and public health professionals stand between us and pandemic pathogens; these individuals are essential for anticipating, discovering, and mitigating future pandemic threats. Yet, scientists and public health professionals have been harmed and their institutions have been damaged by the skewed public and political opinions stirred by continued promotion of the lab leak hypothesis in the absence of evidence. Anti-science movements are not new. However, anti-science has become more virulent and widespread in the internet and social media age. Rejecting evidence derived from independent and controlled studies grounded in the scientific method, while embracing spectacular and unevidenced claims, leaves us in a dangerous position for confronting future threats. If these narratives are left unchecked,*

we become a society that dismisses and vilifies those with exper-tise and experience relevant to the challenges we face. We then base decisions affecting large populations worldwide on specula-tion or chosen beliefs that have no grounding in evidence-based science.[6]

The lab leak hypothesis doesn't just fuel "mistrust in science and public health infrastructures." For WWTI doctors and their supporters, that was the entire point.

Chapter 14: Ultimately, They Failed Us, and We are Left Without Answers and Policies That Caused Significant Harm

A one size fits all maxim about public health is the real problem.
— Dr. Vinay Prasad

Randomized-controlled trials (RCTs) are the gold standard in medicine for their ability to minimize bias. They are truly a remarkable achievement that has greatly benefited humanity. I firmly believe that every intervention that can be studied via RCT should be, and there should have been more of them during the pandemic. My dedication to RCTs is so strong I participated in a COVID vaccine RCT. My contribution was small, but real, and as far as I know, it exceeded any contribution by any WWTI doctor to an actual RCT.

In a fantasy world with unlimited resources, but without ethics, an RCT would yield the optimal answer for nearly all medical questions. However, in the real world, significant practical and ethical limitations prevent us from studying everything via RCTs. Having an idea for an RCT is infinitely easier than actually *doing* an RCT, and every day doctors make countless decisions without the benefit of an RCT to guide our every action. That's a normal part of medicine. As Dr. Vinay Prasad posted in March 2020:

> *For vaccines, the profession has accepted Ab (antibody) titers. For seatbelts in cars, we accept pathophys (pathophysiology) and time trends. But for cancer screening, because of how it works, we need RCTs for all cause mortality. A one size fits all maxim about public health is the real problem.*[1]

He was right. Here is why Dr. Prasad said that at the start of the pandemic:

- The safety of the subjects in RCTs is paramount, as it should be, given the history of Nazi atrocities and the Tuskegee Study.[2] Basic ethics and Institutional Review Boards (IRBs)[3] strictly limit what can be studied via an RCT. RCTs can only be used to study interventions that have a reasonable chance of benefiting patients or when there is true uncertainty about which treatment is better, which is termed *clinical equipoise*.[4] There has never been or will be an RCT showing that smoking harms or that parachutes help.[5] Having said this, there are many fewer "parachutes" in medicine than we often believe. Medicine is full of treatments that everyone "knew" worked until they were found to be useless in an RCT.

- Only the largest RCTs can reliably detect rare treatment harms or benefits. The rarer the event, the larger a study must be to detect it, something termed a study's power.[6] Generally, rare events can only be detected once the studied treatment has been given to large numbers of people outside an RCT. Real-world studies have taught us much more about rare vaccine harms and benefits than the RCTs.

- RCTs are hard to do for rare diseases, as enrolling enough patients is challenging.

- RCTs are of relatively short duration. Any treatment harm or benefit that occurs many years later is unlikely to be detected via an RCT.

- RCTs are slow. A doctor who has an idea for an RCT can't just start one the next day. It takes time to design the trial, to get funding, to have it evaluated and approved by an Institutional Review Board (IRB), to set up the infrastructure, to enroll patients, to run the study, and to synthesize the data. Most RCTs take many years from the time they are conceived to when the final data changes clinical care,[7] which is obviously problematic when a virus arrives like a tornado, demanding that actions be taken without evidence from RCTs. The COVID vaccine trials had several unique features, including the rapid spread of

COVID, that allowed them to proceed faster than most RCTs.

- RCTs are expensive,[8] and funding can be hard to come by, especially for studies where no one can profit based on the outcome. The COVID vaccine trials were unique in that full funding was immediately available.[9]

- An RCT can sound perfect right up until the moment you actually have to enroll patients in it. Those of us who have done this know that recruitment can be very difficult. While some patients are eager to participate in clinical trials, many people don't want to be a "guinea pig." A normally hard process is much harder in a pandemic. One researcher, who has actual experience running an RCT during this pandemic, said:

> *I think of what my clinical research team went through to enroll people in that trial, and I thought my nurses were going to die. One of them got covid and got sick. Imagine trying to do that on a daily basis, multiple patients, some of them facing intubation, none of them have their families. Patients or their families have to be able to give informed consent, which can be impossible for delirious, intubated COVID patients and their distraught families.[10]*

Another researcher said:

> *There was one day our system had 84 deaths. And then you're going to ask me to potentially put them on a placebo? It's just really heart wrenching, talking with families, if your patients are able to communicate—and you're dealing with all these deaths.*

- RCTs require an enormous infrastructure and multiple experts with different skills. Most RCTs occur at multiple locations, and teams have to be in place at every site. One of the mRNA vaccine trials occurred at 152 sites worldwide.[11] The vaccines weren't just a scientific triumph; the RCTs were also a logistical marvel. To get a sense of how complicated RCTs are, one article listed the following costs:

regulatory affairs, site identification and selection, site contracting and payments, site initiation and activation, site management, onsite monitoring, drug safety management, drug logistics, biological sample logistics, clinical supplies logistics, medical writing, site close-out, project management, study files/ document management, data management, statistics, quality control, communication with central CRO/ sponsor, and pass-through costs, which includes, trial insurance policies for each country, shipping: physical files to sites, site contracts, and tumor/blood samples, blood tubes and shipping packages, office supplies: files, paper, and printing, payments to sites per enrolled patient (to cover clinical procedures and laboratory tests), publication fees, ethics committee evaluation fees, site contract fees, regulatory authority evaluation fees, travel costs for selection, initiation, routine monitoring, and close-out visits, central pathology and radiology reviews, translational/ biomarker studies, coordinating investigators, drug manufacturing and testing, drug distribution services, EDC license and service fees, web tools (imaging platforms, eTMF), document translations, and data and Safety Monitoring Board (DSMB).[8]

- Given their complexity, RCTs don't always go smoothly. Serious problems can sometimes arise, and small hiccups are more common than not. Vaccine trials, in particular, have to be close to flawless. Those who enjoy spreading fear about vaccines will magnify the *slightest* imperfection to cast doubt on the whole project. This happened with the original COVID vaccine RCTs,[12] much to the delight of anti-vaxxers. A rushed or sloppy RCT would do much more harm than good.
- RCTs, including vaccine RCTs, commonly exclude key segments of the population, such as pregnant women or immu-

nocompromised patients. Therefore, researchers use other study designs to evaluate the vaccine in these populations. The exclusion of pregnant women from most RCTs is a source of controversy.

- RCT participants, who have to be savvy enough to learn about the trial in the first place, may not be representative of the general population. They are generally healthy and motivated enough to travel back and forth to the study site on a regular basis. The most vulnerable people, those who benefit from the booster the most, would likely be underrepresented in an RCT, thus skewing the results. Racial and ethnic minorities have also been underrepresented in clinical trials.

- An RCT done in one area may not generalize to another area. For example, an RCT of masks in Bangladesh relied on "role-modeling by community leaders." Its results would not be applicable to areas where community leaders oppose masks.

- Unlike any other condition in medicine, the disease being studied changes rapidly during a pandemic. The original vaccine RCTs were done with a variant that is now long gone. Does anyone believe these RCTs, where the vaccine was 95% effective at stopping COVID, have any relevance to our individual and policy choices today? Of course not. These RCTs rapidly became historical relics, and we've learned much more about the vaccines through real-world studies. An RCT of other interventions that was initiated at the pandemic's onset would likely be obsolete due to the more contagious variants that are circulating today.

Given these challenges, it's no surprise that many RCTs fail along the way. The NIH closed a proposed RCT of hydroxychloroquine and azithromycin after enrolling just 20 patients, or 1% of their goal.[13] I'm sure that study looked great on paper. Storage boxes are full of dead RCTs, and there's research into why trials fail. The vaccine trials were unique in that boatloads of volunteers, like me, beat down the door to enter them.

For these reasons, researchers use different types of observational studies to investigate topics that are difficult or impossible to study via an RCT. Though they aren't as rigorous as RCTs, observational studies can provide invaluable information about vaccines/medicines once they've been released in the real world. Because they don't select patients randomly, however, they have greater potential for spurious associations due to random chance and confounding variables. Researchers try to control for these biases, and they acknowledge these limitations in their papers. While these limitations are often magnified out of proportion by those who wish to cast doubt on the validity of studies whose results they don't like, there are *a lot* of really bad observational studies out there.

Randomized trials could have turned political fights into scientific questions. Not running them was a huge failure.
— Dr. Vinay Prasad

While everyone agrees that RCTs are the gold standard, the fact that many things can't be studied via an RCT makes them useful for anyone who wants to create doubt. Those who claim RCTs and *only* RCTs can provide reliable information are guilty of methodolatry, a favorite technique of anti-vaxxers that is currently being used by WWTI doctors to drastically restrict COVID vaccines, including for healthy 64-year-olds and pregnant people.

Disingenuous anti-vaxxers often pretend they would embrace vaccines *only* *if* there were an RCT of the entire vaccine schedule lasting the entire human lifespan measuring every possible health outcome. Obviously, that study will never be done, which is the entire point. Anti-vaxxers just want to spread doubt. For example, prior to the pandemic, anti-vaccine cardiologist Dr. Jack Wolfson said, "To all the pediatricians in the world, please show me the study that found 69 doses of 16 vaccines do not cause cancer, auto-immune disease, and brain injury."[14]

Predictably, anti-vaxxers reject the validity of existing RCTs, which show that vaccines are mostly safe and effective. For example, they often point out there is no RCT showing that the HPV vaccine prevents cancer. This is true. The RCTs of the HPV vaccine used a surrogate endpoint, cervical intraepithelial neoplasia, which can be a cancer precursor.[15] As HPV-related cancers take many years to develop, this outcome would not be possible to study in the time frame of an RCT, nor would it be ethical to let people remain in the placebo group once evidence emerged of the vaccine's safety and efficacy.

Not everyone agrees. An article titled "Will HPV Vaccination Prevent Cervical Cancer?" reviewed the RCTs of the HPV vaccine. It noted that "None of the trials were designed to determine efficacy or effectiveness against cervical cancer. There were no reported cases of cervical cancer in any trials."[16] As such, the authors felt that:

> It is still uncertain whether HPV vaccination prevents cervical cancer as trials were not designed to detect this outcome, which takes decades to develop. […] There are too few data to clearly conclude that HPV vaccine prevents cervical intraepithelial neoplasia grade 3.

The rebuttal to this piece was "Evidence of HPV Vaccination Efficacy Comes from More Than Clinical Trials." It discussed "the huge amount of non-trial research evidence that enables most scientists to conclude that HPV vaccination will prevent most cervical cancers."[17]

These scientists were right. It was never a great leap to surmise that if a vaccine prevents HPV infections and a cancer precursor, it would also eventually be shown to prevent HPV-related cancers. Unsurprising-ly, there is now clear evidence from massive observational studies from multiple countries showing the HPV vaccine is very effective at prevent-ing cervical cancer.[18] Those who reject this evidence because it was not obtained from an RCT are guilty of methodolatry. Countless people are spared HPV-related cancers because we used the HPV vaccine without RCT-level evidence that it prevented cancer.

> **My philosophy is RCT or STFU.**
> — *Dr. Vinay Prasad*

During the pandemic, WWTI doctors weaponized RCTs to spread fear and doubt. They wanted the public to think that we shouldn't do *anything* until we knew *everything*. The formula was mind-numbingly simple:

- I don't like mitigation measure X.
- Mitigation measure X was not studied via an RCT.
- If it was studied via an RCT (e.g., pediatric vaccines, the first booster), that RCT was too small or is now out of date.
- Therefore, we should not do mitigation measure X.

Despite writing on the limitations of RCTs prior to the pandemic, few doctors used methodolatry to spread doubt more than Dr. Prasad, who said, "My philosophy is RCT or STFU."[19] He did not STFU, even though he had not worked on any RCTs himself. Instead, he created long lists of unwanted mitigation measures. claiming they were useless because *other doctors* hadn't demonstrated their value in massive RCTs. One typical social media post read:

In the decades to come post COVID, the greatest failure will be a failure to generate better data. It is forgivable to be ignorant in March 2020, but we failed:

Zero randomized trials of school closure

Zero randomized trials business closures

Zero randomized trials on masking in schools

Zero randomized trials on masking kids

Zero randomized trials on masking in USA

Zero randomized trials of 3 vs 6 ft Zero randomized trials of cohorting

Zero randomized trials of installing HEPA filters

Zero randomized trials of masking, post vaccine

Zero randomized trials testing alternative dosing strategies of vax (post phase 3)

Zero randomized trials of whatever foolishness we are doing on college campuses

Zero randomized trials of asymptomatic testing

Zero randomized trials of quarantine duration

Zero randomized trials of testing for preschool/ school

Zero randomized trials of plexiglass

Zero randomized trials of wearing your mask from the door to table, and table to bathroom, but at no other points during your restaurant experience

Yet many of these things were wrongfully called parachutes by at least some people who should know better. Leaving a pandemic as ignorant as we entered is awful It is also why all of these issues have become political and not scientific Science should be ashamed of itself In 100 years we will look as primitive as the folks who survived the plagues of the middle ages[20]

Dr. Prasad portrayed the failure to do these RCTs as a choice. In one video, he rages against people he calls "pieces of shit" and "fucking liars"[21] while demanding they "admit they didn't run any studies even though people told them to." In Dr. Prasad's vision, "telling people" to do studies was all it took to do them.

When it came to vaccines, Dr. Prasad felt that RCTs had to be repeated for every variant and for every demographic group. In his article, "Covid19 Therapeutics & Boosters All Need New Studies," he wrote:

> *Not a single one of these trials has assessed the value of these medications in the current world where many people have had COVID multiple times, and received multiple boosters. Not a single one of these trials applies to current circulating strains. These data don't apply.*[22]

According to Dr. Prasad, every tweak to the vaccine meant we had to start from scratch with a new RCT that demonstrated its value against COVID's gravest outcomes. He felt that, absent that evidence, we should assume vaccines didn't work, and we shouldn't use them. For example, his article, "No More Covid-19 Boosters Without Evidence," said:

> *The issue with perpetual COVID-19 boosters is what evidence is needed to justify their push? The answer has to be randomized trials powered for reductions in severe disease, hospitalization and death.*[23]

Using a classic influencer technique, Dr. Prasad even asked his followers to "pledge no more shots without RCT." In Dr. Prasad's vision, we'd continually test vaccines but never have the opportunity to actually use them—which was the point.

Dr. Prasad was not alone in this. Dr. Jay Bhattacharya also cast doubt on COVID vaccines by saying, "I have yet to see any RCT data released to the public about the efficacy, side-effects, contraindications, dosing, etc. on covid vax boosters. I'd welcome links in replies if someone has seen these data."[24]

He also complained that *other doctors* didn't do more RCTs, saying, "The Science (tm) threw away randomized trials, control groups, civil rights, informed consent, benefit harm analysis, and scientific debate. We are in a new dark age."[25]

Florida Surgeon General Dr. Joseph Ladapo also recommended against COVID vaccines by saying, "People are pretending that they can continue skating along with the clinical trials that happened four years ago to justify approvals today."[26]

However, Dr. Prasad didn't demand perpetual RCTs to aid medical researchers or because he wanted to do the RCTs himself. Rather, his endless calls for *other doctors* to run RCTs of everything were just another way to spread anger and doubt about common sense measures to control a rapidly spreading virus in a world with finite time and resources. For example, in his article, "How to Save Science from Covid Politics," he wrote:

> Let's say we want to find out if a particular policy—say, mask mandates—actually helps. A randomized trial is a tool that allows us to separate the biases of the world—some states are blue, some people take more precautions, some places have higher vaccine rates—and lets us figure out the actual value of an intervention. By randomly assigning groups to either have the intervention or not, you balance out the variables and isolate the effect of the mandate.
>
> Many experts have called for more randomized trials during the pandemic. But they were ignored. We should have studied whether social distancing works, and how much distance is ideal. We should know a lot more about who to test, why we're testing, and

how often to test. Even school closure and reopening could have been studied. Randomized trials could have turned political fights into scientific questions. Not running them was a huge failure.[27]

This seems straightforward, but it raises a very basic question. What exactly does Dr. Prasad mean by the words "helps" and "works"? He seems to be saying, "We should have done RCTs to investigate whether or not mitigation measures slowed the spread of COVID." He seems to further imply that *if only* we had solid evidence from RCTs that mitigation measures "helped" and "worked," then we would be perfectly justified in using them, and nobody would object to them, as if we all shared the same goal of limiting COVID.

But we didn't all share that goal. WWTI doctors wanted to purposefully infect unvaccinated children to usher in herd immunity, and Dr. Prasad embraced this pro-infection philosophy. For example, in his article, "Should We Let Children Get Omicron?" he wrote:

It is reckless to let children age into a more serious encounter with a disease best dealt with while younger. [...] Shielding kids from exposure only increases their future risk. [...] By rebuilding population immunity among the least at-risk, moreover, we help buffer risk for those most vulnerable. [...] For children, getting sick and recovering is part of a natural and healthy life. [...] Exposures are how we best protect our children against the variants of the future. [...] Immunity is built through illness.[28]

So, let's imagine a fantasy world where it was possible to have every RCT Dr. Prasad imagined. Let's further pretend that these pristine RCTs unambiguously showed that mitigation measures meaningfully slowed the spread of COVID. Would Dr. Prasad then say these measures "helped" or "worked"? Would he have come out guns blazing advocating for these mitigations?

Of course not. His mind was already made up. He didn't need any RCTs to say it was *"reckless"* to even try to prevent COVID in children. When Dr. Prasad wrote the article "Should We Let Children Get Omicron?" he answered not by calling for any RCTs but by saying, *"restrictions in schools must never return."* He also said:

> It is important to emphasise that a more laissez-faire approach to kids and Covid makes public health sense, too. Dropping masks, quarantines, distancing, and all other mitigations will allow children to develop the kind of broad immunity gained by living a normal life.

Once again, WWTI doctors didn't honestly question whether mitigation measures slowed the spread of the virus; they sought to undermine them precisely because they *knew* they slowed the virus. Almost no one, not even Dr. Prasad, sincerely doubted that mitigation measures limited COVID; however, WWTI doctors often feigned ignorance about their impact because they wanted to "allow children to develop the kind of broad immunity gained by living a normal life." In the mirror world, the policies that "helped" or "worked" were, by definition, those that "allowed" unvaccinated children to be repeatedly exposed to SARS-CoV-2.

This is why Dr. Prasad invariably managed to find "flaws" in RCTs whose results he did not like. For example, even though it was 100% effective at preventing COVID infections, he rejected the RCT of the adolescent COVID vaccine because it was not large enough to demonstrate efficacy against rare but grave outcomes.[29] Dr. Prasad felt that even though the vaccine perfectly prevented COVID infections, it somehow might *not* prevent severe COVID. He further argued that until an RCT demonstrated its efficacy on hospitalizations and deaths for *every* variant, we should tolerate these tragedies in unvaccinated children.

Predictably, WWTI doctors' demands for RCTs were applied *very selectively*—only to the mitigation measures they opposed. They didn't demand RCTs before advocating unvaccinated children and young adults contract COVID. They did not demand RCTs before claiming that repeat SARS-CoV-2 infections were harmless to children. They did not demand RCTs before making bold, confident claims that "natural immunity" was powerful and long-lasting. They did not demand RCTs to overhype vaccines in early 2021, claiming they blocked transmission and would end the pandemic. They did not demand RCTs to claim that mitigation measures caused harm. Dr. Prasad's article "The Downsides of Masking Young Students Are Real"[30] wasn't based on any RCT.

WWTI doctors did not portray removing mitigation measures as taking an action, and so they didn't demand RCTs to prove it was safe to take them away. Indeed, they *never* demanded RCTs to support their favored pandemic policies. They never called for an RCT of "focused protection." They conveniently set the baseline, so they were always right by default and never had to prove anything. The burden of proof—the highest level imaginable—always lay with those who wished to limit the virus in any way.

Meanwhile, Dr. Prasad casually dismissed literally all observational studies whose results he did not like. He brushed aside dozens of studies that support the pediatric COVID vaccines by saying, *"Observational data has been used to support vaccines, but is plagued by confounding."*[31] In contrast, he was eager to amplify any observational study, no matter how flawed, that showed a whiff of harm from vaccines or mitigation measures. For example, after his colleagues Drs. John Mandrola and Tracy Beth Høeg inappropriately used data from the Vaccine Adverse

Event Reporting System (VAERS) to claim the COVID vaccine would hurt young males more than help,[32] Dr. Prasad lauded their study as a "bombshell."[33]

Thus, it becomes clear that methodolatrists performatively fetishized RCTs not to advance medical research but rather to sow doubt about unwanted mitigation measures and the entire concept of public health. Methodolatry converts a study design into an epistemological weapon.

> **Ultimately, they failed us, and we are left without answers and policies that caused significant harm.**
> — *Sensible Medicine*

It was a very effective weapon, however, and an article on Dr. Prasad's Substack *Sensible Medicine* titled "Death and Isolation During a Pandemic" shows how methodolatry was used to create doubt and anger. The article discussed the tragedy of people dying alone at the start of the pandemic.[34] As someone who lived through it, I couldn't agree more. Anyone who worked in the hospital at that time remembers patients suffering without their loved ones and aching goodbyes via iPads. It happened to an overwhelming number of families, leaving them forever scarred. I'll never forget one father, consumed by grief, who wailed at us over the phone that we didn't try hard enough to save his 35-year-old son. Had he been there, he would have at least had the comfort of knowing we did everything possible. His son had clots throughout his body, and there was nothing to do. How horrible that he believes his son might still be alive had we only tried a bit harder.

However, the core argument of the *Sensible Medicine* article was this:

> *Now, the empirical question, does limiting visitors reduce the*

transmission of SARS-CoV-2 and thus lower the incidence of COVID-19? The answer to this question is important and can provide a framework for thinking about the risk-benefit calculus of allowing visitors. Unfortunately, we don't have an answer or any high quality data supporting this question, as shown in this systematic analysis. As discussed previously, there are a host of possible upsides to this policy; however, it is unclear if they are true.

*Even with reasonable predictions, we live in a world that is messy and random, and thus require rigorously designed studies to uncover one form of the truth. I imagine that a cluster randomized controlled trial could have provided an answer. This would consist of randomizing hospitals into two groups: ones that allows visitors and others that restrict them. Then, over time, outcomes would be tracked in each group to measure the impact of the policy. I specifically left outcomes vague because the pertinent outcomes are debatable, but I would argue that a good starting point is COVID-19 hospital admissions. Another relevant outcome may be the number of positive COVID-19 cases in the surrounding community – although this would be more difficult to directly link to the policy. The broader point being that there are ways to uncover answers. There are smart people in positions of power with resources that can design and conduct such studies. **Ultimately, they failed us, and we are left without answers and policies that caused significant harm.***

It's worthwhile pondering this *"imagined cluster randomized controlled trial"* to show how obviously unserious these proposals were. These RCTs were conjured out of thin air not to advance medical research but rather to create rage and mistrust.

First, the article implied that *"They"* should have had the foresight to run this RCT in spring 2020. As morgues overflowed with victims of a new virus that lacked treatments and a vaccine, the article claimed *"They"* should have been marshaling their resources to conduct an RCT of hospital visitation policies, as if there were no bigger fish to fry at the time. Of course, this RCT would have sounded utterly absurd at the start of the pandemic, which is why nobody actually suggested anything like it.

Second, the article assumed that *"They"* had the power and resources to run this RCT but chose not to for some reason. According to the *Sensible Medicine* article, someone could have snapped their fingers and ordered an RCT of hospital visiting policies, but they refused. Perhaps there should be an elite RCT Strike Force, but the simple truth is that no government or institution anywhere could have instantly whipped up dozens of rigorous RCTs to answer *every* pandemic conundrum and quandary as WWTI doctors implied. In the real world, politicians meddled with scientific agencies, and the CDC couldn't even get basic tests right.[35] Much of the federal response was in shambles from the pandemic's earliest days. According to one article:

> *Early on, the government went off the rails.*
> *In February 2020, the focus was on containment, with measures such as the travel ban on China and repatriation of Americans, including those stranded on cruise ships. Emergency mobilization efforts "languished," the report noted. There was "confusion and friction about who was in charge of what problems." The government's "crisis action plan" amounted to little more than jargon. "There was little in it about what people would actually do."*

On Feb. 24, 2020, President Donald Trump tweeted from India,
"The Coronavirus is very much under control in the USA ...
Stock market starting to look very good to me!" But according to
the report, that same day, the White House task force concluded
"containment was failing." It was time to shift to mitigation.
The next day, a high-ranking Centers for Disease Control and
Prevention official, Nancy Messonnier, announced that commu-
nity spread in the United States was inevitable. The stock market
dived.

"President Trump was furious," the report recalls. He kept
downplaying the danger. "It's going to disappear," he said on
Feb. 27. "Everything is really under control," he said Feb. 29.
It was not. The authors of the report show, in detail, how feder-
al crisis management "splintered by the third week of March."
HHS Secretary Alex Azar had placed the assistant secretary for
preparedness and response, Robert Kadlec, in charge of the HHS
effort — but at the same time, Vice President Mike Pence's staff
kicked him off the White House task force. The head of the Food
and Drug Administration was not even on the task force for the
first month. The CDC was "fractured into too many missions."
While some officials recognized the urgency of a crash program
of testing and masks, "Kadlec had no money, no real emergency
fund."

"By late April, as a frightened and bewildered country became
more and more confused about continuing business and school
closures, and after some brow-raising comments at a White
House briefing in which he discussed treating the virus with light,
heat, or disinfectant, Trump essentially detached himself from his

own government," the report says. "He moved toward ques-
tioning and challenging what other government officials were
doing."

"The administration abdicated its wartime responsibility to
lead," they add. "It left the battlefield, and the war strategy" to
the states and localities. By April, the White House chief of staff
concluded the task force was "useless and broken."[36]

Even if *"They"* had an elite RCT Strike Force at their disposal and
bizarrely prioritized an RCT of hospital visiting policies as morgues overflowed in April 2020, it would still face many obstacles.

- Would hospital administrators have agreed to participate in this
  RCT? I doubt it. An RCT of hospital visiting policies wouldn't
  have been on their radar at the pandemic's start. They were too
  busy trying to get PPE, staffing, and places to store the dead
  bodies.

- Would multiple IRBs, which helps ensure research is safe and
  ethical, have approved a study that allowed large numbers of
  unvaccinated family members into unventilated rooms full of
  contagious patients? As morgues overflowed and forklifts were
  needed to move corpses into refrigerated trucks, would an IRB
  have *actually* accepted that there was true clinical equipoise
  and that this study needed to be run at that moment? I'm skeptical.

- I work at two hospitals, New York University and Bellevue,
  that are blocks apart in terms of their distance but worlds apart
  in terms of the patients they treat and the communities they
  serve. To control for these discrepancies, this study would have
  to enroll a large number of hospitals. How many would have
  to participate to get meaningful results? What would happen if
  some of those hospitals dropped out?

- What if hospital staff objected? We are packed like sardines in
  the elevators on a normal day. This RCT would have greatly
  increased our exposure to the virus at a time when no one was

vaccinated. I wouldn't have been thrilled to have been randomized to the "visitors allowed" hospital. We had enough sick
healthcare workers as it was, and several of my co-workers
died. Would frontline healthcare workers have had any say in
this study?

- What if other family members objected to this study? It's
easy to imagine family members strongly disagreeing about
whether to visit a dying relative. Consider an elderly couple
living with their two adult children. If Dad gets hospitalized,
his immunocompromised daughter may strongly feel the risk
of anyone visiting is too high. *Does she get a say in this RCT?*
What if her brother visits their dad against her wishes and
brings the virus home? What effect might this have on the
family? He might also regret his decision, especially if anyone
suffers as a result. What if this RCT created great conflict in
people and families?

- What if the general public objected? Allowing hospital visitors
would have meant more people on subways and buses, and
therefore more risk for the essential workers who used them.
Would these workers have had any input into the study?

- Many hospitals were deluged with COVID patients in the
spring of 2020. It's not unreasonable to imagine that large
groups of mourners in a hospital room would have greatly
increased the spread of COVID in the spring of 2020. What
contingency measures would be in place if that happened?

- Might patients and their families choose a hospital that was
randomized to allow visitation? How would this affect the
results?

- While I agree that COVID hospital admissions would be a
reasonable outcome to track, there are some logistical issues.
A woman who visits her sister at Hospital X isn't necessarily
going to be admitted to Hospital X if she contracts COVID
herself. At Bellevue, where I worked, nearly all of our patients
were transferred from other overwhelmed hospitals. As such,
this RCT would require that hospital visitors be followed, and

their hospital admissions tracked. This, in turn, would require informed consent for every hospital visitor. How would a grieving family feel if they lost their mother and only later learned she was infected in a hospital that was part of a medical experiment to which she did not consent?

- Consenting every visitor at multiple hospitals while COVID raged would have been a Herculean task. Obtaining informed consent is a lengthy and formal process, not something that can be done as people walk by in the hallway. What woman, on the verge of losing her husband of 50 years, would listen patiently as researchers explained the nature of this experiment? Much of this would have to be done via translator phones. Many of our patients did not speak English.

- Tracking every visitor at multiple hospitals would also have been an enormous task. People would likely travel great distances to say goodbye to a loved one. Would grieving families be willing to share details of their fate with researchers over the telephone? It's easy to imagine people would just want to be left alone if they got very sick with COVID as part of this experiment.

- Who *exactly* had the resources to do all this? Such expertise can't be created out of thin air in a matter of weeks in the middle of a raging pandemic. There's not an endless supply of clinical research coordinators and staff. Why should these skilled professionals have dropped everything to run this RCT? Thankfully, *"They"* chose to prioritize vaccine RCTs.

- Would a trial conducted in the spring of 2020 have any relevance today? I don't think so. Both the population and the virus itself have changed too much. The original vaccine RCTs became relics in less than a year. Why would this RCT age better?

- How long would the RCT have taken? In New York, one of the states with the strictest policies, hospitals were mandated to allow visitors in June 2021.[37] Would this imagined RCT have yielded actionable results before this? I doubt it.

- Would anyone support visitation restrictions *today* if this study found that hospital visitors increased the spread of COVID? Even RCTs that yield unambiguous scientific results rarely create agreement on what policy should flow from them. They almost never provide a crystal-clear answer to complicated social and ethical questions. Let's pretend this RCT found that allowing visitors increased community COVID infections by 14.3%. Should hospitals allow visitors or not? Would everyone agree with the answer? Might this imagined RCT interject uncertainty and polarization into the rare issue where there seems to be near uniform agreement today? I'm not sure exactly when the policy of restricting visitors should have ended, but like *everyone else*, I'm glad it's gone. So, even if the study was perfectly and rapidly executed at the pandemic's start, for how long would it have held relevance? Everybody made up their mind about this issue long ago, and everyone agrees on it today. So really, what would have been the point of this study?

Any one of these factors would have doomed an RCT of hospital visiting policies, but the *Sensible Medicine* article didn't consider a single one of them. It was an entirely unserious proposal

A calamitous error that will leave a stain on public health's reputation for decades.
— Ben

The *Sensible Medicine* article concluded by saying:

It seems as if our hyper-focus on the virus blinded us to the negative implications of certain policies – a calamitous error that will leave a stain on public health's reputation for decades. Even in times of crisis, we must be able to weigh all the pros and cons of a policy – especially those that are less obvious.[34]

Communicating this message— "*a calamitous error that will leave a stain on public health's reputation for decades"* —was the article's true message, and it succeeded. The comment section was a cesspool of rage and revenge fantasies against *"They"*:

- *I will never forgive the staff that had become so brainwashed with their own needs to mask up, Mask my Mom up over her O2, which she really didn't need, yet got sent "home" with. Now I realize the incentives to keep C19 monies moving into these hospitals. To the MD that wouldn't let her go "home" on her birthday, may he be forever riddled with guilt. May he suffer the loss of a loved one in the same manner. May he die alone.*[38]

- *The whole thing was soooo inhumane.*[39]

- *The powers that be messed up big time during the Covid pandemic. I hope we never forget how death was dehumanized. It was criminal in my mind.*[40]

- *These people need to be held accountable*[41]

- *Maybe COVID will open our collective eyes to see the disaster of having clueless and/or spineless administrators in charge everywhere.*[42]

- *There's an element within the medical system that is deeply inhumane. COVID allowed that element free reign over all of our lives.*[43]

- *So many of our policies seemed inhumane at the time, and even more inhumane in retrospect.*[44]

- *It was a maniacal focus on eliminating the virus above all other goals.*[45]

- *We did know from the beginning how awful most of these policies would be. […] If improvement is to be made then start with questioning WHY did the medical community ever go along with such inhuman policies?*[46]

- *Many of us, knowing the horror stories of dying alone as told by friends or family, will avoid hospitals in the future, unless unconscious and transported to one.*[47]

- *It was a purposeful dictate designed to wreck humanity.*[48]

- *The senseless cruelty of those policies can never, ever be forgiven.*[49]

- *Just....it would have been nice if actual doctors could have located their Ethics Balls 3 years ago when all this was happening *because even then they knew it was wrong*, instead of waiting until now when the dust has more or less settled and it's suddenly safe to be critical of "things that were well-intentioned but ultimately turned out to be less than helpful." No. They knew it was wrong then. They had an ethical duty to speak up. And if they're unwilling to apologize for failing in that duty, then I'm uninterested in 2020 (ha!) hindsight.*[50]

- *To isolate people who are sick enough to be near death is so cruel I can barely think about it. No, it didn't prevent the spread of covid.*[51]

- *We should all be angry. The masks were bad enough (depersonalizing us), but the lockdowns were cruel, inhumane and completely unnecessary.*[52]

- *Mistakes were not made; the herd was culled. Well into the pandemic no course corrections were allowed, early treatments were banned, natural immunity was scorned.*[53]

- *Thank you for this. No one I know of had to die alone during this time, but every time I read accounts and am reminded of it I am filled with rage and sorrow, and try to connect in my mind and soul to those people left alone and cut off. The inhumanity is deplorable. I hope more and more is publicized about this so it's never ever ever again.*[54]

Dr. Adam Cifu, one of the founders of *Sensible Medicine*, also showed up in the comments to say, *"wonderful! Thank you so much"*[55] to the article's author. Dr. Cifu wasn't the slightest bit disturbed by the threats and rage his publication engendered.

It's impossible not to feel enormous sympathy for anyone who lost a relative early in the pandemic. However, *Sensible Medicine* readers weren't comforted by what they read; they were furious and vengeful. In the real world, during a raging pandemic with a brand-new virus, *"They"* had to make many difficult decisions, in an instant, without the benefit of a rigorous RCT to guide them at every turn. Right or wrong, the decision to ban hospital visitors was made to limit mass illness and death, not out of wanton indifference, as the article on *Sensible Medicine* implied. After all, the best way to have prevented people from dying without their families in 2020 was to have prevented them from dying in the first place.

Moreover, hospitals were full of people who were kind and compassionate to the people who died there. It's no substitute, but anyone who lost a loved one to COVID should know this and perhaps feel some consolation. Of course, too many of these kind and compassionate hospital workers died of COVID too. Perhaps those in mourning today might have received a sliver of solace had they been reminded of any of this. But that was not the purpose of the *Sensible Medicine* article.

It also wasn't written to *actually* advance medical research. The *Sensible Medicine* article did not encourage its readers to enroll in an RCT. Being part of an experiment is scary for a lot of people, yet medicine couldn't advance without *trusting* volunteers. Being a "guinea pig" is a derisive term, when it should be a compliment. I've tried to enroll patients in many different studies over the years, and it's not always easy. Many patients don't trust *"They."* Unfortunately, articles that needlessly denigrate *"They"* give the general public every reason to distrust researchers who *actually* try to enroll patients in RCTs. *Sensible Medicine* readers won't be signing up for an RCT anytime soon.

In contrast, I genuinely care about RCTs and want them to succeed. The first article I wrote about this pandemic was titled "I'm a Neurologist Who Happily Volunteered for the AstraZeneca Vaccine Trials," which discussed my experience in a vaccine RCT. In it, I said:

Having argued for years that vaccines are properly tested, I jumped at the chance to participate in a vaccine trial myself. I've always believed that people who participate in medical research are doing a noble thing. If no one volunteered for such research, medicine would never advance.[56]

Like Dr. Prasad, I too asked my readers to take a pledge in an article, "Take a Pledge to Enroll in a Randomized-Controlled Trial."[57] WWTI doctors never did this. They never promoted real-world RCTs that were trying to recruit volunteers or exhorted their audience to enroll in them. They glorified RCTs not to advance science research but to spread their core message of doubt.

"Randomized controlled trials are not always necessary" — *Dr. Vinay Prasad*

Dr. Prasad excoriated his predecessors for not doing RCTs of every COVID mitigation measure for every variant and demographic group. In 2023, he blasted scientists who recognized that RCTs were sometimes "not possible, not practical, or not useful," he said in his article titled "The Scientists Who Undermined Randomized Trials."[58] "All of these arguments are false."

However, he drastically changed his tune once he gained power and responsibility and might be expected to generate evidence himself. On his first day as the Center for Biologics Evaluation and Research (CBER) director, he said that "randomized controlled trials are not always necessary,"[59] and in a conversation about talc with Dr. Marty Makary, he said that RCTs are not necessary for "risk factor mitigation."[60] This was a "simple teaching point," he said. In another discussion about rare diseases, he said, "We know that randomized trials are not always feasible, possible, or practical."[61] During a discussion on stem cells he added:

> *Trials vs. real world evidence? The answer to that is both. We will always have a place for controlled clinical studies, but we will also leverage the incredible promise of real world data.*[62]

Despite these reasonable sentiments, Drs. Prasad and Makary are intent on restricting updated COVID vaccines for healthy people under age 65[63] using a lack of RCTs as their justification. Though they rejected the first booster—which was found to be 95% effective against COVID in an RCT[64]—they are now demanding subsequent vaccine doses again demonstrate their efficacy via new RCTs. They feel the vaccine should be unavailable to millions of Americans until these trials are done. Once again, the possibility that someone might receive a vaccine dose they don't need bothers them much more than the certainty that people are missing vaccines they do need.

In an *NEJM* article explaining their position, Drs. Prasad and Makary wrote that because of COVID boosters, "public trust in vaccination in general has declined,"[65] and in one interview, Dr. Makary again invoked trust as a reason for his decision. He said:

> *The day of rubber-stamping covid vaccines for young healthy kids is over. You cannot send us an application for a new covid booster each year with no new updated clinical trial data and expect the FDA to just blindly rubber-stamp it ... people don't trust us.*[66]

It is destabilizing, frustrating and enraging to feel like my daughter, who wasn't even 18 months old, has done more for public health than some people who are now currently in charge of it.
— Nick Giglia

Dr. Makary was right that people don't trust our current medical establishment. Shortly after his announcement, the headlines read, "Top CDC COVID Vaccine Adviser Quits After RFK Jr. Ended Recommendations."[67] Understandably, parents who had previously volunteered their children for COVID trials, which involved "literal blood and tears," were livid that their prior contributions were so casually discarded.[68] According to the article "A 'War On Children': As US Changes COVID Vaccine Rules, Parents Of Trial Volunteers Push Back":

> When Nick Giglia got the call asking if he still wanted to enroll his one-year-old daughter in the Pfizer pediatric vaccine trial, he immediately said yes.
>
> For eight visits, extending over nearly a year, he would drive an hour each way to a trial in New Jersey. In all, his daughter received seven shots – three saline placebos, three vaccines and a booster. [...]
>
> "It is destabilizing, frustrating and enraging to feel like my daughter, who wasn't even 18 months old, has done more for public health than some people who are now currently in charge of it," Giglia said.
>
> "It is very frustrating to hear that sacrifice that we volunteered to make for the country, and frankly, the world, belittled."
>
> At the end of the trial, Giglia's daughter was given a stuffed teddy bear in a sweater that said "Covid-19 vaccine study hero".
>
> "I don't care what anybody says. That's what she is," Giglia

*said. "I look forward to one day being able to tell my little girl
all about how she helped save the world. And it's hard to hear
that many people think that we did the exact opposite."*

Methodolatry is also being used to limit vaccines for pregnant women, even though they have an elevated risk of severe COVID and their newborns depend on maternal antibodies. In 2023, Dr. Makary spread doubt about the vaccine in pregnancy, writing articles such as "Was the COVID Vaccine Safe for Pregnant Women?"[69]—spoiler alert, it was.[70] However, as FDA commissioner, Dr. Makary didn't blame articles like this for low vaccination rates in pregnant women. Rather he said this was "probably because they want to see randomized trial data."[71] Dr. Makary presented no evidence that obstetricians' offices are full of skeptical patients demanding RCTs. Nonetheless, in May 2025, Kennedy, flanked by Drs. Bhattacharya and Makary, announced the COVID vaccine was being removed from the CDC vaccine schedule for healthy children and pregnant women. Dr. Bhattacharya said this was "common sense and it's good science," though he presented no science at all.

Kennedy announces the COVID vaccine is being removed from the vaccine schedule for healthy children and pregnant women.

While our medical establishment fought for people who wanted to avoid mandated vaccines, they are eager to withhold vaccines from people who want them. Although many people are satisfied with the dozens of observational studies supporting the vaccine's benefits, our current medical establishment doesn't feel people should have the right to choose for themselves. They are perfectly fine using government power to impose their will and personal standards of evidence on millions of Americans.

Naturally, many people are not happy about this. According to a news report titled "FDA's Plan to Limit Covid Vaccines Worries Some Who Won't Be Eligible":

> *Allison Flynn, 56, of New Jersey would probably be considered low risk, but she stays up-to-date on her shots to protect her 72-year-old husband and reduce the risk of debilitating long covid symptoms that could put her out of work.*
> *"I don't want to bring that home and kill him," Flynn said.*
> *"They are not letting me make a choice."*[72]

Ms. Flynn faces essentially no risk from the vaccine beyond a sore arm. The rate of myocarditis from the booster is 8 per one million and, as always, "tends to resolve quickly."[73]

Predictably, there is no indication anyone in our current medical establishment is planning on doing new vaccine RCTs themselves. In fact, there is no indication that our new medical establishment is planning on doing any RCTs at all, though they do plan to dredge medical records to "discover" the cause of autism.[74] Once they became the medical establishment, WWTI doctors held themselves to different standards than their predecessors. "RCT or STFU" was for other doctors. It didn't apply to Dr. Prasad or anyone in the current administration.

By saying RCTs were not needed to mitigate risks, Dr. Prasad was giving himself and the current medical establishment the permission structure—which they denied to those who tried to control COVID—to make drastic policy changes without RCTs or even consulting experts. According to the article "CDC Blindsided as RFK Jr. Changes Vaccine Recommendations":

*Health and Human Services Secretary Robert F. Kennedy Jr.'s
surprise announcement Tuesday ending coronavirus vaccine recommendations for healthy children and pregnant women blindsided the agency that offers that advice, according to current
and former federal health officials. Officials at the Centers for
Disease Control and Prevention are scrambling to understand
Kennedy's decision, announced in a 58-second video on X on
Tuesday morning, which took agency staff by surprise.*[75]

Instead of leading the way with new RCTs, our medical establishment is demanding that vaccine companies do all the work, even though
prior to taking office, they told the public not to trust their research. One
of the oldest and most effective ways to spread doubt about vaccines is to
spread doubt about the companies that make them. Dr. Prasad, for example, made inflammatory comments such as:

*These corrupt doctors are the ones who decided that babies
need covid shots. If you run vaccine trials for Pfizer, the conflict
doesn't go away when the trial ends, because you're going to run
another one after you ram through their garbage products.*[76]

Today, our medical establishment claims that these pharmaceutical
companies should test their own "garbage products" and that only they
can generate reliable evidence for the American public. As they did
throughout the pandemic, they are again making videos "calling on"
other people to do RCTs under the pretense of wanting the "gold-standard
science," a new MAHA buzzword. Their real goal, of course, is to sabotage vaccines, and thanks to their efforts, even if Pfizer was able to successfully complete a new RCT, many people would distrust the results.
Why would anyone trust the "corrupt doctors" who work there?

However, since WWTI doctors are now the medical establishment, we can hold them to the same standards they created for their predecessors. We can tell them "RCT or STFU." We can call on them to run innumerable RCTs and expect that their every decision and utterance will be backed by large, high-quality trials. If they don't do this, we can all say, **"They failed us, and we are left without answers and policies that caused significant harm."**

Chapter 15: The Fact Check Genre Is a Lie

Scott Atlas lawyer threatens defamation suit over critical Stanford open letter.
— News Headline, September 2020

Doctors who claimed that COVID would kill 10,000 Americans, that it was mild for people under 70, or that mass infection would lead to herd immunity can't make the affirmative case that they were right. Although WWTI doctors can't or won't defend their words, this does not mean that they are defenseless. For them, the best defense is a good offense.

Though WWTI doctors claimed to value "civil debate and discussion," they vigorously defended themselves in the public sphere. They almost never engaged with their critics in good faith; instead, they launched an avalanche of childish attacks against anyone who corrected their disinformation. Much of this occurred on social media, which, like it or not, is how much of the public consumes scientific information and how journalists find "experts" to interview. As such, it's vital to discuss the techniques WWTI doctors used to shield themselves from criticism and put their critics on the defensive.

In addition to denying their own words, WWTI doctors adopted several techniques to distract from their disinformation and to shut down discussion about it. The primary function of this was to intimidate and discredit their critics. According to WWTI doctors, those who disagree with their plans for herd immunity via mass infection are unqualified fearmongers, lying idiots beset by groupthink, and greedy grifters.

Though WWTI doctors claimed to be against ad hominem accusations and all for the actual substance of the disagreement, this was just an act. In reality, many of them unleashed a firehose of bad faith attacks against their critics, all while casting themselves as victims. This technique is known as DARVO (Deny, Attack, and Reverse Victim & Offender), and it's how WWTI doctors tried to spread doubt about anyone who corrected their disinformation. If people like me can't be trusted, then the disinformation spread by WWTI doctors might not be disinformation after all.

None of their techniques were new. Rebecca Goldberg and Dr. Laura Vandenberg described them all in their article, "The Science of Spin: Targeted Strategies to Manufacture Doubt with Detrimental Effects on Environmental and Public Health."[1] History shows that the tobacco, coal, and sugar industries also used strawman arguments and personal attacks to discredit their critics. What may appear to be just petty behavior was in reality a valuable tool to sway public opinion and intimidate potential critics. WWTI doctors borrowed from their playbook.

I will discuss my experience because I am familiar with it, not because there was anything special about it. It was completely ordinary. Anyone who openly pushed back on anti-vaccine disinformation was treated this way, though I was accustomed to it from my pre-pandemic vaccine advocacy. I still have a t-shirt from 2015 celebrating my being placed on a list of pro-vaccine "trolls."

Countless doctors could write their own personal versions of this chapter, and many of them had it *much* worse than I. Other doctors were targeted by online mobs, had their employers contacted, or were threatened by frivolous lawsuits–a fact celebrated by Robert F. Kennedy Jr.[2] Some doctors received vile death threats, needed bodyguards, and had anti-vaxxers film them at their homes. The purpose of this bad-faith engagement and harassment was to wear people down, silence them, and send a message to potential critics. It was successful. While WWTI doctors have been catapulted to power, several doctors who fought passion- ately against their disinformation at the start of the pandemic have since vanished from the public sphere. They will be forever scarred by their experience.

> **The public is watching this spat and has lost trust in science, medicine, and public health.**
> — *Dr. Jay Bhattacharya*

In their telling, WWTI doctors wanted nothing more than civil debate and the free exchange of scientific ideas. Dr. Jay Bhattacharya, for exam- ple, said:

> *For science to work, you have to have an open exchange of ideas...If you're going to make an argument that something is misinformation, you should provide an actual argument. You can't just take it down and say, 'Oh, it's misinformation' without actually giving a reason...Let's hear the argument, let's see the evidence that YouTube used to decide it was misinformation. Let's have a debate. Science works best when we have an open debate.*[3]

That sounds nice, and, indeed, WWTI doctors demanded such courte- sy when they were criticized. Dr. Bhattacharya also portrayed himself as someone who was open to the possibility that he might be wrong. In an interview with *Reason*, he said, "I want to treat ideas that I disagree with respectfully because I might be wrong."[4]

While Dr. Bhattacharya claimed to be open and courteous, he felt that his critics had been unkind and unwilling to have good-faith debates with him. In one interview he lamented ad hominem accusations. He said:

*So I think that if somebody is arguing against a policy idea or
a set of scientific hypotheses in this ad hominem way, that is a
position of weakness that they're arguing for. Because if you
really want to engage with somebody, you have to engage with
their ideas. And I think that it's very easy for the press or others
to look and see that fight that's nasty. Okay, this group is making
ad hominem accusations against another group and just report
the ad hominem as opposed to reporting the fact about the actual
substance of the disagreement.[5]*

Again, that sounds nice.

In an article he wrote, Dr. Bhattacharya painted a dark picture of
pandemic discourse, one where he was a victim. He stated:

*University professors and students who publicly questioned the
mainstream consensus were censored on social media, vilified
by their colleagues, and, in the case of Covid vaccine mandates,
fired by administrators. Social pressure was harsh – almost
Stalinesque.[6]*

As a reminder, Joseph Stalin murdered his critics *en masse*. Dr. Bhattacharya continued:

*Universities failed in their mission to promote academic debate
and freedom during the most significant domestic policy issue
of this century. This abdication of responsibility encouraged the
climate of groupthink and censorship that predominated among
much of the intelligentsia during the Covid years.*

*During these years, colleagues and students with critical, scepti-
cal viewpoints and countless members of the public approached
us, asking why institutions of higher education were not hosting
reasoned debate. They were right: few such events took place.*

*Public health officials sacrificed the understandable desire for
an open exchange of ideas on an altar of infection control; it was
supposedly too dangerous to let the public see that there were
qualified experts who disagreed on the wisdom of lockdowns,
school closures, mask mandates, social distancing, and vaccine
mandates. Now, of course, the evidence increasingly questions
the effectiveness of these measures and draws attention to their
harms.*

*The pandemic taught us a valuable lesson for those interested to
hear. We need more freedom of expression and academic debate
during crises and emergencies, not less.*

*Yet a small sub-culture of scientists and journalists who support-
ed destructive policies like school closures and vaccine mandates
continue to denigrate efforts to promote thoughtful debate about
the pandemic. They fear an honest appraisal of these ideas.*

Dr. Bhattacharya felt his critics were to blame for the loss of trust in
public health. He said:

*The scientists clamoring about misinformation and the rise of
anti science, and endorsing censorship or worse to combat it,
should familiarize themselves with Friedrich Nietzsche. They are
to blame for the collapse in public trust in science.*[7]

Elsewhere, he wrote:

*Scientists should be able to disagree on public health policy with-
out being branded monsters. The public is watching this spat and
has lost trust in science, medicine, and public health.*[8]

I agree with that last sentence.

The Misinformation Police Strike Out.
— Dr. Vinay Prasad

Indeed, the *public was watching this spat*, and WWTI doctors sought to spread doubt about the entire concept of fact-checking. Dr. Bhattacharya, for example, repeatedly tried to discredit unnamed "fact checkers." Instead of saying *where* he felt they had erred, he impugned their motives, claiming they were intent on "censoring dissident voices."[9] The following are a few examples of where he expressed his disdain for fact checkers:

- *Fact checking organizations privilege partisan analysts, often with inadequate training, to take sides on thorny scientific questions on which there is no scientific consensus. The fact check genre is a lie.*[10]

- *Just because 'fact checkers' in and out of the government say they check 'facts' does not mean they actually do so. They often get facts wrong and they cherry pick which 'facts' to check to fit their ideological agenda. Ironically, the industry is based on a lie.*[11]

- *The 'fact' checking industry has no interest in the discovery of true things, a noble goal. Its main purpose is the enforcement of the taboo against saying socially or politically inconvenient true things.*[12]

- *Free speech is most important when hard public decisions must be made, such as election season and during a public health crisis. What follows? The censorship complex and selective, fatuous fact 'checking' is most harmful when free speech is most needed.*[13]

- *Through the @CDCFound, pharmaceutical companies funnel money to the @CDCgov. The money is used to fund "fact checking" organizations, which promote pharma propaganda and lies in the media, and aid government in censoring dissident voices.*[9]

- *Selective, politically motivated "fact" checking was a major problem during the pandemic. It led to a lot of bad policies being implemented and persisting long after they should have been rubbished.*[14]
- *I know the "don't be evil" motto never really worked in practice, but @Google and @youtube actively funding the anti-science "fact-checking" and censorship regime after its catastrophic failures of the last ~three years is just too much. Bad fact-checking harms public health.*[15]
- *"For some odd reason, Big Fact-Check decided that natural immunity doesn't exist... Why checking organizations dismissed the basic biology of natural immunity has never been made clear, but this is exactly what they did." -- A devastating takedown of Big Fact-Check by @thackerpd.*[16]
- *If fact checkers were serious about their mission, they would be checking themselves and other fact checkers. They would worry about errors of omission and commission by fact checkers. I'm afraid that they do not as a whole give the impression of being serious about their mission.*[17]

These criticisms were entirely devoid of content and were meant to trigger emotions.

Dr. Vinay Prasad also tried to spread doubt about those who corrected his disinformation. He wrote an article in which he said his critics lacked the qualifications to disagree with someone of his stature. He said:

The COVID19 pandemic reveals the limitations and arrogance of science influencers... But these 'experts' were woefully unprepared for the pandemic. Lockdowns, the possibility of lab leak, school closure, masking adults, masking kids, 5 vs 10 days of quarantine, and who should get how many doses of vaccine and when— are complex technical questions that require deep knowledge of biomedicine, trials, trade-offs, statistics, and more.

> *Science debunkers and influencers—who often don't work at universities, don't publish research, don't understand statistics, don't peer review for journals, don't have a good sense of the pre-test probability of interventions, and/or don't have deep technical understanding of drug regulation—tried to crusade against misinformation, but they made many mistakes. This would be okay if they were merely debating, but repeatedly they sought to use the tools of the platform to extinguish ideas they disliked.[18]*

Again, this wasn't a reasoned explanation of why these "science debunkers and influencers" were wrong. Dr. Prasad was making emotional accusations to spread doubt about his critics.

In another article Dr. Prasad wrote about masks and vaccines and said:

> *We are living in a world where the CDC director can say something that is false, made-up and no institution will say otherwise. At the same time, major, venerable fact checking institutions are literally asserting as fact something which is at best unproven. No matter how you feel about these issues; these are dangerous times. Truth and falsehood is not a matter of science but cultural power— the ability to proclaim and define the truth. If this continues, dark times lie ahead. Someday soon, we may not like who defines the truth.[19]*

Did the flu kill more children than COVID? The answer is no,[20] but Drs. Bhattacharya and Prasad claim that basic facts like this are up for "debate" and those who answered this question correctly were unqualified and dishonest.

In addition to calling fact checkers "liars," WWTI doctors sought to discredit their critics via cries of censorship, straw arguments, fake book reviews, tone-policing, ad hominem attacks, and poisoning the well.

> **You seek to silence discussion by slander and innuendo and abusive language rather than open it. The damage you have done to science and public health by your bullying is incalculable.**
> — *Dr. Jay Bhattacharya*

Though they claimed to value open debate, WWTI doctors reflexively framed all criticism as "harassment," "propaganda attacks," and "slander." Dr. François Balloux, for example, said I was "threatening"[21] him when I even considered writing an article disagreeing with him. When my article was finished, he called it a "hit piece"[22] and said I had "harassed" him.[23] It was impossible to disagree with WWTI doctors without triggering this reaction.

Dr. Prasad moaned about "@MonicaGandhi9 hit pieces,"[24] a "one sided hit piece,"[25] and a "hit piece on RCT."[26] Dr. Bhattacharya also said that every article that disagreed with him was a "hit piece." A few of the numerous examples are listed here:

- *An incoming **hit piece** by @latimes columnist Michael Hiltzik.[27]*
- *Hiltzik is now threatening (if I may paraphrase him) to write another **vapid hit piece** about the conference.[28]*
- *Hiltzik had written an earlier **hit piece** attempting to get the conference canceled.[29]*
- *In October 2020, Business Insider wrote a **hit piece** about the @gbdeclaration.[30]*
- *Please issue a correction to Hiltzik's **hit piece** or better yet retract it.[31]*
- *A Buzzfeed News "journalist" wrote a **hit piece** to create a scandal out of Prof. Ioannidis' doomed delegation. She abused her perch as a science communication writer to create the*

> *illusion of consensus in favor of lockdowns that did not exist then and does not exist now.*[32]

- *I wonder how many people's lives were harmed by intellectually incurious reporters, who viewed their job as conducting **hit pieces** on anti-lockdown scientists?*[33]

- *@WalkerBragman has sent a follow up email for the **hit piece** he's writing.*[34]

- *I mean the piece is an insult to **hit pieces**. I've had puff pieces written about me during the pandemic that hit harder with more substance than that.*[35]

- *The **hit piece** is so odd. She seems fixated on the fact that, as a public health professional, I have an obligation to speak to everyone respectfully, not just the people @kieraevebutler likes.*[36]

- *A senior editor of @MotherJones (@kieraevebutler) is apparently writing a **hit piece** about @VPrasadMDMPH and his take on the lack of human clinical data on the bivalent booster. Since when did Mother Jones join forces with Pfizer?*[37]

- *@kieraevebutler's **hit piece** is already up!*[38]

- *Their **hit piece** quotes Fauci, Deepti Guradsani, & Rochelle Walensky, but no one who actually signed it. This was not balanced reporting -- it was narrative enforcement of Fauci & Collins' illusion of consensus in favor of lockdown. Propaganda.*[39]

- *That was a **hit piece** based on lies, Bryan. Part of a coordinated disinformation campaign to silence dissident scientists.*[40]

WWTI doctors claimed all criticism was "slander" or part of a "smear campaign." Anyone who tried to argue facts was met with an emotional response. In a typical example of self-pity, Drs. Bhattacharya and Martin Kulldorff wrote an article titled "The Smear Campaign Against the Great Barrington Declaration." It said:

> *In October 2020, along with Professor Sunetra Gupta, we authored the Great Barrington Declaration, in which we argued for a 'focused protection' pandemic strategy. We called for better*

protection of older and other high-risk people, while arguing
that children should be allowed to go to school and young adults
should be free to live more normal lives. We understood that it
might lead to vigorous and heated discussions, but we did not ex-
pect a multi-pronged propaganda campaign that gravely distort-
ed our arguments and smeared us. We are just three public-health
scientists, after all. So how and why did this slanderous counter-
attack emerge?[41]

In reality, the GBD called for herd immunity via mass infection, but
instead of engaging with the substance and arguments of their critics,
WWTI doctors *always* dismissed criticism as "propaganda" and "slanderous counterattack." It was impossible to have good faith disagreements
with them. They were too busy parading their victimhood and accusing
anyone who corrected their false claims of "slander." Here are some
examples from Dr. Bhattacharya on social media:

- *Why did public health bureaucrats mischaracterize http://*
  gbdeclaration.org as a "let it rip" strategy? Though given
  responsibility to protect the old they lacked the creativity to do
  it without lockdown, which failed. Rather than admit inade-
  quacy, it was easier to **slander** *the GBD.*[42]
- *You are a coward. By attacking me with a false* **slander** *behind*
  a block, you have demonstrated an incapacity to engage in
  good faith discussion. Your support of lockdown and covid
  fear-mongering has done harm to children, to the poor, and
  to the working class (to the extent you have had any influence
  whatsoever). You should be ashamed of yourself.[43]
- *.@BusinessInsider should best be seen as a* **propaganda** *outlet*
  whose business model is **slander** *of people who pose a threat*
  to powerful elites. They and their ilk did tremendous damage
  to public health during the pandemic.[44]
- *How to be anti-vax, a primer:* **Slander** *everyone pointing at*

> the scientific evidence of waning covid vax efficacy vs. infection or side-effects "anti-vaxxers".[45]

- *As someone involved in public health, I view it as a professional obligation that I engage civilly and constructively even with people who I do not agree with. It's hard when some people vilify or **slander** me or attribute positions to me that I do not hold. I'm trying my best![46]*

- *It's in the country's interest that, no matter who is elected, the administration get the best scientific advice. It's shocking that naked partisanship so motivates some academics, that they would **slander** other scientists for the crime of advising politicians they don't like.[47]*

- *Atomsk, whoever you are, the paper was not retracted when I spoke about it. You are a bad, anonymous troll who traffics in innuendo and **slander**. Your behavior and demeanor are antiscience.[48]*

- *Three steps to lockdown: 1. Put a man in charge of science funding who thinks of himself as 'science itself' 2. Have that man as the government's primary advisor on pandemic policy 3. Have the government collude with big tech and media to **slander** anti-lockdown voices.[49]*

- *You seek to silence discussion by **slander** and innuendo and abusive language rather than open it. The damage you have done to science and public health by your bullying is incalculable.[50]*

That last comment was directed at Dr. Angela Rasmussen, who responded by saying:

> *It's not slander, innuendo, or abusive to factually state that you have made numerous false claims about vaccines, immunity, & the invented harms of invented lockdowns.[51]*

Dr. Rasmussen emphasized facts. Dr. Bhattacharya emphasized feelings.

This weaponization of legal terms wasn't just all idle chatter. Dr. Scott Atlas threatened to sue the 98 Stanford faculty members who wrote a letter criticizing him.[52] According to one article by Dr. Mallory Harris:

> *The threat — penned by Marc Kasowitz of the firm Kasowitz Benson Torres LLP, who served as an outside counsel to President Donald Trump during the investigation into Russian election interference — gave the letter signers until the end of the day Friday to withdraw their claims or face legal action.*
>
> *"[Y]our letter, which you wrote and sent with no regard for the truth, maliciously defames Dr. Atlas," Kasowitz wrote. "We therefore demand that you immediately issue a press release withdrawing your letter and that you contact every media outlet worldwide that has reported on it to request an immediate correction of the record."*
>
> *Kasowitz's letter was posted on Twitter by Michael Fischbach, a professor of microbiology and immunology at Stanford who signed onto the missive criticizing Atlas.*
>
> *"I stand by everything we said," Fischbach wrote. "More facts, more science. Less Kasowitz."*[53]

Fortunately, Dr. Fischbach didn't back down, but it's understandable why many people kept silent rather than subject themselves to accusations of "slander" and legal threats.

You are entering into a phase of countries that we used to criticize severely like the USSR, like communist China...I mean, this is almost the end of our civilization if we have this sort of censorship, I'm afraid
— Dr. Scott Atlas

In the summer of 2024, I was invited to give a talk on the WWTI movement by a health agency in a red state whose governor was under consideration for the vice-presidential nomination. I was instructed to keep politics out of my talk, and I agreed. My plan was to merely show videos of WWTI doctors' pro-infection comments from 2020. Reality didn't seem political to me.

However, upon reviewing the videos, my invitation was rescinded as this health agency didn't want to upset politicians in their state and jeopardize their funding.

I was not pleased, but I didn't center my identity around this canceled talk. I also understood where the conference hosts were coming from. They were worried I might upset important politicians in their state, and I would have felt horrible had my talk negatively impacted their vaccine outreach. Although I was silenced, censored, and canceled for purely political reasons, no WWTI doctors came to my defense. However, WWTI doctors were not so shy when it came to their own "cancellation."

There are reasonable debates to be had about content moderation, as well as the government's role in requesting disinformation be limited. It's true that YouTube and Twitter removed or deprioritized some content produced by WWTI doctors. Perhaps that was wrong. Legal cases involving potential government censorship and WWTI doctors—namely Dr. Bhattacharya—made it up to the Supreme Court. Dr. Bhattacharya lost his case. The majority opinion said that:

> *Neither the timing nor the platforms line up... so the plaintiffs cannot show that these restrictions were traceable to the White House officials. In fact, there is no record evidence that White House officials ever communicated at all with [the social media platforms in question].*[54]

In an article about the SCOTUS ruling, Mike Masnick wrote:

> *Bhattacharya responded to this ruling on his X account, without acknowledging what the Supreme Court actually said. Instead, he said that "free speech in America, for the moment, is dead." Except anyone who actually read the ruling would see that's not what was said at all. Instead, the court pointed out that internet companies, as private entities, have the right to moderate as they see fit, and without actual traceable evidence of government coercion, there was no evidence of a First Amendment violation. Indeed, as (Justice Amy Coney) Barrett wrote, the evidence showed that the platforms were all moderating similar content "long before" anyone in the government spoke to them about anything, and further that the evidence shows that moderation actions from the platforms appeared to be exercises of "independent judgment." She further noted how even when some White House officials later flagged content to review, the platforms were quick to push back and respond that the content in question "did not violate company policy."*
>
> *Basically, this was all an example of the marketplace of ideas at work, not censorship.*[55]

I never followed this legal drama very closely. The fate of a few YouTube videos and tweets did not seem that important to me, especially considering the doctors who made them were loud, famous, influential, and wrong about life and death matters. I also know that doctors killed by COVID—including several I knew—were truly silenced.

However, social media content became the central part of the pandemic for some WWTI doctors. They wanted more attention and more influence, and they felt YouTube had robbed them of the platform to which they were entitled. In the mirror world, tweets were more important than COVID's victims, and celebrity doctors who advised world leaders were silenced and censored. For example, while I quoted a snippet of this previously, consider the entire press release from April 2021:

> *Govenor Ron DeSantis Holds Roundtable with Public Health Experts to Discuss Big Tech Censorship.*
>
> *Tallahassee, Fla. – Today, Governor Ron DeSantis held a roundtable with renowned doctors and epidemiologists to discuss Big Tech censorship and the COVID-19 pandemic. Today's meeting follows the recent decision by Google to remove video footage of a previous roundtable the Governor held with these experts from its video-sharing platform, YouTube.*
>
> *"YouTube's decision to remove the video of our previous roundtable is just another example of unabashed overreach and bias by Big Tech," said Governor DeSantis. "Silicon Valley and the corporate media have drawn a line in the sand: they don't care about the facts. They only care about pushing their agenda and will do so by whatever means necessary, the truth be damned. That's why we are taking action here in Florida to hold Big Tech accountable and call out their hypocrisy."*
>
> *Watch the Governor's roundtable by clicking HERE.*
>
> *The following individuals participated in the roundtable with Governor DeSantis:*
>
> - *Dr. Scott W. Atlas, MD, Robert Wesson Senior Fellow in health care policy at the Hoover Institution of Stanford University*
> - *Dr. Jay Bhattacharya, professor of medicine at Stanford University and research associate at the National Bureau of Economic Research*
> - *Dr. Martin Kulldorff, PhD, biostatistician, epidemiologist, and professor of medicine at Harvard Medical School*

"There's nothing more dangerous than being able to censor what is said in a country, because then you are simply not ever going to even hear the truth. And you are entering into a phase of countries that we used to criticize severely like the USSR, like communist China...I mean, this is almost the end of our civilization if we have this sort of censorship, I'm afraid," said Dr. Scott Atlas.

"For science to work, you have to have an open exchange of ideas...If you're going to make an argument that something is misinformation, you should provide an actual argument. You can't just take it down and say, 'Oh, it's misinformation' without actually giving a reason...Let's hear the argument, let's see the evidence that YouTube used to decide it was misinformation. Let's have a debate. Science works best when we have an open debate," said Dr. Jay Bhattacharya.

"We need to have debates, rather than censoring...When we do censoring and slandering, even if we are willing to continue to speak out, there are many other scientists that I know, including junior scientists, who do not want to speak out because they see what's happening to us. They don't want to have to go through the same thing. So, we really need a debate," said Dr. Martin Kulldorff.[56]

In April 2021, after hundreds of thousands of Americans had already died of COVID and with hundreds of thousands more deaths yet to come, WWTI doctors centered on their "censorship" because YouTube had removed one of their videos. They considered themselves pandemic victims and were utterly indifferent to what had happened in hospitals for the past year. WWTI doctors and their supporters produced an overwhelming amount of content bemoaning their "censorship" and experience with social media. Some examples of their speeches and podcasts include:

- Stanford's **Censorship**: An Interview with Dr. Scott Atlas[57]
- Free Speech is in Dire Shape[58]
- Dr. Scott Atlas: On **Censorship**, Academic Freedom, and the Pandemic[59]
- Dr. Scott Atlas on COVID Failures and How **Censorship** Kills[60]
- SARS2 Pandemic & **Censorship** | Scott W. Atlas, Martin Kulldorff, Jay Bhattacharya[61]
- Free to Investigate: Dr. Scott Atlas on the Freedom in the Sciences[62]
- Twitter **Censors** Famed Epidemiologist Martin Kulldorff[63]
- Stanford's **Censorship**: An Interview with Dr. Jay Bhattacharya[64]
- The Twitter Blacklisting of Jay Bhattacharya[65]
- The Biden Administration Tried to **Censor** This Stanford Doctor, But He Won in Court[66]
- Dr. Jay Bhattacharya: The Supreme Court Thinks Government Can Threaten Social Media Companies[67]
- Scientist Who Battled for Covid Common Sense Over Media and Government **Censors** Wins Top Award[68]
- How Scientific 'Groupthink' **Silenced** Those Who Disagreed with Covid Lockdowns[69]
- Biden's Covid **Censorship** STRUCK DOWN in Court: Jay Bhattacharya INTERVIEW[70]
- Jay Bhattacharya: Free Expression and Unsettled Science[71]
- The End of Free Speech is the End of Science with Jay Bhattacharya[72]
- How Stanford Failed the Academic Freedom Test[73]
- COVID 19 **Censorship** | Dr. Jay Bhattacharya & Dr. Gigi Foster[74]
- Social Media **Censorship**: Jay Bhattacharya vs. Kate Klonick[75]
- Dr. Jay Bhattacharya: This Was **Censorship**[76]

- Dr. Jay Bhattacharya: The Dangers of Big Tech **Censorship** on Public Health[77]
- Universities Shred Their Ethics to Aid Biden's Social-Media **Censorship**[78]
- The Government **Censored** Me and Other Scientists. We Fought Back—and Won.[79]
- Free Speech on Trial[80]
- Dr. Bhattacharya: Francis Collins DESTROYED Scientists Who Favored Covid Lab-Leak Theory[81]
- SCOTUS Versus Free Speech[82]
- The Contagion of Covid Policy: Dr. Jay Bhattacharya on Freedom of Speech[83]

Meanwhile, when talking about young people killed by COVID, WWTI doctors could only ever say, "The old have a thousand-fold higher mortality risk than the young."[84] They treated the fate of a very small percentage of a massive volume of online material with more gravitas than any of COVID's young victims.

These complaints of censorship predictably provided another opportunity to bash public health. During one interview, Dr. Bhattacharya said, "It's not like public health is infallible."[4] Dr. Bhattacharya also spoke about the "censorship industrial complex"[85] endlessly on social media. To pick one example amongst many, he said:

> If you f**king love science, you should oppose the censorship industrial complex. The censors are bad at science and they make it impossible for actual science on important topics to get done.[86]

He also frequently pretended that he was a victim of a fictional "Ministry of Truth," sending multiple tweets such as:

> The American medical and public health establishments threw away public trust in them during the covid era. Their support for a government Ministry of Truth is a sign of weakness. And what

makes them think they would control the ministry forever?[87]

Dr. Bhattacharya even mentioned his imagined "Ministry of Truth" 13 times in his opening statement to the U.S. House of Representatives Select Subcommittee on the Coronavirus Crisis, accusing it of not saying enough nice things about the virus. Dr. Bhattacharya said:

> *The Ministry has consistently downplayed or censored the truth about lasting and robust immunity after COVID recovery, despite overwhelming evidence in the scientific literature documenting this fact.*[88]

Noting that the "Ministry of Truth" existed only in the mirror world, several Congressmen mocked Dr. Bhattacharya for pretending it was real.

> ***Congressman Jamie Raskin:*** *And I just want to be clear about this. The Ministry of Truth was one of four government ministries in Oceana in Orwell's fictional 1984. It does not exist in the United States or anywhere on earth. Do you disagree with that?*
>
> ***Dr. Jay Bhattacharya:*** *No, I've referred to it, as I said, as a joking shorthand.*
>
> ***Rep. Jamie Raskin:*** *Okay. Well, I just never heard a scientist refer to a fictional entity so repeatedly and so consistently as something real in the world.*
>
> ***Congressman Raja Krishnamoorthi:*** *Sir, you quote something called the Ministry of Truth, which you jokingly refer to in your expert witness, I'm sorry, in your opening testimony. Are you aware of something called the, quote, publicity department of the Chinese Communist Party?*
>
> ***Dr. Jay Bhattacharya:*** *No.*
>
> ***Congressman Raja Krishnamoorthi:*** *Okay. I presume that you would never want to talk to an organ of the publicity department*

Jonathan Howard 615

of the Chinese Communist Party, right?

Dr. Jay Bhattacharya: *I don't know anything about it.*

Congressman Raja Krishnamoorthi: *Sir, you gave an interview on May 5th, 2020 to China Global Television Network, which is owned by the publicity department of the Chinese Communist Party. And you know what they did with your interview? They posted it on their Facebook page. You became a mouthpiece of the publicity department of the Chinese Communist Party. This was pure propaganda.*[89]

Dr. Bhattacharya would later say this "attack" was "among the lowest moments of the pandemic for me."[90]

Now, in 2025, with WWTI doctors in power, the headlines read: "RFK Jr. Threatens to Bar Government Scientists from Publishing in Leading Medical Journals,"[91] "Medical Journals Hit with Threatening Letters from Justice Department,"[92] and "Top NIH Nutrition Researcher Quits, Citing Censorship Under Kennedy."[93]

There needs to be a quick and devastating published take down of its premises.
— *Dr. Francis Collins*

WWTI doctors did more than claim they were censored because of the loss of a YouTube video and some tweets. They claimed that they were censored and silenced if anyone even *considered* disagreeing with their *premises*. Shortly after the GBD was signed in October 2020, Dr. Francis Collins sent an email that read:

> *This proposal from the three fringe epidemiologists who met with the Secretary seems to be getting a lot of attention- and even a co-signature from Nobel Prize winner Mike Leavitt at Stanford.*

There needs to be a quick and devastating published take down
of its premises. I don't see anything like that on line yet- is it
underway?[94]

This email was intended for three people, and it became public only
after a Freedom of Information Act request by the American Institute
for Economic Research (AIER). However, this email became the defin-
ing moment of the pandemic for several WWTI doctors, the same way
watching a healthy 23-year-old die of COVID in April 2020 was the
pandemic's most enduring memory for me. Dr. Bhattacharya shared a
screenshot of the email on social media and said:

So now I know what it feels like to be the subject of a propagan-
da attack by my own government. Discussion and engagement
would have been a better path.[95]

Dr. Bhattacharya, who is alive and well, fortunately, lamented being
called fringe endlessly on social media. He posed with a t-shirt about it[96]
and recorded a long, somber video titled "Stanford Prof. Jay Bhattacharya Responds to Being Called 'Fringe' in Collins, Fauci Emails."[97] He
even read the email in his testimony before Congress and said:

In the following days, I was subjected to what I can only describe
as a propaganda attack. Though the GBD called public health
authorities to think more creatively about how to protect vulnera-
ble elderly people from covid, reporters accused me of wanting to
let the virus rip.[98]

Dr. Bhattacharya felt that being called fringe was a great affront, and
he wanted others to be angry on his behalf. After all, if he can be called
fringe in an email, then anyone could be called fringe in an email. Even
on his first day as NIH director, when over 1,000 employees were fired,
Dr. Bhattacharya gave an interview to Bari Weiss where he complained

that he was called fringe four and a half years previously.[99] Dr. Bhattacharya said he should receive a public apology from Dr. Collins.

Dr. Bhattacharya was not alone in treating this email and the word "fringe" as the pandemic's seminal moment. In his article "Public Health Should Lose Your Trust," Dr. Prasad said the "FDA and NIH and CDC engaged in lies and propaganda."[100] His top reason as to why was:

Lack of debates/ smearing scientists who disagreed

We were making unprecedented massive decisions and we had ~zero debates. Worse, any dissent was punished. Francis Collins, NIH director, famously emailed Anthony Fauci calling for a "quick and devastating" take down of the "fringe" epidemiologists who opposed lockdowns...

It's one thing to act in times of uncertainty. It is another thing to stifle dissent and dialog [sic]. In many ways talking with the "fringe" epidemiologists could have helped us. We might have reached a compromise, with schools opening sooner than they otherwise would.

If I got together with a couple of my buddies and wrote a 1-page declaration under the watchful eye of a pro-tobacco, child-labor advocate, I would not feel this action alone entitled me to an audience with top government officials and to have them enact my policies.[101] In contrast, Dr. Prasad believes that our nation's public health leaders *were obligated* to meet with and "compromise" with advocates of herd immunity through mass infection. He said that anything less "shuts down" debate. We'll see if he invites his critics for public debates now that he is in power.

WWTI doctors frequently misrepresented Dr. Collins' email. For example, Dr. Kulldorff said:

And the NIH director, Francis Collins asked for a published

take-down on me and Sunetra Gupta and Jay Bhattacharya after
writing the Great Barrington Declaration calling us fringe epide-
miologists.[102]

Dr. Bhattacharya tweeted about a "Ministry of Truth can't tell right
from wrong, and organizes devastating takedowns of government critics,"[103] and Dr. Prasad accused Dr. Collins of calling for a "'quick and
devastating' take down of the 'fringe' epidemiologists."[104]

In reality, Dr. Collins did not ask for a "take down" of anyone. He
felt the plan for the mass infection of unvaccinated youth was unwise,
and a strongly worded rebuttal of its *premises* might be of value. He
wanted public debate, which is totally fine. Scientists strongly disagree
with each other's *premises* all the time. The *premises* of the GBD are not
sacrosanct and above criticism as WWTI doctors implied.

This hypersensitivity to being called "fringe" and to having one's
premises challenged was obviously absurd, but it was not benign. First,
it served as a distraction technique. Time spent discussing the word
"fringe" was time not spent discussing the tragic real-world consequences
of pro-infection policies.

Second, it sent a clear message to potential critics of WWTI doctors:
Be very careful. If you're not courteous and circumspect at all times,
even in emails, we'll accuse you of stifling "dissent and dialogue."[100] If
you slip and call someone "fringe," that will be treated as public health
failing #1.

In the mirror world, WWTI doctors were owed a safe space and anyone who even considered publicly disagreeing with their *premises* was
guilty of censorship. In the real world, this is normal and appropriate. As
one social media commentator rightly put it:

Seems to me that debate about the Barrington Declaration wasn't quashed at all. The declaration was signed and released and many scientists responded, mostly to argue that it was based on false premises and was not a workable solution. That's not censorship any more than subjecting journal articles to peer review is censorship. Just because your argument doesn't hold up well under scrutiny, you don't get to cry "censorship". Come up with a better argument.[105]

Indeed.

The bigger problem is that lockdowners [...] think that living your life is an irresponsible act. Sending your kids to school is an irresponsible act. The implication is that unless you comply with his prescription -- lockdown with no logical endpoint -- you are irresponsible.
          — *Dr. Jay Bhattacharya*

It's dishonest to put your words in someone else's mouth and then declare victory over your own creation. I always quote people accurately and fully. I don't want to misrepresent anyone's views. I have a small YouTube channel that is nothing but videos of WWTI doctors. You can hear Dr. Bhattacharya claim that COVID is milder for people under 70 or that children don't spread COVID. My writing is full of accurate quotes with references so readers can check my work.

This basic courtesy was never repaid to me, however. Most doctors mentioned in *We Want Them Infected* ignored it, which is their perfect right. No one owes me their time or a response. However, of the doctors who chose to respond to it, none of them did so in good faith. None of them quoted a passage and explained why they disagreed. None of them laid a glove on the content. They didn't even try. Instead of disagreeing with what I wrote, they made things up.

The month after *We Want Them Infected* was published, Dr. Bhattacharya blasted the following message to his 500,000 social media
followers:

> *I wasn't going to comment on the inane Jonathan Howard*
> *(@19joho) book on the pandemic, but I ran across an unhinged*
> *claim by him that illustrates perfectly a certain covidian mindset*
> *that is too perfect to pass up...*
>
> *Let's also leave aside his deep lack of understanding of the idea*
> *of herd immunity, which is a biological fact and the endpoint of*
> *any strategy we follow, whether lockdowns, focused protection,*
> *or let-it-rip. California and NY followed lockdowns, and every-*
> *one got infected anyway!*
>
> *(Free advice for you, Jonathan: maybe take an epidemiology*
> *class if you don't want to keep embarrassing yourself in public*
> *further?)*
>
> *The bigger problem is that lockdowners like Howard (an NYU*
> *doctor, I think), think that living your life is an irresponsible act.*
> *Sending your kids to school is an irresponsible act. The implica-*
> *tion is that unless you comply with his prescription -- lockdown*
> *with no logical endpoint -- you are irresponsible.*
>
> *But he's wrong. Living your life is not irresponsible. Absent*
> *tremendous laptop class privilege, there is and was no way to*
> *hide away from the virus forever without harm to your physical,*
> *psychological, and economic health.*
>
> *The unspoken root idea of his is that the general public owed it to*
> *doctors to not get covid because it would place doctors at risk of*
> *getting covid. Of course this is an inversion. Medical profession-*
> *als serve the public, not the other way around.*[106]

Dr. Bhattacharya, who did not treat any COVID patients, signaled he was too important to even google my name—*"Howard (an NYU doctor, I think.)"* In addition to featuring many accurate quotes from Dr. Bhattacharya, I described my experience working at Bellevue Hospital during NYC's 2020 COVID nightmare in *We Want Them Infected.* Indeed, after someone suggested he actually read my book, Dr. Bhattacharya shared his "review" of it and responded:

> *You mean this guy? I don't think I'll learn much from his book Richard. It seems you've learned all the wrong lessons.*[107]

Dr. Bhattacharya wrote a completely fake review of *We Want Them Infected*, only to later reveal that he never read it. He put his words in my mouth, making me sound like both a jerk and a moron while ignoring what I actually wrote. The same doctor who said, "The public is watching this spat and has lost trust in science, medicine, and public health,"[8] called me "inane" and "unhinged." The same doctor who said he treats ideas that he might disagree with "respectfully because I might be wrong,"[4] conjured a fantasy of *We Want Them Infected* and presented it to the world as fact. That's wildly dishonest, but it was not uncommon.

Dr. Balloux also wrote a fake review of *We Want Them Infected*, saying:

> *The inane thesis of Howard's book, a turgid lament that had medics/scientists been less complacent, no one would have gotten infected.*[108]

Again, I accurately quoted Dr. Balloux, who said in a now deleted tweet, "If the objective were to send SARCoV2 into endemicity, then healthy kids have to be exposed to the virus, ideally earlier than later,"[109] and explained why I disagreed with this. In return, he made things up about my book to make me look like a moron and erase my writing.

Dr. Joseph Fraiman wrote a bizarre screed that read:

Hi @19joho your book "we want them infected" I'm one of the handful of people who bought it, ...wow it is really bad. It's painful to read the words of a self-proclaiming scientist so out of touch with reality who has no idea how out of touch he is.

Were you surprised your book sales have been so poor?

Your tweets were getting so much attention, you maybe got fooled given your tweets were artificially throttled up for extra viewing by being pro-government narrative and pro- pharma (they used to get to push that Twitter throttle and de-throttle.). But sadly for you they can't throttle up book sales.

It is shocking you don't realize, but most Americans now know they were lied to by our government and scientists like you. They know lockdowns hurt more than they helped, those school closing you supported destroyed our children, as did the worthless masking you supported. Also most realize the vaccine is worthless at best & are upset, they got fooled into taking it. Your track record for pandemic recommendations has been 100% harmful.

I'm sure your book isnt selling. Most Americans have learned better, despite being fed the government propaganda you gladly parroted the last couple of years.

Your book is a going to live in history as testament to the thoughtless and harmful government recommendations scientist's embarrassing didn't oppose for fear of losing their jobs and some like your self stupidly supported.

You book is being judged poorly today by nearly all Americans (your book sales are the example) but even worse you will be judged more harshly by generations to come. As now nearly all realize the ideas you promoted were wrong and harmful, yet you could not see this and published a book doubling down on your own hubris...I actually feel bad for you, as I don't think you realize how silly you look right now.[110]

Deceptive strawman arguments were exceedingly common, and they served a valuable purpose. Anyone who acknowledged COVID's toll was blamed for it, which obviously discouraged people from acknowledging COVID's toll. For example, anyone who recognized that overwhelming COVID outbreaks could affect schools was told, "Those school closings you supported destroyed our children." Meanwhile, what I actually wrote didn't matter at all to WWTI doctors. They misrepresented and silenced my words, all while claiming that "science works best when we have an open debate."[3]

We need more civil discourse.
— *Dr. François Balloux*

Some WWTI doctors treated manners and decorum as more important than COVID itself. However, their complaints about indecorous behavior were only made in defense of certain voices, and they had no problem dishing out a deluge of immature insults themselves.

On April 27, 2020, Drs. Jeffrey Flier and Prasad wrote a defense of "independent thinkers, like John Ioannidis," titled "Scientists Who Express Different Views on Covid-19 Should Be Heard, Not Demonized."[111] Though the pandemic had just started, Dr. John Ioannidis had already made *many* obviously wrong claims. For example, on April 9, 2020, he said:

If I were to make an informed estimate based on the limited testing data we have, I would say that covid-19 will result in fewer than 40,000 deaths this season in the USA.[112]

Though the death tally would be surpassed in just eight days, Drs. Flier and Prasad weren't concerned that his overly optimistic predictions might cause some people to underestimate a very dangerous virus. Instead, they were concerned that critics might hurt Dr. Ioannidis' feelings. They wrote:

> *At the same time, academics must be able to express a broad range of interpretations and opinions... We think it is important to hear, consider, and debate these views without ad hominem attacks or animus... We believe that the bar to stifling or ignoring academics who are willing to debate their alternative positions in public and in good faith must be very high...*
> *Society faces a risk even more toxic and deadly than Covid-19: that the conduct of science becomes indistinguishable from politics. The tensions between the two policy poles of rapidly and systematically reopening society versus maximizing sheltering in place and social isolation must not be reduced to Republican and Democratic talking points, even as many media outlets promote such simplistic narratives. These critical decisions should be influenced by scientific insights independent of political philosophies and party affiliations. They must be freely debated in the academic world without insult or malice to those with differing views.*[111]

They worried Dr. Ioannidis would be deprived of a platform to which he was *entitled.* They concluded:

> *Scientific consensus is important, but it isn't uncommon when some of the most important voices turn out to be those of independent thinkers, like John Ioannidis, whose views were initially doubted. That's not an argument for prematurely accepting his contestable views, but it is a sound argument for keeping him,*

and others like him, at the table.

On social media, Dr. Prasad explained why he cared so much about someone calling Dr. Ioannidis mean names, writing:

> *If someone says the IFR (infection fatality rate) is low and 1000 people call him an idiot or worse, yes that is chilling and silencing and dangerous and what we discuss.*[113]

Dr. Prasad thought it was *dangerous* if anyone called Dr. Ioannidis an idiot.

As bodies piled up, Dr. Flier continued to claim that mean words might be worse than a virus that killed and disabled many millions of people. In March 2021, he expressed concern for the feelings of economist Emily Oster after she was criticized for her article, "Your Unvaccinated Kid Is Like a Vaccinated Grandma."[114] Dr. Flier said:

> *I don't know @ProfEmilyOster but her writing in this area has been a valuable addition, subject to appropriate discussion/debate in areas of ongoing uncertainty. Vitriolic attacks against her reflect a moral sickness that may rival COVID19 in its ultimate harm to public health.*[115]

Dr. Prasad also worried about hurt feelings and bad manners. He wrote an article titled "The Tragedy of COVID19," which didn't lament the loss of life. Rather, Dr. Prasad wrote again about mean words toward Dr. Ioannidis and said:

> *Yet, during the pandemic, COVID19 policy issues became extremely heated and politically polarized. I was shocked and dismayed...What I view as the tragedy of COVID19 is that medicine had no way to have a dialogue about any important issue without devolving to ad hominem.*[116]

Drs. Prasad and Ioannidis also wrote an article, "Constructive and

Obsessive Criticism in Science," that lamented harassment and scientific bullying with "ad hominem aspects," saying:

> *Typical behaviors include: repetitive and persistent comments (including sealioning), lengthy commentaries/tweetorials/responses often longer than the original work, strong degree of moralizing, distortion of the underlying work, argumentum ad populum, calls to suspend/censor/retract the work of the author, guilt by association, reputational tarnishing, large gains in followers specifically through attacks, finding and positing sensitive personal information, anonymity or pseudonymity, social media campaigning, and unusual ratio of criticism to pursuit of one's research agenda.*[117]

They never responded to the substance of their critics and instead wrote that "ignoring obsessive critics may be the most effective way to cut their blood line."

Several other WWTI doctors were also concerned about decorum. Dr. Balloux said, "we need more civil discourse,"[118] as well as:

> *I appreciate everyone is a bit tense by now, but a modicum of rigour, respect and civility may be helpful to allow the scientific community to get through the tail of the pandemic and its aftermath reasonably unscathed.*[119]

That was in September 2021, right after the Delta wave peaked and just before Omicron arrived.

Dr. Stefan Baral similarly said:

> *At the beginning of covid, I was worried that academics personally attacking other academics with whom they didn't agree would undermine the respect for academia and ultimately the power of evidence in driving policy. But that ship has long since*

sailed and the respect for academics and academia has been permanently diminished. I don't know the way forward as many of the self-professed misinfo or disinfo specialists are amongst the worst perpetrators of this.[120]

Dr. Bhattacharya put out an impassioned plea for civility in his article "The Scientific Establishment Is Turning 'Science' Into a Dogmatic Tool of Oppression." He described the Great Barrington Declaration (GBD) as being about the "focused protection of the vulnerable elderly, for opening schools, and for lifting lockdowns"[8] and said:

Scientists who do choose to participate in debates about science or public health policy are met with slanderous attacks, not just by social media companies but by scientist bruisers who lobby accusations of racism, sexism, antisemitism, false allegations of conflicts of interest, and even mass murder at us rather than engage in good faith debate. The public, who would benefit from sober, reasoned discourse, is instead presented with bluster from scientific bullies who intimidate their targets into silence... Science thrives on skepticism, on challenges to the status quo. When the pursuit of scientific truth is sacrificed on the altar of ideological conformity, science ceases to be a beacon of enlightenment and instead becomes a tool of oppression.

Fair enough. While it is ludicrous to suggest that "vitriolic attacks" against sheltered doctors might rival COVID's carnage, I won't argue that tone and decorum is unimportant. I try to engage with doctors' words and ideas, and I never want to bully anyone into silence. Quite the opposite. WWTI doctors claim to be censored, and I do my best to amplify and preserve their words. While I can be blunt and snarky, I hope my writing is free of juvenile japes and content-free insults. After all, I also know what it's like to be on the receiving end of "bluster from scientific bullies."

@19joho is a B-list Covid Twitter influencer and a grifter with no domain expertise, who wrote noxious blogposts and even a silly book.
— *Dr. François Balloux*

Indeed, WWTI doctors who treated civility as the highest virtue when they were critiqued responded to my writing with childish insults. They called me "objectively anti vax" because I presented accurate information on the pediatric COVID vaccine. The fact that *We Want Them Infected* was for sale was used as "evidence" that it was worthless, which of course would invalidate every book. They called me "dishonest, nasty, and woefully ignorant" and ignored or insulted anyone who asked for examples of my dishonesty, nastiness, and woeful ignorance.

While Drs. Prasad, Baral, Flier, Balloux, and Bhattacharya extolled the virtues of civilized scientific debate, here is some feedback they gave me for the sin of accurately quoting them and explaining why I disagreed.

- *I blocked Howard a long time ago. He is dishonest, nasty, and woefully ignorant in his prior writing. No reason to think that has changed. An exemplar of the failings of medical twitter.*[121]
- *I've been frequently 'harassed' on social media including by @medpagetoday contributors. @19Joho is the worst. He's deeply dishonest, unhinged and vile. Then, I appreciate it's just part and parcel of his grift and he's got a book to flog. The two people who wrote proper hit pieces about me are @19Joho and @AlexBerenson. This may look like 'horseshoe theory', but it's actually easier to explain by greed. Both were prepared to cause major damage to childhood vaccination programmes to push sales of their shite books...His behaviour was*

bit of a mystery to me, until I realised he was trying to cash in on a Covid book. Then it all started to make sense....[23]

- *Here you are already, shouty as always. Intellectually, I rank you on the level of antivaxx cranks such as such Wakefield, Yeadon, Berenson and Malone, and you're equally damaging vaccine stewardship with your dogmatic idiocy.*[122]

- *@19joho_is a B-list Covid Twitter influencer and a grifter with no domain expertise, who wrote noxious blogposts and even a silly book. His shtick is to cite scientists and doctors out of context and misrepresent their views.*[123]

- *@19joho approaches everything through the lenses of conspiracy theory, and seems incapable to engage with any argument even marginally in variance with his dogmatic and often uninformed views. He reminds me of Alex Berenson, just with polar opposite opinions.*[124]

- *Joseph you can't indulge someone just trying to make money from selling a book.*[125]

- *In fairness Dr Howard is just hawking his book so can't blame the man for trying to line his pockets during a pandemic when he saw so many of his friends doing the same.*[126]

- *But what he does have is nine truly terrible books on Amazon. The man clearly doesn't earn enough wherever he works and I sincerely hope it's all been worth it.*[127]

- *It won't since no one cares enough to actually worry about a person like him. But I do feel pity for how sad his life must be and do wish him better days ahead.*[128]

- *Twitter's biggest book-selling shmuck...*[129]

- *Is this about Jojo? It took a while for me to get there. But indeed, he's a stain on the academy.*[130]

- *Just asked you to leave me alone... Still praying that*

happen one day.[131]

- *At this point, twitter is just about driving people to his book and their blog. I have actually thought about this--if I arrive at the pearly gates and am told that if I read just one of these blog posts I could spend eternity in heaven... It's not clear to me what I would do.*[132]

- *I pity him,@surrealtruther. He seems like a man broken by an extended encounter between deeply held (but false) ideas about the way the world works and the way the world actually works.*[133]

- *It's amazing. He's objectively anti vax.*[134]

Scientists who treated zero COVID patients told doctors who worked in hospitals throughout the pandemic that they lacked "domain expertise."

I was nothing special. Dr. Prasad routinely called people "idiots,"[135] "STUPID,"[136] a "bunch of fools,"[137] and "total morons."[138] He often said those who disagreed with him were "mentally ill" and "off their rocker."[139] He said doctors who didn't treat vaccine side effects more seriously than COVID were "motherfuckers" and "fucking morons."[140] He said they were "just as stupid as the people shooting ivermectin in their ass." The Cancer Letter even wrote an article titled "Vinay Prasad Describes His Vanderbilt Colleagues As 'Despicable,' Raising New Questions About Physicians' Conduct on Social Media" that said:

> *A Google search for the words "Vinay Prasad" and "despicable" will yield evidence of the UCSF faculty member's fondness for the d-word. Applying it to colleagues at another academic institution—in this case, Vanderbilt—is, of course, a breach of decorum most physicians and scientists would avoid.*[141]

In fact, Dr. Prasad often said things like:

- *Ashish is full of shit. There is no evidence to tell a 20-year-old man who had covid to get the shot. It is probably net harmful. No evidence that benefits any third party. Totally derelict drug regulation. Pfizer gets money. No randomized data. Total failure.*[142]

- *Medhi Hasan is an idiot. Of course we have to learn to live with covid. Everyone is living with it. That is precisely what happened. No one gives a shit about COVID anymore & no one sane is taking any precautions. It even bores me & I know fully how wrong the establishment was.*[143]
- *Laurie Garrett is a lot like James Watson. She won the Pulitzer, and he won the Nobel prize. Then both of them started saying crazy shit.*[144]

Dr. Flier never criticized Dr. Prasad for this. He only felt that critics of Professor Oster and Dr. Ioannidis had to watch their every word.

Dr. Bhattacharya also launched a flood of childish insults against anyone who disagreed with him. He said Dr. Fauci was "probably the number one anti-vaxxer in the country"[145] because he didn't treat vaccines as a perfect panacea in 2021, and according to an article by Dr. Mallory Harris:

Bhattacharya amplified Twitter threads that doxxed student researchers at the Stanford Internet Observatory.[52]

Dr. Balloux called a frontline doctor "dickhead,"[146] and Dr. Baral called those who disagreed with him "online trolls,"[147] "a bunch of clowns,"[148] and a "mediocre twitter gang."[149] Dr. Baral also defended Dr. Ioannidis by saying:

I'm just saying that John Ioannidis remains a leader in the field no matter what the twitter morons say.[150]

Incredibly, some of this behavior even made its way into medical literature. Although he later removed it, Dr. Ioannidis published a paper titled "Reconciling Estimates of Global Spread and Infection Fatality

Rates of Covid-19: An Overview of Systematic Evaluations,"[151] which included a lengthy tirade against several people—namely epidemiologist Gideon Meyerowitz-Katz—who criticized him. Dr. Ioannidis said:

> In multiple main media interviews and quotes Meyerowitz-Katz is presented professionally as an "epidemiologist", but apparently he has not received yet a PhD degree as of this writing and he is still a student at the University of Woolongong in Australia. Neither he nor his co-author of the evaluation (apparently another PhD student) had published any peer-reviewed systematic review or meta-analysis on any topic prior to the pandemic...
>
> At that time, the name of the Twitter account owner was not obviously visible (the photo showed an unrecognizable figure with big glasses and a cat), but Meyerowitz-Katz seemed to use the Twitter account prolifically to promote his own work and criticize work contradicting his work. The identity of the Health Nerd Twitter account has become transparent now, since the owner has added a photo of him (wearing a T-shirt that writes "Trust me, I am an epidemiologist"). The identity of the reverberating Atomsk's Sanakan Twitter account is still unclear (to me at least) and its relationship to Meyerowitz-Katz, if any, is unknown.[152]

Dr. Ioannidis also authored a paper titled "Citation Impact and Social Media Visibility of Great Barrington and John Snow Signatories for Covid-19 Strategy" to undercut signers of the John Snow Memorandum, a rival to the GBD. In it, he calculated the "Kardashian index," a satirical metric of social media prominence, of the respective signers and concluded:

> Both GBD and JSM include many stellar scientists, but JSM has far more powerful social media presence and this may have shaped the impression that it is the dominant narrative.[153]

Rather than discuss the arguments of the John Snow Memorandum, Dr. Ioannidis chose to belittle and cast doubt on its authors and their credentials.

> **At the beginning of covid, I was worried that academics personally attacking other academics with whom they didn't agree would undermine the respect for academia and ultimately the power of evidence in driving policy.**
> — *Dr. Stefan Baral*

Dr. Bhattacharya was not wrong when he worried about "bluster from scientific bullies who intimidate their targets into silence."[8] Dr. Baral was not wrong when he worried that:

> *Academics personally attacking other academics with whom they didn't agree would undermine the respect for academia and ultimately the power of evidence in driving policy.*[120]

Dr. Prasad was not wrong when he said that childish name-calling is "chilling and silencing and dangerous."[113] Indeed, WWTI doctors used insults and personal attacks because they wanted to chill and silence their critics.

As with disingenuous exhortations that *certain* doctors should not blend politics and medicine, WWTI doctors applied their high standards of decorum, not to themselves, but rather *only* to those doctors who objected to the mass infection of unvaccinated youth. Those doctors had to be the epitome of decorousness and sobriety with their every utterance. After all, "critical decisions should be... freely debated in the academic world without insult or malice to those with differing views."[111] Meanwhile, they launched a tsunami of nastiness against their critics while ignoring their actual arguments.

Tone policing is almost always about content, not tone, and it serves several functions.

First, it shields *certain* doctors from criticism. Anyone who corrects disinformation spread by WWTI doctors will be accused of "vitriolic attacks" and forced to defend themselves against charges they are acting unprofessionally. However, by framing their criticisms with regards to tone, the tone police seek to silence potential critics and make them feel like they are walking on eggshells. Of course, strident criticisms are not "vitriolic attacks." As long as they are based in reality, they are part of a healthy discussion and debate.

Second, the tone police seek to preemptively destroy the reputation of anyone who corrects their disinformation. WWTI doctors falsely portrayed fact checkers as overwrought and not worth listening to.

Finally, tone-policing is a distraction technique. Every moment discussing manners is a moment not spent discussing the consequences of anti-vaccine disinformation.

Doctors who sincerely believe in the value of civil tone apply their standards equally and consistently. WWTI doctors did not. Their hypocritical admonitions to avoid personal attacks were nothing more than a tactic to shame and discredit unwanted voices and preemptively discredit unwanted opinions, all by doctors who claim to value "free and open debate."

> **The groupthink in this country has been so painful.**
> *— Dr. Monica Gandhi*

"Poisoning the well" is an informal fallacy where adverse information about a target is preemptively presented in order to mock and discredit the target's positions and ideas.[154] WWTI doctors made liberal use of this technique to falsely portray their critics as hysterical and blinded by conformity. In so doing, they not only spread doubt about their critics but also avoided dealing with the substance of their arguments.

Nearly all of the quotes below come from social media; however, WWTI doctors used identical language in their articles, podcasts, and YouTube videos. I share these quotes to demonstrate the uniformity and consistency of their messaging. It's important to pay attention to the linguistics of the pandemic. WWTI doctors sounded very much alike as they repeatedly inundated the public with the same words and phrases, all carefully chosen to signal in-group loyalty and to spread doubt and mistrust.

Ironically, one of their messages was that everyone else was guilty of groupthink. According to *Psychology Today*:

> *Groupthink is a phenomenon that occurs when a group of well-intentioned people makes irrational or non-optimal decisions spurred by the urge to conform or the belief that dissent is impossible. The problematic or premature consensus that is characteristic of groupthink may be fueled by a particular agenda—or it may be due to group members valuing harmony and coherence above critical thought.*[155]

Everyone wants to consider themselves an independent thinker, and according to WWTI doctors, everyone except for them was blinded by groupthink. Only they were able to see the world objectively, as it really was. Yet, they all sounded the same as they robotically accused others of groupthink.

- **Dr. Martin Kulldorff, April 2021:** *"Academics must urgently counter the very real danger of **groupthink** ... At least politicians are explicit about their disagreements. ...The world is a crazy place when an academic is extoling [sic] the honesty of* *politicians." -@profpauldolan*[156]

- **Dr. Martin Kulldorff, May 2021:** *"The short circuit of the pandemic has led to a dramatic tightening of **groupthink** among public health pundits." -@michaelbd*[157]

- **Dr. Monica Gandhi, June 2021:** *Yes, the **groupthink** in this country has been so painful @MartyMakary because I know we all are colleagues, all trying to work on the COVID problem together, all trying to help, but seems like it has to be done the same way here.*[158]

- **Dr. Martin Kulldorff, October 2021:** *"Researchers in a particular field can be so paralyzed by .. **groupthink** that only those outside of their field, .. other scientists and the public, can aid in the .. corrective process of science .. to get closer to the truth." - immunologist @stemplet74*[159]

- **Dr. Martin Kulldorff, December 2021:** *Picking weak spokespeople undermines debate and encourages **groupthink**. It is a cheap mainstream media tactic. -@VPrasadMDMPH_in@ brownstoneinst*[160]

- **Dr. Martin Kulldorff, December 2021:** *"The emails suggest a feedback loop: The media cited Dr. Fauci as an unquestionable authority, and Dr. Fauci got his talking points from the media .. This is how **groupthink** works." -@WSJ*[162]

- **Dr. Lucy McBride, January 2022:** *This clip of @ZDoggMD on tribalism/**groupthink**/social media is spot on.*[162]

- **Dr. Lucy McBride, January 2022:** *I have teenage kids. I see teens as patients. Like adults, teens can be vulnerable to myriad things *at once*: COVID-19, isolation, fear, **groupthink** ... They also can be smarter than adults! They are our future. We need to empower them w education & critical thinking skills.*[163]

- **Dr. Vinay Prasad, January 2022:** *Many are true believers, others may be financially biased by specific for-profit products Most may not be familiar with the underlying evidence, but subscribe to **groupthink**. After all, it is natural we cannot think about all topics ourselves, and must trust others interpretaton*

[sic].[164]

- **Dr. Marty Makary, February 2022:** *Amen, grateful to the many physicians who kept their scientific objectivity &stood up to the estab bullying.* **Groupthink** *hurt us bad: Surface transmission, barbaric hosp visitation policies, closing schools, narrow dosing interval, cloth masks, ignoring nat immunity, boosting kids.*[165]

- **Dr. Marty Makary, February 2022:** *One of the most devastating conseq of medical* **groupthink** *for which many were complicit: shutting out family from visiting dying loved ones. Great piece by @MartinKulldorff. Thank u @DrJBhattacharya @VPrasadMDMPH et al for speaking against this human rights violation at the start!*[166]

- **Dr. Vinay Prasad, April 2022:** *My disappointment with my fellow progressives centers on restrictions done on kids (a huge error), our failure to push for randomized trials so we remain ignorant, and the* **groupthink** *that kept us from reconsidering.*[167]

- **Dr. Marty Makary, May 2022:** *NIH's failure to fund rapid research on the big Covid questions early (Airborne vs surface, cloth vs quality mask, distancing, nat immunity, etc.) resulted in an evidence void. Opinions filled that vacuum, resulting in Covid policy guided by* **groupthink** *opinion rather than science.*[168]

- **Dr. Jay Bhattacharya, July 2022:** *"Prasad spoke on...the failure of lockdowns, ... mask & vaccine mandates, & school closures and restrictions on children. Says that* **'groupthink'** *overtook the medical establishment early in the pandemic" Great interview of @VPrasadMDMPH.*[169]

- **Dr. Vinay Prasad, October 2022:** *This was from March of 2022. Now it is Oct and no one does it, and no one laments that Just remember the "health experts" the media prefers-suffer from* **groupthink**.[170]

- **Dr. Marty Makary, December 2022:** *Organizations spread-*

ing Covid misinformation ==> the NYT &NPR. Both blindly parrot the dogma of govt doctors just like as they did with govt declarations of WMDs in Iraq. They forgot their job to question as journalists. Instead they became activists for the medical **groupthink**.[171]

- **Dr. Vinay Prasad, January 2023:** *One thing that sticks with me from this article is that Stanford never asked Jay to present his views at Grand Rounds You can't be a place of learning and be unwilling to hear and discuss reasoned points of view in times of crisis and uncertainty.* **Groupthink** *run rampant.*[172]

- **Dr. Vinay Prasad, January 2023:** *"Common sense advice" = not supported by any data whatsoever in the last 20 years, and never previously advised. The irony is that the authors are the partisans, struck in* **groupthink***, incapable of reading the evidence.*[173]

- **Dr. Vinay Prasad, February 2023:** *An unimaginable crisis These kids are lost They all got covid anyway Had school never closed, they would have graduated high school Their lives were ruined b/c of* **groupthink** *Prepandemic guidance said not to close schools 4 virus like this Sad.*[174]

- **Dr. Marty Makary, February 2023:** *Natural immunity (first observed during the 430BC Athenian plague) worked against Covid severe disease. The totality of data has proven wrong Public Health officials and the medical* **groupthink***, just as it did on their dogma that myocarditis was more common after Covid infection than after the vaccine. Great video by Dr. Prasad.*[175]

- **Dr. Martin Kulldorff, March 2023:** *"An illuminating conversation on the dangers of* **groupthink** *and herd mentality in science and the solutions to preventing such thinking for future crises." -@ScottAtlas_IT.*[176]

- **Dr. Vinay Prasad, April 2023:** *There are huge issues here beyond this appointment. If monumental public Health choices are made in a feedback loop between elites on Twitter, political* *parties, and the media, we are doomed to* **groupthink**, *cheer-leading, and bad choices.*[177]

- **Dr. Marty Makary, May 2023**: *Just amazing. The establishment* **groupthink** *bypassed the scientific method of using data and instead arrogantly used political absolutism as they decreed medical dogma and censored respected physicians with different opinions (who ended up being correct). The science is now clear.*[178]

- **Dr. Scott Atlas, June 2023**: *"[C]enters of academic scholarship, ideological tolerance, & intellectual discipline have degenerated into cesspools of partisanship, anti-intellectualism, &* **groupthink***. [O]n full display…when Scott Atlas, a public expert who happened to be right about everything on Covid, was heckled by graduating students at New College of Florida."*[179]

- **Dr. Vinay Prasad, July 2023:** *Scott Atlas was pro school opening and anti toddler masking. He was guilty of touching Trump's hand and generally being correct Treated unfairly by crazed,* **groupthink** *faculty.*[180]

- **Dr. Vinay Prasad, September 2023:** *During the spring of 2020, I had many private conversations with faculty across the globe critical of the school closures that were going on. And yet, zero debates at universities on this topic. That's a testament to how spineless they have become. Run by* **groupthink***.*[181]

- **Dr. Vinay Prasad, September 2023:** *Wow, what a quote. US policy on masking kids down to 2 yo could only happen w/ incompetent leaders who suffer from* **groupthink** *can't read data are ignorant of behavioral interventions low success & lack common sense truly crazy times.*[182]

- **Dr. Jay Bhattacharya, March 2024:** *But it is important to know what you went through. Your experience points to the fact that our academic institutions need reform if they seek to be places where science can thrive. The purpose of the non-*

*sense you faced was to create **groupthink** and an illusion of consensus in favor of bad science. Thank you, Tracy. You are a hero.*[183]

In reality, this is what groupthink looks like, and it is not the only example of WWTI doctors using similar phrases to manipulate their audience.

The Pandemic Has Created a Market for Gloom and Doom
— *Dr. François Balloux*

By August 2021, 610,000 Americans had died of COVID,[184] and the Delta variant was ravaging many parts of the country. According to an article that month:

> *The state is experiencing its worst surge of the pandemic. Last week, it was averaging nearly 25,000 new cases every day. The previous high, in January, was about 18,000. More than 17,000 Floridians are hospitalized with Covid-19, another record; around 230 people are dying every day. Florida leads all states in the number of hospitalizations and deaths per capita.*
> *The city of Orlando has urged residents to limit their water use, because the same liquid oxygen used to treat the water supply is being used to provide air to Covid-19 patients. The Florida health department asked the federal government to send more ventilators as the number of hospitalized patients spiked.*[185]

Yet, that same month, an article appeared titled "Prof Francois Balloux: 'The Pandemic Has Created a Market for Gloom and Doom.'" It said:

> **Can you explain what you mean by "scientific populism"?**
> *As the pandemic has advanced the mood of the public has be-*

come darker and more fearful and this has created a market for
gloom and doom. It's as bad as the effects of the super-optimism
at the beginning – stay at home for two weeks, it's a mild disease
or wear a mask and it will be gone.[186]

To be fair, Dr. Balloux's comment about "doom and gloom" was not *entirely* off-base. There were a handful of doctors who gained prominence by sending out FIVE-ALARM RED ALERTS!!! about every variant and purported COVID sequelae. I never did that, and I won't defend it. False alarms likely numbed some people to COVID's real risks.

Yet, doom and gloom were often an appropriate response to mass death, while the death toll of excessive COVID fear is probably zero. However, by portraying nearly all concerns about COVID as "doom and gloom," even in 2020, WWTI doctors sought to spread doubt and signal that anyone more cautious than they was hysterical and not to be taken seriously. Dr. Balloux was deeply offended that not everyone shared *his* personal standard of concern. He felt cautious people should keep quiet, and they were as bad as people who completely denied the pandemic at its start.

Several WWTI doctors even attempted to shame cautious people by claiming that anyone who was "doom and gloom" was hurting vaccine uptake. In a March 2021 article, Dr. Monica Gandhi said:

The second concern translating to "doom and gloom" messaging
lately is around the identification of troubling new variants due
to enhanced surveillance via viral sequencing.[187]

Delta and Omicron would arrive within the year. Perhaps more people would have been vaccinated had they been more concerned about these variants. Yet WWTI doctors told them not to worry in interviews such as "Pandemic Exit Interviews: Stop Panicking About the Covid-19

Variants, Says UCSF's Monica Gandhi," from February 2021.[188]

- **Dr. Zubin Damania, March 2020:** *Guess what? It's not all* ***gloom and doom*** *people, we can do this. Our latest update, re-corded live. #covid19.* [Editor's note: Dr. Damania's Twitter/X account has since been deactivated.]

- **Dr. François Balloux, August 2020:** *Some countries dealt competently with their #COVID19 public communication. For instance, Switzerland did well, no excessive* ***doom & gloom*** *and a focus on the uncertainties. This may explain why the Swiss population feels comparably untraumatised, despite significant cases/deaths.*[189]

- **Dr. François Balloux, September 2020:** *I had never fully realised until now that the reason pandemic brought down so many empires and kingdoms in history, wasn't the death toll, but the fear, the sense of* ***doom***, *the irrationality and the disunion they unleashed.*[190]

- **Dr. Zubin Damania, October 2020:** *Welcome to the show, we're heading into fall and the media all over the place is banging the drums of* ***doom***.[191]

- **Dr. François Balloux, October 2020:** *#COVID19 is a severe health crisis, which adds to this burden in multiple ways but pretending it should dictate the way we live our lives long-term is misleading if not sinister.*[192] *Such* ***doom-mongering***, *besides being uninformed is deeply unhelpful. Spreading the myth of a dystopian future ahead of us undermines public engagement in pandemic mitigation measures that are essential for us to get to the other end of #COVID19 as unscathed as possible.*[193]

- **Dr. François Balloux, January 2021:** *A refreshingly opti-mistic article on the way out of the #COVID19 pandemic. @ rwjdingwall makes a strong case against condemning society to a dystopian future of endless* ***doom and fear***, *whilst recog-nising the severity of the current situation.*[194]

- **Dr. Monica Gandhi, January 2021:** *Try not to* ***doomscroll***, *seriously. Think of that cloud dissipating over the earth; has* *been such an incredibly hard time and I am sorry for every single person on this planet (including those talking about **doom**) because we are all having such a hard time. Light is so so close.*[195]

- **Dr. François Balloux, January 2021:** *The pandemic has unleashed a vision of an apocalypse bordering on the religious at times. Once it will become clear this is not the end times, I expect the addiction to pandemic **doom and gloom** will recede, with people resuming more meaningful lifes.*[196]

- **Dr. Monica Gandhi, January 2021:** *The best way to do this is to not message on **doom/gloom** now that we have the vaccines but do everything in our power to get everyone access to these vaccines which are so so protective!*[197]

- **Dr. Monica Gandhi, January 2021:** *So, this is too important not to stress. Vaccines will get us out of this pandemic- anger/ quibbling/**doom** can lead people to doubt vaccine and decline it. This reminds me of the @mask debate actually. Remember some fought against the message it "protects you and others".*[198]

- **Dr. Monica Gandhi, January 2021:** *Until this journalist @ CodyBroadway did this story, I am not sure I understood the addictive power of **gloom** messaging. Please watch addiction expert (I was just hyper; coffee; skip that). If **doom** messaging addictive, networks put doom messengers on TV.*[199]

- **Dr. Monica Gandhi, January 2021:** *I am completely confused by it. the reason we should be excited by vaccines is to get us out of this. Addiction to **doom and gloom**?*[200]

- **Dr. Monica Gandhi, January 2021:** *Well, I don't think people would be so elated about vaccines (and concerned about slowness) if they didn't know it was to get back to 'normal'. Maybe addiction to **doom/gloom**?*[201]

- **Dr. Monica Gandhi, January 2021:** *I think it's complicated- there is something addictive about **fear and doom** apparently to humans so addiction "sells". But with these amazing vac-*

cines, I see nothing else to concentration upon but hope.[202]

- **Dr. Monica Gandhi, January 2021:** *you only have to live like this until summer. Please listen to all of the optimism and try to phase out the **doom**.*[203]

- **Dr. Monica Gandhi, January 2021:** *There will be an end... soon. And oh yes, I should have mentioned overweight problem and non-healthy eating during a time of **doom**.*[204]

- **Dr. Monica Gandhi, January 2021:** *What will happen with vaccines is that - when we see the hospitalizations go away (100% effective for this dire outcome so far, still marveling)- all arguments on messaging and who can be the most **doom-filled** will go away.*[205]

- **Dr. Zubin Damania, February, 2021:** *Radiant joy, positivity, laughter, and a cute dog... countdown to the Twitter COVID **doom-bags** taking a s**t on us? w/ the amazing @Monica-Gandhi9 #variantschmariant, The End Of The Pandemic (w/ Dr. Monica Gandhi).* [Editor's note: Dr. Damania's Twitter/X account has since been deactivated.]

- **Dr. Monica Gandhi, February 2021:** *Yes, these vaccines expected to decrease infections. Many have tweeted extensively on it and I wrote a thread on this with all sorts of IgG/IgA references! But the **doom/gloom** is persisting and that is okay.. it will lift by itself because the results will be clear with roll-out.*[206]

- **Dr. François Balloux, February 2021:** *To get to the other end of the pandemic as unscathed as possible. The world needs more: - cautious optimism - realistic endpoints - empathy / compassion - acknowledgment of uncertainty And less: - **doom & gloom** - dystopian predictions - blame / ostracism - dogmatism / ideology.*[207]

- **Dr. Monica Gandhi, February 2021:** *Right, that is exactly what we want to combat by messaging hope, optimism and excitement about these vaccines getting us out of this! It will happen definitively now that we see the data from the trials* *(**doom sayers** can mutter all they want then).*[208]

- **Dr. Monica Gandhi, February 2021:** *This is something I wrote that summarizes the points I have been making by tweets. Good to have optimism; not good to message **doom.***[209]

- **Dr. Monica Gandhi, February 2021:** *Want to Motivate Vaccinations? Focus on Optimism, Not **Doom.***[210]

- **Dr. Monica Gandhi, February 2021:** *Yes, I somehow didn't blame the media before but I should have - they get the same people to comment on **doom** as they can't believe the good news and maybe want to keep us on the **doom** hamster wheel for as long as they can.*[211]

- **Dr. Monica Gandhi, February 2021:** ***Doom & gloom** seems to be part of the narrative from many in the scientific community because they got politicized in the last administration and they are sticking to it. But it is okay; all of this will fall away when we watch what happens (like is happening elsewhere) w/ mass vax.*[212]

- **Dr. Monica Gandhi, February 2021:** *They were so **doom-y** for so long (and yelled at me & other) for not being **doom-y**. But that's okay; as long as they come around, great. I just hope CNN/MSNBC who have a lot of influence put on people who are not talking about **doom** too much moving forward.*[213]

- **Dr. Monica Gandhi, March 2021:** *Really important article. I know we say "we will deal with that later" but the anxiety provoked by the pandemic (and by too much **doom** messaging) is real and has real-world consequences for patients. Please message optimism. Vaccines are here; we will get through this now.*[214]

- **Dr. Monica Gandhi, March 2021:** *I think it's an addition to fear, an addition to **doom**, and perhaps an addiction to being on TV or in the paper. It will pass.*[215]

- **Dr. Lucy McBride, March 2021:** *Agree- I don't subscribe to the notion that fear motivates. I also think **doom & gloom** messaging doesn't reflect the facts...my point here is that people* *are often motivated by witnessing someone's humanity...as a physician (and human) myself, I was moved by her words in this clip.*[216]

- **Dr. Lucy McBride, March 2021:** *The **doom and gloom** message is off - I agree. The real world data is extraordinarily hopeful. And most humans are not motivated by fear. But I do think that by showing us her humanness and by being REAL she might motivate people to get vaccinated.*[217]

- **Dr. Monica Gandhi, April 2021:** *Well, I know I keep on showing the evidence but here is the evidence and here is a thread. Don't worry, even the most pessimistic, variant-discussing, **doom-steeped** people are no match for the vaccines!*[218]

- **Dr. Monica Gandhi, April 2021:** *That's okay if I haven't convinced anyone - the vaccines will persuade even the most **doom-based** messenger eventually.*[219]

- **Dr. Monica Gandhi, April 2021:** *I see, well, the **doom & gloom** reporters & experts are no match for these vaccines. So, wait it out & the vaccines will win even the most **doom/gloom** messengers over!*[220]

- **Dr. Lucy McBride, April 2021:** *I thoroughly enjoyed my live convo w/ @MonicaGandhi9_last week on #vaccine efficacy & optimism; replacing fear w/ facts; & shifting the public narrative from **doom and gloom** to hope. The vaccines are the clear path forward; let's sing it from the hilltops!*[221]

- **Dr. Zubin Damania, April, 2021:** *"Impending **doom** for COVID," says the CDC. More people like Michael Osterholm going on TV and saying we're in for a fourth surge, things are really scary. Aaaaah! Okay can we have a rational discussion about things like the fourth surge, variants, vaccines, and what we should do because I think we're all tired of the fear mongering... And we're done with the pandemic. All this talk about there's an impending sense of **doom**, don't jump the gun, don't do all this. How about this, shut up and get the vaccines out there in as many arms as you can.*[222]

- **Dr. Monica Gandhi, May 2021:** *As I have always said, the most **doom-based**, variant-focused, non-T-cell based person in the world is no match for the power of these vaccines![223]*

- **Dr. Monica Gandhi, June 2021:** *And cases continue to go lower despite 20% being delta, so it is okay to want to motivate vaccination, but please don't continue the **doom/gloom** messaging, please.[224]*

- **Dr. Monica Gandhi, June 2021:** *keep schools restricted instead of following metrics-based approach where restrictions for kids cease when @CDC metrics of low hospitalizations (<5/100K in population reached); 4) **doom based** messaging so common but can paradoxically decrease vax uptake.[225]*

- **Dr. Monica Gandhi, June 2021:** *Know we are all delta variant right now but look- plummeting cases since April 14 when we passed 40% 1st dose, cases continue to go down, deaths reached <300, this is the impact of vaccines on the US epidemic. Instead of **doom**, celebration that we have means to end epidemic in US.[226]*

- **Dr. François Balloux, July 2021:** *those who seem to be most easily terrorised by 'bad covid news' already tend to follow dedicated doomsday accounts, but their daily dose of **doom & gloom** is unlikely to affect much their already prudent behaviour.[227]*

- **Dr. François Balloux, August 2021:** *There is a massive international surveillance effort for SARSCoV2 Variants of Concern (VoC). The next VoC should be flagged early and rapidly reported by reputable sources (e.g. PHE, ECDC). Thus, I recommend everyone try to ignore twitter **doom-mongers** announcing end-times VoCs.[228]*

- **Dr. François Balloux, September 2021:** *Announcing new SARSCoV2 variants is an unbeatable strategy in epi-game theory. The chance of being right is tiny - there has been no variant of concern that emerged in 2021 until now.[229] Though, if you hit the jackpot with your SARSCoV2 variant, you can*

smugly look down on everyone until the end times. If you're
wrong, you just delete the thread, and no one really cares, as
*the attention has moved on to the latest 'variant of **doom**'.*[230]

- **Dr. François Balloux, December 2021:** *The reason I tend to*
favour a hopeful and uplifting messaging is due to a sense of
moral responsibility towards others.[231] *Spreading terror, **doom***
and gloom from a position of authority, however well intend-
ed the underlying objectives may be, is not something I can
condone. There needs to be hope and clear endpoints for any
public health measure to be justifiable.[232]

- **Dr. Jay Bhattacharya, January 2022:** *Another enormous*
study of long-COVID in children with a control group finds
that the syndrome is vanishingly rare. It is far past time for
***doom-mongering** doctors & public health officials, who are*
causing parents to panic for no good end, to desist.[233]

- **Dr. François Balloux, July 2022:** *Maybe because many are*
fearful and traumatised, and we have become accustomed to
*the constant **doom & gloom** nonsense that grifters relish, feed*
on, and fuel.[234]

- **Dr. Monica Gandhi, August 2022:** *I wrote a piece February*
*2021 of messaging optimism about the vaccines (not **doom &***
***gloom**) if we wanted better uptake like Europe; I feel failing to*
infuse confidence in the vaccines is one of the greatest failure
of (mostly Democrat) messaging on them over past year.[235]

- **Dr. Monica Gandhi, September 2022**: *I also thought they*
were important in 2020 but I think places that signaled life
would return to normal (e.g. not wearing masks) with vaccines
*had higher vaccine uptake. we signaled **doom** & said nothing*
would change with vaccines in US, not good messaging.[236]

- **Dr. François Balloux, May 2023**: *Most of those measures*
rapidly stop making sense outside a 'forever pandemic' mind-
*set. The despair and **doom mongering** was the necessary fuel*
for public health overreach, not just a symptom.[237]

- **Dr. François Balloux, August 2023:** *The pandemic's over*
now, and it's actually been over for a while, whatever metric

we may choose to use. That doesn't mean everything's great, but the pandemic provides no excuse anymore for any of us not to try to engage with life.[238] *There are endless pandemic grifters and ghouls who have a vested interest in pretending the pandemic isn't over, and won't be over ever, and as they're getting increasingly desperate because they realise their grift/abuse is over, their claims are getting increasingly baroque.*[239] *As the livelihood, relevance and control over peoples' lives of those grifters and ghouls entirely depend on them spreading never-ending* **gloom** *and* **doom***, and misery, them being ignored, laughed at, or scolded, will just make them go away into the irrelevance they deserve.*[240]

- **Dr. Jay Bhattacharya, November 2023:** *The Hopkins Map of* **Doom***, made to look like a real-life video game, was an irresponsible misrepresentation of disease risk.*[241]
- **Dr. Jay Bhattacharya, March 2024:** *We are approaching the three year anniversary of former cdc director @RWalensky's infamous video in which she shared her sense of "impending* **doom***." If there is a more irresponsible piece of public health communication out there, I don't know what it is.*[242]

According to WWTI doctors, a lack of cheerfulness was a significant problem during the pandemic.

Some zero covid people are apparently appearing on some propaganda show on MSNBC, saying that school is bad for kids.
— *Dr. Jay Bhattacharya*

It's true that some doctors advocated for zero COVID early in the pandemic, though it soon became clear that totally eliminating the virus was an impossibility. I certainly never argued for it. Nonetheless, well after most people realized zero COVID was a fantasy, WWTI doctors created doubt about their critics by saying *anyone* who disagreed with them as being a zero COVID zealot. In so doing, WWTI doctors portrayed their critics as deluded while ignoring the substance of their criticisms.

- **Dr. Martin Kulldorff, December 2020:** *We do know that there is more than a thousand-fold mortality risk between old and young. **Zero-COVID** is impossible in US/UK, and focused protection minimizes #COVID19 mortality irrespectively of R0, IFRs and herd immunity thresholds.*[243]

- **Dr. François Balloux, February 2021:** *An excellent read. It gives a good feel for what will likely be the major societal conflict ahead of us. At the risk of being blunt, **#ZeroCovid** is not compatible with the individual rights and freedoms that characterise postwar democracies.*[244]

- **Dr. Vinay Prasad, February 2021:** *Every week in the hospital, IRL, docs who lurk tell me that the worst part of twitter is: COVID absolutism Shame & blame doom & gloom failure to understand tradeoffs failure to understand prob/ risk illogical testing recs & of course **#zerocovid**.*[245]

- **Dr. Vinay Prasad, February 2021:** *Indeed Covid **zero** is not going to happen, but normal life still can--- correction will.*[246]

- **Dr. Martin Kulldorff, September 2021:** *#ZeroCovid is, and always was, a pipe dream. Let's focus on zero #Polio instead. That's doable.*[247]

- **Dr. Jay Bhattacharya, September 2021:** *The **zero-COVID** movement is dangerous misinformation. If I were not in favor of free speech, I would demand censorship. Instead, I think more & better speech is the answer.*[248]

- **Dr. Martin Kulldorff, December 2021:** *Among politicians and journalists ignorant about infectious disease epidemiology, **Zero COVID** was a prevailing 2020/2021 view, with the unrealistic and destructive aim for complete containment.*[249]

- **Dr. Martin Kulldorff, January 2022:** *"**Zero Covid** was finally rejected as the guiding principle. Canadian politicians and experts had to admit that we do not have the technology to stop Covid. It was a tragic mistake to base policy on an* *unrealistic fantasy." -@MikkoPackalen.*[250]

- **Dr. Martin Kulldorff, April 2022:** *"As zero Covid advocates recover from Covid, we may eventually reach herd sanity." -@ VPrasadMDMPH.*[251]

- **Dr. Jay Bhattacharya, April 2022:** *Zero covid was a destructive utopian fantasy in March 2020 and it still is. The difference is that now only the naive and credulous still believe in the ideology. Unfortunately for the people of Shanghai, this includes the government of China.*[252]

- **Dr. Francois Balloux, April 2022:** *"Zero Covid is not compatible with the individual rights and freedoms that characterise post-war democracies," says Prof Francois Balloux, director of University College London's Genetics Institute.*[253]

- **Dr. Jay Bhattacharya, July 2022:** *Zero-covid logic: the only way to prevent a lockdown is to have a lockdown.*[254]

- **Dr. Jay Bhattacharya, July 2022:** *If only we had had Shanghai style drones on our streets reminding people to control their 'desire for freedom' while people run out of food, locked into their apartments. Then the laptop class could have had zero covid. At least we should have died trying.*[255]

- **Dr. Jay Bhattacharya, January 2023:** *People who believe in a flat earth do no harm to others by their false belief. People who believe in zero-covid, on the other hand, did so much harm...*[256]

- **Dr. François Balloux, May 2023:** *A difficulty in the #COVID19 discussion lies in many failing to acknowledge trade-offs in any pandemic mitigation measure. This is rarely explicitly stated. One exception is the 'zerocovid' CAG group whose first mission statement states "There is no trade-off".*[257]

- **Dr. Jay Bhattacharya, August 2023:** *Some zero covid people are apparently appearing on some propaganda show on msnbc, saying that school is bad for kids, and so closing schools was good & maybe we should keep schools closed. I am stunned it needs to be said. School is good for kids. Covidian-*

ism is a cult.[258]

- **Dr. Vinay Prasad, August 2023:** *The only people who thought covid caused type 1 diabetes were the **zero COVID** zealots who cannot read research. All of the papers making such claims were laughable. Many used icd10 codes.*[259]
- **Dr. François Balloux, March 2024:** *I don't know what fraction of the population those 'Covid-terrorised' represent, but given the traction some insane, irrational and totally 'non-scientific' **Covid-zero** tweets still attract it may be a non-trivial number of people who are suffering for no good reason.*[260]
- **Dr. Jay Bhattacharya, May 2024:** *I wonder if the @washingtonpost regrets publishing this bit of anti-science invective in Dec. 2020. Thinking like this pushed harmful school closures and other destructive policies into 2021 and beyond. Neither then nor now did we have the technology to get to **zero covid**.*[261]

Draconian mitigation efforts to delay the time to meet the virus make no sense.
— Dr. Vinay Prasad

Doctors who warned of "doom and gloom" when it came to COVID embraced doom and gloom when it came to measures to contain it. They routinely used frightful, histrionic language to scare people about mitigation measures, describing them all as "draconian."

- **Dr. John Ioannidis, March 2020:** ***Draconian** countermeasures have been adopted in many countries.*[262]
- **Dr. Marty Makary, January 2022:** *Great article by Georgetown student Jacob Adams about the university's **draconian** Covid protocols & conflicting policies, which now include a booster mandate--I'd love to see ANY data that boosters in young people lower hospitalization risk. @freebeacon.*[263]
- **Dr. Vinay Prasad, January 2022:** ***Draconian** mitigation ef-

forts to delay the time to meet the virus make no sense. Makes no sense for a vaccinated person to wear an n95 or equivalent. Certainly makes no sense, and is borderline insane, to make a child wear such a mask.[264]

- **Dr. Lucy McBride, February 2022:** *Thank you. I fully realize that people are suffering a lot more than he is. Everyone is exhausted & worn out It's just that it doesn't make sense any longer. I honestly cannot figure out for the life of me how these colleges can justify the* **draconian** *measures. It's not adding up.*[265]

- **Dr. François Balloux, August 2022:** *Also mitigation measures should have been enforced in a much kinder, smarter way. I'm still shocked that pandemic policies that had such high public support were primarily enforced through arbitrary,* **draconian,** *repressive and oppressive means.*[266]

- **Dr. Monica Gandhi, February 2023:** *Interesting thing, @ BallouxFrancois , is that I lived in US city/state with most* **draconian** *measures (latter associated with liberal politics, which confused me since #harmreduction in HIV went other way politically): think my arguments for school openings helped moderate SF a bit.*[267]

- **Dr. Jay Bhattacharya, May 2023:** *It was the Canadian truck drivers who forced Trudeau to relax his* **draconian** *mandates. So grateful for all truckers. #honkhonk.*[268]

- **Dr. Martin Kulldorff, September 2023:** *"One of the most disturbing images of the Covid-19 pandemic was when a teacher .. forced a mask on a crying toddler .. In some ways, the U.S. government .. treated all of us like toddlers, compelling us to endure* **draconian** *Covid measures" - @HRaleighspeaks.*[269]

For WWTI doctors, there was no such thing as a "non-draconian" measure to control COVID.

Public Health = COVIDian. That's why no one trusts them.
— *Dr. Vinay Prasad*

Some WWTI doctors made frequent use of the phrases "covidian cruelty," "covidian zealots," "covidian tyranny," "covidian madness," and "covidian authoritarian overreach" to discredit their critics and avoid the content of their arguments.

- **Dr. Martin Kulldorff, July 2021:** *It is an article of faith contrary to scientific evidence that recovery from COVID does not provide long lasting immunity. Hence, if you have had COVID and do not want to abide by vaccine mandates, you can claim a religious exception for not belonging to the **Covidian church**.*[270]

- **Dr. Vinay Prasad, January 2022:** *This is still going to get worse for the CDC as the goals & mother nature keep clashing Zero covid/ **covidian zealots** will not be happy to accept reality.*[271]

- **Dr. Jay Bhattacharya, February 2022:** *I thank the folks who shared their stories of grief & loss amidst **covidian cruelty** with me. @MartinKulldorff collected your stories & published them here. No one should have to die alone. Healing starts with an unflinching devotion to the truth.*[272]

- **Dr. Martin Kulldorff, April 2022:** *"Shanghai's lockdown has held up a mirror to the West's **Covidian zealots**. .. The era of lockdownism started with shocking footage from China, and so it should end." -@galexybrane in @compactmag_*[273]

- **Dr. Vinay Prasad, January 2023:** *I am also worried about this. The only really challenging commentary in any med journal was Offit/ vax/ NEJM and just b/c E. Rubin is annoyed by Marks (see CNN quotes) BMJ series awful **covidian bias** Top journals intolerant of debate Science mag is just a DNC superpaC now.*[274]

- **Dr. Vinay Prasad, February 2023:** *Public Health = COVIDi-*

***an*. That's why no one trusts them.**[275]**

- **Dr. Jay Bhattacharya, October 2023:** *WIth the whole world watching, the Canadian truckers won an enormous civil rights victory for all Canadians. They struck an enormous blow against **covidian authoritarian overreach**.*[276]

- **Dr. Jay Bhattacharya, November 2023:** *If lockdowns, school closures, mask and vax mandates, and **covidian tyranny** work to protect human life, why don't they?*[277]

- **Dr. Jay Bhattacharya, January 2024:** *I am grateful to everyone who has stood up at any point in the last four years against **covidian tyranny**, especially those who did so at personal cost. There may be issues and times in future where we disagree, but you will always have my deep respect and admiration. Thank you!*[278]

- **Dr. Jay Bhattacharya, January 2024:** *Good news out of Canada. The Ontario group that oversees doctors there has dropped its persecution of Dr. Jean Marc Benoit for the crime of tweeting true things it didn't like. The illusion of consensus in favor of **covidian insanity** was created by such persecutions.*[279]

- **Dr. Jay Bhattacharya, January 2024:** *Justin Trudeau violated the basic civil rights of the hero Canadian trucker protestors, who freed Canada from Trudeau's **covidian tyranny**. Glad to hear of this new court ruling.*[280]

- **Dr. Jay Bhattacharya, January 2024:** *Apparently, the **covidian cult** thinks 'we' had to destroy the health and well being of children, the poor, and the working class to fail to protect the elderly from covid. There was another way for those with eyes to see…@gbdeclaration. Lockdown = let it rip among the poor.*[281]

- **Dr. Jay Bhattacharya, January 2024:** *It's a complicated set of motives. Some had financial motives. Others, professional jealousy. Still others personal covid panic. There were also some true believers in **covidian tyranny**. The university itself* *was focused on brand protection.*[282]

- **Dr. Jay Bhattacharya, March 2024:** *I got to meet my good friend, Br. @NahasNewman in real life today! Over the years, he has taught me more about the mysteries of the* **covidian faith** *than I ever wanted to know.*[283]
- **Dr. Jay Bhattacharya, June 2024:** *@ZubyMusic, it was wonderful to finally meet! Even more fun to discuss the psychology of what made some people stand up against the* **covidian madness**, *while others stayed silent.*[284]

This was all meant to signal in-group bias and trigger emotions.

> **I can understand why BioNTech and Pfizer wanted to deny immunity after covid infection.**
> — *Dr. Jay Bhattacharya*

Vaccines are made by pharmaceutical companies, and these companies are often unpopular for good reasons. However, WWTI doctors often made gratuitous criticisms of these companies to spread doubt about the science behind vaccines and public health in general.

- **Dr. Marty Makary, November 2022:** *The cozy relationship between gov't health agencies and* **Pfizer & Moderna** *evidenced by closed door meetings and the lack of transparency around clinical trial outcomes data has damaged public trust. It's clear why the top 2 vaccine experts at the FDA quit last year in protest.*[285]
- **Dr. Scott Atlas, May 2023:** *Speaking at Friday's Academia's COVID Failures symposium...Atlas claimed that [university hospitals, funded by]* **Pfizer**, *a key in COVID vaccine development, used infants and toddlers in clinical trials for a disease from which they faced little to no danger.*[286]
- **Dr. Vinay Prasad, July 2024:** *Scott Gottlieb moved from FDA to the* **Pfizer** *board of directors, and then allegedly coordinated with social media companies to suppress criticism of the*

vaccine. Doesn't get more unethical than that.[287]

- **Dr. Jay Bhattacharya, August 2024:** *I can understand why BioNTech and Pfizer wanted to deny immunity after covid infection. I mean, look at what immunity is doing to BioNTech's bottom line! But why did governments, scientists, and public health deny such a basic biological fact for so long?*[288]

- **Dr. Martin Kulldorff, October 2024:** *With only emergency authorization, Pfizer and Moderna ads had to declare that their COVID vaccines were not fully tested. They did not! Nor did their ads follow the law of reporting side effects.*[289]

As usual, none of this is new. As the meme shows, anti-vaxxers have long depicted doctors as nothing more than pharma shills, even though vaccines keep people healthy and out of the hospital.

TRUTH
Mainstream "Doctors" are simply
Big Pharma Sales Reps
in White Coats.
Pushers for a Cartel
whose profits depend upon sick people.

Making you Healthy
is not
part of the Equation

Keeping a
Customer Base

The unyielding push to vaccinate kids with a COVID19 vaccine.
— *Dr. Vinay Prasad*

Several WWTI doctors sought to spread mistrust about COVID vaccines by describing recommendations to vaccinate children as an "unscientific, unyielding push." They used this emotionally manipulative language to dissuade people from getting the vaccine.

- **Dr. Marty Makary, April 2022:** *Very bizarre behavior that smells of politics and collusion. It's no wonder that the FDA's 2 top vaccine experts quit the agency in protest last September--over this very issue: Political pressure to **push** boosters beyond what the science supports.*[290]

- **Drs. Leslie Bienen and Tracy Beth Høeg, July 2022:** *With its unscientific **push** to vaccinate all infants and toddlers against COVID, the agency will harm vaccine uptake for more significant diseases.*[291]

- **Dr. Marty Makary July 2022:** *Important data from overseas (sadly not from the CDC) that is informative to people wondering what their risk of Covid infection is ahead of the government's/big Pharma's hard **push** for everyone to get re-vaccinated this fall with a new omicron BA1/2 based vaccine.*[292]

- **Dr. Marty Makary, August 2022:** "Before We **Push** the New Omicron Vaccine, Let's See the Data"[293]

- **Dr. Marty Makary, April 2023:** "The CDC Keeps **Pushing** Covid Boosters On Kids Despite Real Health Risks" *The Centers for Disease Control and Prevention and Dr. Anthony Fauci keep **pushing** hard for all healthy children to have four doses of the COVID vaccine despite the lack of clinical outcomes data to support the recommendation.*[294]

- **Dr. Vinay Prasad, November 2023:** *I'm not the only one who has noticed that Ashish Jha continues to make up fabrications about the new COVID vaccine in order to **push** it. Just shameful behavior.*[295]

- **Dr. Vinay Prasad, November 2023:** *I worried that the unyielding push to vaccinate kids with a COVID19 vaccine that has never shown reduction in severe disease or hospitalization in a randomized trial at any age, and certainly not against prevailing variants, was a huge mistake, and would lead the public to doubt all vaccines, rather than an embrace of all.*[296]

> **I detail how the CDC, in a series of publications and proclamations, abandoned science to push propaganda.**
> — *Dr. Vinay Prasad*

WWTI doctors claimed that no one could disagree with them in good faith. They repeatedly claimed that anyone who disagreed with their plans for mass infection or tried to limit COVID in any way was guilty of propaganda.

- **Dr. Martin Kulldorff, May 2021:** *Those arguing that the fully vaccinated must wear masks and socially distance are the true anti-vaxxers, insinuating that vaccines do not work well. Surprising that the media spreads such anti-vaccine propaganda.*[297]
- **Great Barrington Declaration, May 2021:** *"Unfortunately, herd immunity became a propaganda tool to push for endless lockdowns." - @MartinKulldorff and Jay Bhattacharya in @Telegraph*[298]
- **Dr. Martin Kulldorff, August 2021:** *When commenting, neither the UK government nor Dominic Cummings denied their propaganda campaign against the Great Barrington Declaration, with @Dominic2306 stating it "was almost all decentralized", as one would expect from a master political strategist.*[299]
- **Dr. Martin Kulldorff, August 2021:** *On COVID: "It wouldn't be an underestimation to say that this is probably one of the biggest propaganda operations that we has seen in history." - @PiersRobinson1 , co-director of the Organisation for*

Propaganda Studies[300]

- **Dr. Jay Bhattacharya, December 2021:** *Wikipedia has been an active participant in the pro-lockdown government* **propaganda** *campaign. Every prominent anti-lockdown figure's page has been vandalized, violating wikipedia's neutral point of view policy.*[301]

- **Dr. Jay Bhattacharya, December 2021:** *On TV today Francis Collins doubled down on his lies and* **propaganda** *attack and on the Great Barrington Declaration. If you read the GBD, you will not find the words "let it rip" because the central idea is focused protection of the vulnerable.*[302]

- **Dr. Marty Makary, February 2022:** *CDC has repeatedly weaponized science--we need to stand against it, increase public accountability. Our health agencies need radical reform "the brave new world of science as political* **propaganda***" Incredible piece by @VPrasadMDMPH . Article of the year IMO*[303]

- **Dr. Vinay Prasad, February 2022:** *Now out in @tabletmag I detail how the CDC, in a series of publications and proclamations, abandoned science to push* **propaganda.**[304]

- **Dr. Marty Makary, May 2022:** *This study demonstrates how the CDC was cherry-picking data to support their school mask dogma. The article states that CDC's MMWR journal rejected publishing this re-analysis. Most likely because it exposed the CDCs salami-slicing of data & use of science as political* **propaganda**[305]

- **Dr. Vinay Prasad, May 2022:** *It's always worth remembering that the reason we didn't run any credible studies--- Zero trials in kids Zero cluster trials in high income nations. ---is because people took scientific uncertainty and turned it into* **propaganda**[306]

- **Dr. Marty Makary, June 2022:** *Most of the media today* *blindly parrot government **propaganda** like this, without ask-ing key questions. Why did it take a senate hearing for anyone to ask Dr. Fauci the simple quest: Are you paid Moderna roy-alties? Over 2 yrs of thousands of media interviews, somehow no one asked??*[307]

- **Dr. Vinay Prasad, June 2022:** *If the FDA/ CDC makes vac-cine decisions based on false, misleading, and fear-mongering **propaganda**, and that is revealed.... Should the decisions be revisited?*[308]

- **Dr. Vinay Prasad, July 2022:** *It's really shameless **propa-ganda** to disguise the cold reality that there will be very poor uptake for this vaccine that was pushed through for political purposes.*[309]

- **Dr. Vinay Prasad, October 2022:** *You* [Biden administration] *pretended there was a big rush to approve this booster, so you omitted human trials prior to EUA. Then nobody wanted your product. Duh. And now you put out **propaganda**. The two best people at FDA quit because you pressured them Fire ur covid advisors. They're bad.*[310]

- **Dr. Vinay Prasad, October 2022:** *The media coverage of the new booster is negligent. They just keep pushing white house **propaganda**, they don't even mention that peer nations in Western Europe do not follow our delusional lead.*[311]

- **Dr. Vinay Prasad, July 2023:** *Great to see it out and thanks to @TracyBethHoeg If you extend the time range on NEJMs paper on masking kids, the effect becomes zilch Non random-ized kids masks studies are essentially **propaganda** NEJM should have published this if they care about the record.*[312]

- **Dr. Vinay Prasad, September 2023:** *This is an important article that directly refutes former CDC director Rochelle Wal-ensky. Her legacy will be extremely poor. Many mistatements, and no generation of credible evidence. Basically a leader of a* *propaganda regime and not a scientific agency.*[313]

- **Dr. Vinay Prasad, October 2023:** *It's important to remember the CDC is a steady stream of **propaganda**. Not really a scientific organization.*[314]

- **Dr. Jay Bhattacharya, July 2024:** *For most of my scientific career, I worked in a high trust field, where critiques were focused on ideas and only incidentally at scientists. Science needs that assumption of good faith to work. This is why corporate capture or government censorship and **propaganda** destroy science.*[315]

- **Dr. Jay Bhattacharya, July 2024:** *This is an opportunity to bring the whole world together for a common mission: tear down every bit of remaining covid **propaganda** everywhere. Mr. Fauci, tear down this wall!*[316]

- **Dr. Jay Bhattacharya, July 2024:** *The fully unredacted version of the RKI files in Germany is now available. The reacted version suggested no consensus among scientists for lockdown, despite **propaganda** to the contrary. It will be interesting to see what the new materials show.*[317]

- **Dr. Jay Bhattacharya, September 2024:** *If you define 'misinformation' as everything your political opponents believe, then 'studies' will find that your political opponents are misinformed. This kind of partisan nonsense gives science a black eye. **Propaganda** is its proper name.*[318]

There it is. This is how WWTI doctors were able to—and are still seeking to—convince the world that only they can be trusted. *Everyone else is lying to you.*

Conclusion

Do Basic Facts Even Matter?
— *Dr. Jonathan Howard*

My interest in the anti-vaccine movement began in 2010, and by 2018, I knew enough about it to write a book chapter with law professor Dorit Reiss titled "The Anti-Vaccine Movement: A Litany of Fallacy and Errors."[1] In addition to working at Bellevue Hospital throughout the pandemic, I was very familiar with anti-vaccine rhetoric and techniques when COVID arrived.

In October 2022, well after it was clear the COVID vaccine limited rare but grave harms in children, Dr. Vinay Prasad published an article on Bari Weiss's website titled "Covid Vaccines Shouldn't Be 'Routine' for Kids."[2] All of his arguments were very familiar to me. Dr. Prasad's article was a more polished version of the nonsense I had read about the MMR and HPV vaccines before the pandemic on quack sites like Green-MedInfo and Natural News. However, just as they did, he too used bogus statistics and logical fallacies to trick people about vaccines.

Dr. Prasad's core argument was that unvaccinated children should contract COVID because measles and polio were "truly dangerous," while COVID was not. This was absurd. Measles last killed American children, 9 of them, in 1990–1991,[3] while polio hasn't killed a single American child in my entire life. Meanwhile, COVID killed 2,000 American children and hospitalized 234,000 of them in the first four years of the pandemic. Moreover, these vaccines are not in competition with each other. Children can and should be vaccinated against any virus that threatens them. Babies do not arrive with immunity, and they have the highest COVID risk of all children, equal to that of adults 50-64 years old,[4] a fact Dr. Prasad himself later recognized in a *NEJM* commentary.[5]

Dr. Prasad provided no reason why unvaccinated infants should contract COVID forevermore. However, Dr. Jeffrey Flier, the former Dean of Harvard Medical School, found Dr. Prasad's arguments compelling. Dr. Flier shared his article on social media and said:

> *The arguments made here are quite reasonable, and whether COVID vaccines should now be "routine" for kids should be the subject of discussion and debate within the pediatric, medical and public health communities. We have the responsibility to do so.[6]*

Dr. Prasad was making standard anti-vaccine arguments, and the former dean of Harvard said they were "quite reasonable."

Dr. Flier's comment also implied that pediatric vaccines had not been discussed and debated previously. In reality, the CDC had held multiple public meetings on the topic,[7] and countless people had been discussing and debating pediatric vaccines since before they first came out. My first article on *Science-Based Medicine*, from May 2021, was on the pediatric COVID vaccine,[8] and I'd written dozens more articles by October 2022. The data clearly showed the vaccine was safer than the virus for children. Dr. Flier was both unaware of this and uninterested in learning about it. I accepted his invitation to discuss and debate the topic with him, and he refused.

However, in November 2024, after Robert F. Kennedy Jr. was nominated to be the Secretary of Health and Human Services, Dr. Flier developed a sudden intolerance for anti-vaccine propagandists. Dr. Flier published an essay, also on Bari Weiss's website, titled "The Case Against RFK Jr."[9] Although it was perfectly adequate, it was too late. While many of us saw it coming, Dr. Flier was blindsided. Indeed, the day Trump announced Kennedy's nomination, he said:

> *Over the edge. Down the rabbit hole. Completely insane. Would not have believed this possible until right now. Completely independent of politics, this must be seen as unacceptable in 2024.*[10]

Dr. Flier had no excuse to be so surprised. From Lysenkoism in the Soviet Union to AIDS denial in South Africa, not only is history littered with examples of quackery triumphing over science, but many people tried to warn Dr. Flier that it was *dangerous* for prominent figures like him to normalize Dr. Prasad's anti-vaccine disinformation.

> ***Dr. Frank Han****: A former medical school faculty member should show a little more enthusiasm for protecting kids from severe disease, but @19joho* (Dr. Jonathan Howard) *is ready to debate you if you really insist.*
>
> ***Lydia Green****: What is debatable about preventing suffering in children?*
>
> ***@gardengirl778****: Covid is much more prevalent than the other illnesses you listed. Being opposed to Covid vax for kids will cause less vax for other illnesses. People who doubt Covid vax for kids already are doubting other vaxes and we are going to see resurgences of preventable illness. You use Vinny Prssad, famous anti Covid mitigation minimizer who has consistently pushed to end Covid protections and pushed false ideas about the dangers Covid and long Covid?*

I told him at the time:

> *Right off the bat this is misinformation. Measles hasn't killed kids since the 90s. Covid killed 180 in January 2022, nearly all unvaccinated. Do basic facts even matter?*[11]

Dr. Flier didn't care a bit. He hurled juvenile insults—*"dishonest, nasty, and woefully ignorant*"[12]—at those of us who provided accurate information, recognized the threat before he did, and tried to warn him about it. I asked the question, *"Do basic facts even matter?"* and two years later I provided the sad answer: "Basic facts no longer matter."[13]

At times, it can be hard to know where brave, independent thinking stops, and disinformation begins. Charges of "misinformation" should not be thrown around carelessly. However, doctors who claimed that the flu was worse than COVID[1] or that the worst was over in April 2020[15] didn't just have "different views,"[16] as Dr. Flier claimed. They were wrong, and people suffered as a result.

When an emperor is naked, honest brokers don't compliment his beautiful clothes. Yet, that's exactly what Dr. Flier did. Dr. Prasad told the world that Kennedy was *quite reasonable,* and Dr. Flier told the world that Dr. Prasad was *quite reasonable.* In this important way, Dr. Flier did his part to bring us to this dangerous moment, finding the "courage" to speak out only after it was too late. Even then Dr. Flier refused to criticize Dr. Prasad and other WWTI doctors who gushed over Kennedy.

Meanwhile, Dr. Prasad celebrated Trump's war on Dr. Flier's university. Dr. Prasad called Harvard "Woke University" in an essay titled "Harvard Will Not Comply-- Well, At Least That's What Garber Has to Say."[17] He predicted Harvard would "bend the knee." "To be perfectly honest: many of these reforms are needed to make sure the set point of Universities mirrors the set point of America," he said.

Dr. Flier was hardly the only "leader" of American medicine to either praise or turn a blind eye to obvious disinformation and those who wanted to demolish academic medicine. Many deans, presidents, and esteemed professors, seeking to avoid controversy and fearful of being accused of "censorship," said nothing as anti-vaccine charlatanism took root in their institutions. When science and medicine were under attack, they either sat on the sidelines and twiddled their thumbs or scolded those who sounded the alarm.

Their self-imposed silence sent a dangerous message: *basic facts are up for debate, and the most important thing is not to hurt anyone's feelings*. These "leaders" also numbed the American public to disinformation and paved the way for Kennedy. Dr. Flier was nothing special. He was rather typical, and as a result, here we are.

Countless doctors and people with no medical training did incredible work on multiple platforms exposing disinformation. We all tried to warn people about its dangers. It was never easy. There's no support for it, and it's draining to receive schoolyard taunts from celebrity doctors and their online hordes simply because you had the audacity to accurately quote them and explain why you disagree.

I had it easy. People called me silly names, and that's it. Other doctors had fake tweets attributed to them, generating a torrent of online abuse.[18] Several doctors faced unpleasant and frivolous legal threats because they corrected disinformation. Others received death threats and were stalked at home.[19]

Yet they persisted. Many people showed great courage. They stuck their necks out, knowing the vitriol they would receive in return. Many students showed more fortitude than their university leadership, bravely calling out their professors. These young people recognized that some of their esteemed professors were actually naked emperors.

I know that those of us who warned of the dangers of disinformation are disappointed that, for whatever reason, our message was not taken seriously until it was too late. But at least we left a record of what doctors

668

Everyone Else is Lying to You

said, the policies they pushed, and how they brought us to this sad moment. Future generations will know that at least some of us tried to resist the intrusion of quackery into medicine, and they'll gain some semblance of insight into a confounding reality—*after a pandemic that killed 1.2 million Americans, with a vaccine that saved millions, misinformation doctors and the anti-vaxxers they empowered are more trusted and powerful than ever.*

I can only hope that future medical leaders learn from these mistakes and show some backbone. Silence is not a virtue when doctors spread rank disinformation, and no one should ever again have Dr. Flier's surprised reaction—*would not have believed this possible until right now.*[10]

Presently, I have no words of comfort or solutions to offer. The good guys lost. My only prediction is that things are likely to get much worse before they get any better. If Kennedy succeeds, then vaccinations will plummet under a sea of disinformation and legal barriers. Measles and pertussis will come roaring back, flu and COVID are still here, and we are not safe from another pandemic. The actions of our federal health officials will have real consequences for decades to come, and, unlike during COVID, no one will ignore WWTI doctors. They are now officially the medical establishment, and they are responsible for everything that happens under their watch. Those of us outside the medical establishment need to hold them accountable.

I will not be resting. I plan to continue documenting it all, the whole time keeping in mind the words of Oliver Willis, who said:

> *People are going to be hurt, and they are going to die. Liberalism tried to avert this situation but thanks to docility by the Democratic Party, dishonesty by the mainstream media, and thuggery from the right, we are here anyway. Our role? To tell everyone involved, including the public who went along with it, that we told you so.*[20]

Acknowledgments

My wife, Robin Broshi, gave me the idea to write *We Want Them Infected*. Though I initially brushed off her suggestion, it soon occurred to me that the 100 articles I had written on Science-Based Medicine provided the basis for telling the story of the failed quest for herd immunity via mass infection. The same happened with this book when she suggested I should write not just about individual doctors, but also about systems and institutions that had failed us. Again, I initially brushed off this idea too, only to realize that my next 100 *Science-Based Medicine* articles provided the basis for this book.

Robin and I don't always see the world the same. She is a bleeding-heart liberal, while I still count Ayn Rand as a positive influence. A is A after all, and it's good for individuals to stand against groups. However, this book exists because Robin forced me to think about the world in deep and important ways.

The only other people who have (possibly) read all of my articles are my parents. I am grateful to them for their constant support and thoughtful discussions.

I would like to again thank Drs. David Gorksi and Steven Novella for founding *Science-Based Medicine* and showing the world the value of refuting medical misinformation. I am grateful they have allowed me to express my ideas there.

I am indebted to Patty Thompson and Robert Canipe at Redhawk Publications for taking a chance on a largely unknown author writing controversial books that are often received with anger and vitriol. They told me that authors at Redhawk become part of the family, and that is how I feel.

As always, Cindy Harlow turned my rough pages into an organized,

Everyone Else is Lying to You

referenced work. She's a gem, I am lucky to have found her. I am grateful to Walker Bragman for allowing me to share his entire articles in this book and for writing the foreword. Please support his valuable work. I also appreciate Jeff Kunzler's valuable feedback and insights. Steven Blake and Rebecca Caldwell both made invaluable suggestions to improve the book. I am grateful to them both.

I am grateful to Wendy Orent for being my podcast partner on this topic. Talking to her is a highlight of my week, and she's taught me a ton.

I considered creating a list of other doctors and amazing people who did invaluable work refuting medical misinformation. However, invariably I would leave someone off and feel terrible about it. So to the many brave people who stuck their necks out only to receive taunts and threats in return, you have my gratitude. You made a difference, and one day everyone will realize that.

Never give up.

To access the NOTES and INDEX for this book, please follow this QR Code to the Redhawk Publications website where you can download the materials.

This was done to reduce the amount of pages in the book and reduce the cost of the book.

Thank you!

www.ingramcontent.com/pod-product-compliance
Lightning Source LLC
Chambersburg PA
CBHW071012280326
41935CB00011B/1321